PRAISE FOR

LETHA HADADY

"As rare, unique, and potentized as are the herbs in her brilliantly researched book, so too is the personality of one of America's foremost herbalists."

—GARY NULL

"*Asian Health Secrets* is a valuable and thorough compendium of Asian healing perspectives and techniques. This book belongs in the home of every person who strives for optimal health and happiness."

—ISISARA BEY,
Director of Corporate Affairs,
Sony Music Entertainment, Inc.

"Hadady has treated people in hospitals, royal palaces, and jungle huts. . . . With a little education and experimentation, she says we can become our own best health care providers."

—*DELICIOUS!* MAGAZINE

"She unearths the wisdom of the ancients."

—*NEW YORK POST*

"The best-known blonde in Chinatown."

—*NEWSDAY*

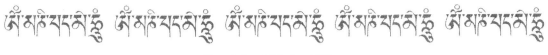

Om Mani Padmi Hum

"Secret" not to be revealed to unsuitable students with the wrong attitudes, which are:

❧ *having a mind like an inverted pot, i.e., not paying attention to the teaching:*
the student cannot hear or does not listen;

❧ *having a mind like a defiled, impure pot, i.e., with the wrong motivation or preconceived ideas;*

❧ *having a mind like a leaky pot, i.e., forgetting everything straightaway.*

From a Tibetan medical text

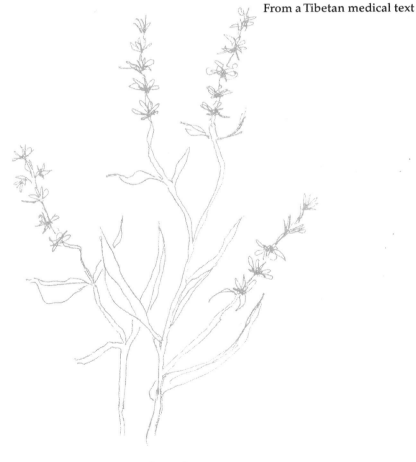

Lavender

ASIAN
HEALTH
SECRETS

The Complete Guide to Asian Herbal Medicine

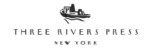

LETHA HADADY, D.Ac.

THREE RIVERS PRESS
NEW YORK

FOR THE HEALER IN YOU

Author's note: Although the information herein is drawn from many medical and traditional herbal sources, the author is mindful that each person is unique and complex. For that reason, the reader is advised to consult qualified health professionals regarding the individual use of herbal treatments when treating illness. If you are currently using any medication, please consult with your doctor before altering your program.

The descriptions and identities of the patients discussed herein have been altered.

Published by Three Rivers Press, New York, New York.
Member of the Crown Publishing Group.

Originally published in hardcover by Crown Publishers, 1996.
First paperback edition printed in 1998.

Random House, Inc. New York, Toronto, London, Sydney, Auckland
www.randomhouse.com

THREE RIVERS PRESS is a registered trademark and the Three Rivers Press colophon is a trademark of Random House, Inc.

Printed in the United States of America

Design by June Bennett-Tantillo

Library of Congress Cataloging-in-Publication Data is available upon request.

ISBN 0-609-80105-8

20 19 18 17 16 15 14 13

ACKNOWLEDGMENTS

I could never have written this book without the love and guidance of Michael Foster. He is the father of the book. I am delighted to have had many beautiful herb illustrations done by my mother, Letha Elizabeth Hadady of Albuquerque. Her love is boundless.

The entire staff at Crown Publishers, from the publisher, Chip Gibson, and executive editor, Ann Patty, to the Art, Production, Publicity, and Sales departments have all given me marvelous support. My wonderful editor, Sharon Squibb, has offered much help and tremendous enthusiasm for this project. Special thanks go also to June Bennett-Tantillo for the book's design and to Joanna Roy for the jacket illustration. Many thanks go to my literary agent, Ms. Ellen Geiger at Curtis Brown Ltd., for her support.

I owe a great deal to my teachers, including His Holiness Tenzin Gyatso, Drs. Yeshe Dhonden of Dharamsala, Sogyal Rimpoche, Yves Requena of France, and Vasant Lad in Albuquerque as well as Drs. Chen Han-Ping and Chao of Shanghai's Institute of Acupuncture and Meridien and Ted Kaptchuk, Subhuti Dharmananda, and Lonny Jarrett in America. I thank Dr. Mark Seem and the Tri-State Institute of Traditional Chinese Acupuncture and especially my Chinese doctor friends in New York City, Susan and Frank Lin and Dr. Lili Wu.

I am very grateful to Dr. Rudolph Ballentine of the Center for Holistic Medicine in Riverdale, New York, for his professional comments on the manuscript. Warm thanks go to my dear friend Elma Meyer for her help, and to my chiropractor brother, Dr. Eric S. Hadady, for his advice. I owe kind thanks to Dr. Albert and Rosa Crum and Naomi Christian for their enthusiasm; also to Michael Romano of the Union Square Cafe, who commented on my recipes. I thank Mama Bear, who lent me her genius.

I am blessed to have had the opportunity to help many clients and friends. I owe them more than I can say for their confidence and love. The encouragement I've received from my beautiful sister, Michelle Noeding, has meant a great deal to me. I am grateful to my dear friend of many years, Gail Christensen, for her inspiration and support. Luke Yankee is a light in my life that I can feel all the way from the Hollywood Hills. Molly McBride and Juan Bererra have helped sustain my spirit and energy. Lew Stowbunenko has healed me with laughter, and Jean-Claude van Itallie with love songs. James Peter Martin and Bob Abplanalp have healed me with their art. My adopted family has sustained me—among them Gad Cohen, François Vallee, Peter Schlosser, William Williams, Frederick Hodgkins, Scott Hoyt, Prestin Pitman, Claudia Patrone, Sharlot Batton, Kim Gremaud, Sandi Levine, Susan Heckler, Cathy Curtin, Ferruccio Rossi-Landi, Jon Naar, Laura Kaplan, Ira Swain, Albert Minns, Gary Null and my friends at the New York Open Center, the New York Botanical Garden and the Brooklyn Botanic Garden, the 92nd Street Y, and the Sierra Club.

CONTENTS

FOREWORD

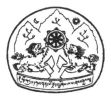

THE DALAI LAMA

I always believe that while humanity must move towards more scientific and technological progress, we must never ignore the knowledge and wisdom of our forefathers. In fact, while we inevitably move forward and make new discoveries, we must preserve and promote our ancient wisdom. In the light of this, I am confident that this book by Letha Hadady on Asian herbal medicine will bring the ancient knowledge of the great cultures of Asia to a larger public.

I am also happy to note that the author of the book has included an examination of Tibet's traditional medicine. The foundation of Tibetan medicine is that mind and body are closely related. Therefore Tibetan physicians have always considered a sound mind as a prerequisite for a healthy body.

His Holiness Tenzin Gyatso,
the Fourteenth Dalai Lama

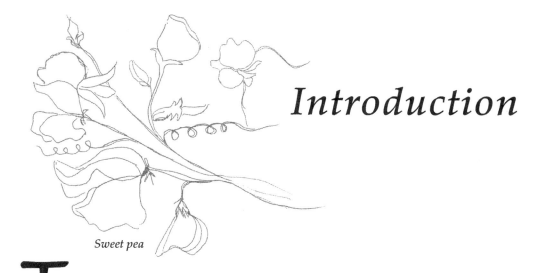

Sweet pea

Introduction

This book opens the door to a secret world. You have lived among Asian herbal medicines your entire life without knowing how they prevent and cure illness, suffering, and aging. Herbs can change your life. They are able to increase your beauty and vitality because they are filled with sunshine and nourishment. Some are as familiar as teas and spices used in cooking; others are the exotic stuff of quaint Oriental shops. No matter what their form, natural herbal medicines increase your life force and immune strength.

Asian herbs are foods, but they also make up the pharmacopoeia of the oldest living medical tradition. Today in every Chinese hospital a traditional medical department uses dried herbs, powders, tinctures, plasters, and herbal pills along with acupuncture to treat a variety of illnesses ranging from arthritis to stroke, many of which are termed incurable by Western medicine. China provides a wonderful laboratory to observe such remedies firsthand with a testing population of about 1.4 billion people. India has provided us with a rainbow assortment of cooking spices that, when used correctly, become potent medicines. All you need to know is how and when to use herbs to unlock this ancient wisdom from the East.

We need herbal medicine now more than ever before. Modern health care has become too expensive and even dangerous. Staph infections have become difficult to control in our hospitals. New strains of malaria and tuberculosis have become as easy to catch as the common cold. Government budget cuts have reduced insurance coverage and threaten to close patient care facilities. The time has come when you must learn how to protect yourself against illness. Prevention is always the best medicine. Besides, it costs less and is more enjoyable.

A few sophisticated American doctors realize we have a great deal to learn from Asian medicine. Dr. Andrew Weil, among others, has become a spokesman for the efficacy of herbal tonics, including several he grows in his garden. In his book on spontaneous healing, he highly recommends them to prevent illness. This is possible because in the Asian tradition, doctors and mothers use herbs according to their observed ener-

getic effects—that is, how they bolster vital energy. In a similar manner, *Asian Health Secrets* will enable you to choose the herbs best suited for your individual needs in order to build your health and longevity daily.

I am happy to share my knowledge and passion for natural remedies with you. They have saved my life numerous times, and have been at the root of many years of world travels and self-exploration. I have conducted research in hospital pharmacies and in street markets, steamed during South China's rainy season, crossed the Thai jungle by elephant, and peered over the cloudy edge of the Himalayas from Dharamsala to Ladakh, finding herbs widely used in Asia that have remained secret in the West. I've watched my American health clients miraculously cured with Asian herbs. There is no excuse for keeping this information privileged, understood only by a few experts. Therefore I am sharing the secrets with you.

Americans spend nearly $20 billion yearly on so-called unconventional therapies, including vitamins and dietary supplements. Herbs account for at least one quarter of that amount. This book makes it possible for you to be very specific in your use of herbal remedies. This is important because in the popular press we are bombarded daily with health advice that is based either on generalities or on laboratory animal studies. But we are not biologically the same as animals, and such studies are not necessarily valid for us.

Our sources for herbal information are often ambiguous. You may have opened a book and read such a statement as "This herb is traditionally used for . . ." or "This herb has been used for centuries to cure . . ." The trouble with such an approach is that it does not apply to you. You have no clue to whether you really need to take a given herb today. You aren't told when to start taking it or when to stop. This is because the typical modern herbal is based on a Western medical model. The author assumes, given a certain malady, that *everyone* can take the same remedy at any time. Such generalized information is totally insensitive to the individual differences that are the basis of Asian medicine. We need to *personalize* herb choice and establish criteria to check whether the herbs are working correctly.

Books concerned with Asian medicine usually either teach traditional theory or list herbs in encyclopedic fashion. Few books teach diagnosis, so that the gulf between your discomfort and the correct herbs to use is never bridged. You need a method of interpreting your own health, to make sure that your choice and use of herbs are appropriate.

It is your present condition and vital energy that must determine your choice of herbs. Those factors always vary according to diet, stress, age, fatigue, emotions, lifestyle, and attitudes. *Asian Health Secrets* demands active participation by you, the reader. Throughout the book you will learn how to choose medicines taken from your supermarket, herb shop, or mail-order sources. You will be able to communicate directly with herbal practitioners and distributors by using the Herbal Access appendix at the back of this book.

This book engages you in healing practices for treating the body, mind, and spirit. It is a vehicle for your personal empowerment, an invitation to enhance vitality with diet, herbs, and guided visualizations. In that way your herbal knowledge will become personally relevant. Applying traditional Asian diagnostic methods, you will realize that your health is ultimately your own responsibility. Your body belongs to you.

Asian Health Secrets enables you to choose your best treatment for weight loss and aches and pains such as headaches, arthritis, allergies, and injuries. The Not for Women Only section of Part Four contains chapters on blood building and on cleansing herbs for beautiful skin and hair, and offers safe remedies for fertility and menopausal discomforts. The Herbs for Vitality section contains chapters for prevention and treatment of devitalizing illnesses such as colds, flu, and insomnia. It also offers an individualized approach for finding your best remedies for conquering fatigue, sexual weakness, and immune deficiency. Part Five, Herbs and the Mind, concludes the book with chapters that treat depression, poor memory, and concentration. The final chapter contains a useful method of employing herbs to enhance your performance at work, in the concert hall, or anywhere you require emotional calm, clarity, insight, and spiritual awareness.

The health issues covered here are most often termed chronic. What is a chronic condition, really? Insurance will not cover its treatment, and doctors cannot cure it, but only possibly palliate it. Your discomfort, however, can be severe, recurrent, and long-lasting. In other words, the term "chronic" is a declaration of the failure of modern medicine. In the herbal tradition we do not recognize illnesses that are incurable, because we treat the person rather than the illness. Any illness or attitude will improve as your circulation, energy, and blood production improve because your total life force is engaged. This is the ultimate mission that herbs can accomplish: they ensure the healthy connection of your body, mind, and spirit.

Some of my Asian health secrets come from field study. In 1993, at Shanghai's College of Traditional Medicine, I treated patients for several diseases that ranged from obesity to schizophrenia.

Much of my approach toward balance in diet, as well as psychology, stems from my work with Ayurvedic and Tibetan doctors in North India. However, my recommendations and case studies from around the world come from many years of experience in a private health practice in New York using herbs, diet, acupuncture, and other healing modalities. This book contains secret knowledge both because it took some pains to acquire—Asian travel is not easy—and because herbs can cure those everyday discomforts to which Western medical doctors respond either with a shrug or by prescribing drugs that often possess harmful side effects.

I have delayed writing this book for a long time because I consider helping people to become aware of their innate capacity for healing to be an act of love. I hesitated to codify herbal information, but the time has come to share my years of experience. The public is faced with a wide information gap, in that more people are using herbs than ever before, but on the basis of less reliable information. Since I started writing this book, an explosion of new American-manufactured Asian herbal products has appeared on the supermarket and health-food store shelves with little or no explanation of their use or dosage. Given such limited information, this herbal treasure remains secret.

Imagine the following scenario: You have a cough and sore throat. You don't smoke, but throat irritation has been bothering you for weeks. You need something stronger than over-the-counter cough drops but can't stand the drowsy feeling caused by drugs. You're not willing to waste half a day at the doctor's office, nor pay an expensive bill, so you try your local health-food store.

The shelves are stocked with rows of bottled herbs, both single and in combinations. Their names, whether in English or Latin, mean little to you. By law, the labels can offer no suggestions concerning use or dosage. The person behind the counter says the store has a special this week on garlic pills, but you don't think garlic has anything to do with your throat. Besides, the employee has a bad cold. You look into one of the shop's herb books and find a variety of herbs traditionally used to alleviate sore throat. Which remedy is the correct one for you? You feel abandoned in a forest of plants that don't speak your language. In truth, your communication with Eden has been severed.

The mislabeled Nutrition Labeling and Education Act of 1990 gives the Food and Drug Administration the right to define specific vitamins and herbs as potentially dangerous and to hinder dissemination of research and even historical information about their health and curative properties. That means the government, under the guise of protecting us from ourselves, has limited the labeling of herbs so that we have less information on home remedies than our grandmothers did.

Asian Health Secrets will initiate you into the methods of traditional Asian diagnosis, after which you will observe your symptoms throughout the book as you study many common ailments. I have explained how the appropriate remedies work, listing their ingredients so that you can find or duplicate them in health-food stores or Asian herb shops, or from mail-order sources. You may want to fax some of my herbal recipes or illustrations of herb boxes to distributors I have listed. In the appendix I have listed qualified herbal practitioners who can assist you.

The herbal pills, soups, and brews I describe can become an easy way to remain strong and vibrant. They come from trusted ancient sources, but I have modified them to suit our times. In cases where certain ingredients are animal sources or are endangered or undesirable, I have offered vegetarian alternatives.

Our lives have changed drastically since the medical classics were written. We are living longer and faster-paced lives than our ancestors did. Many women choose to pursue careers, and have children much later than our mothers did. We strive to remain young and beautiful (not just fertile) as long as possible. Our sexual problems are

most often related to fatigue and stress, not to the "shyness" described in traditional Oriental medical books.

Both men and women need to improve their immune strength because illnesses now exist that did not in preindustrial times. Some have been generated by the abuse of medical or street drugs or by environmental toxins. For these reasons, I have translated the principles of Asian medicine into easy-to-read explanations and examples, usually without relying on esoteric concepts or terminology.

A number of words in the text have been italicized, such as *internal cold, wind, bile,* and *phlegm,* when they have special meaning as Asian medical terms. Proper names of herbal products such as pills and extracts are displayed in bold print, for example, **Tang Kuei Tablets,** although the ingredients in Chinese, Sanskrit, or Latin are not in bold.

How to Use This Book

The book is organized into five major parts: Herbal Secrets from the East; Diagnosis and Diet; Bringing You into Balance; Practice; and Herbs and the Mind. If you are interested in using specific Asian herbs to cure chronic problems, you can find help in appropriate chapters. But if you wish to prevent illness, pain, and aging while improving your beauty, general health, and immune strength, it is better to read the book from cover to cover; it will serve both as an encyclopedic resource book and as a vehicle for self-exploration.

The first several chapters tell the story of my personal involvement with the herbal tradition, and offer historical and cultural background to Eastern and especially Chinese medicine. New York's Chinatown is provided as an experiential field where important concepts such as *chi* and *yin* and *yang* are explained and illustrated. In a chapter covering the many kinds of Chinese tea, I take you on a train ride through the tea-growing country of South China. There are chapters providing practical information on how to find, prepare, and store medicinal herbs, and how to use them in cooking. We explore the Asian concept of a balanced diet based on the Five Tastes.

Part Two explains diagnosis, and makes it easy and fun. By observing yourself with the aid of questionnaires and a map of the tongue, you will become skilled in a most important aspect of traditional Asian medicine. The diagnosis section offers you a means of evaluating your own vitality and immune strength so that you will be able to monitor your wellness according to changes in the seasons or in your level of stress, fatigue, or emotional upset.

The questionnaires and tongue analysis present a dynamic rather than a static profile of your health. Any sensitive vehicle of observation must reflect *changes* in energy.

Part Three provides actual experience in bringing your energy and healing powers into balance with a detailed, multilayered health routine, including diet, herbal remedies, activities, and visualizations. I refer to the information in this section throughout the rest of the book when dis-

cussing appropriate remedies for specific health problems.

In Part Four, my friends and clients serve as examples to guide you in the treatment of everyday problems of the sort we have all experienced, ranging from injuries, weight loss, depression, and sexual dysfunction to the common cold. For example, in the weight-loss chapter, you will learn *why* we crave certain foods and how to enhance digestion and reduce addictive cravings in order to lose weight. Slimming is achieved by growing stronger!

In the chapters on pain and injury, you will learn about a secret remedy that is nothing less than an Asian miracle cure. In the event of an auto accident or mugging, this herbal remedy could save your life.

In the Not for Women Only section we explore the role of blood-building tonics to beautify skin and hair, calm nerves, regulate menstruation, and aid in a healthy approach to menopause. I offer herbal remedies for those who wish never to take synthetic hormones. Using traditional diagnosis, you will decide if you have adequate blood production, and will be provided with examples of the remedies you need. This book will make it possible for you to see and understand the results of your diet and lifestyle and, if necessary, reverse their negative effects.

A section called Herbs for Vitality covers individual reasons for exhaustion, including poor circulation, inadequate digestion, shortness of breath, or mental and emotional stress. Your herbal remedies should address the specific cause. Vitality is threatened by variable factors, including overwork, imbalance, insomnia, and colds or flu.

In a chapter titled The Yin and Yang of Love, you will find out how herbs that build *yin* can also ensure beauty, calm anxiety, and promote depth of feeling, while herbs that build *yang* produce sexual strength. Which do *you* need more? Which cooking spices enhance sexual satisfaction for you and your loved one? Which so-called aphrodisiacs are just irritants? These and other questions will be answered.

Part Five, Herbs and the Mind, explores the illnesses and growth issues pertaining to the mind and spirit. For example, herbs that treat depression create an opportunity for emotional growth. Western drugs affect a few brain chemicals without touching the underlying causes of depression, which can include problems with metabolism, hormones, and aging, not to mention malnutrition, poverty, and drug addiction. But herbs used to counter depression work by enhancing your vitality. They increase your energy and mental clarity, not just sedate you in hopes your problem will go away.

Herbs can also improve memory and promote high performance. Such remedies can facilitate the calmness and insight necessary to improve your work and your love relationships and to attain your personal goals. They can provide emotional support for periods of stress such as divorce, grief, and loss, and aid in passing through important life transitions.

Tibetan doctors believe that to achieve balance and inner harmony, we must devote our body, mind, and spirit to higher purposes—compassion and helping others. Although no person ever stands completely alone, we need to understand who we are individually in order to develop fully.

This book offers personal analysis combined with the individual choice of herbs. It is a revolutionary approach to a time-honored tradition. With this ancient tool, you can attain your highest goals and best health.

Consider the plant: It is perfect. Its roots, stem, and leaves treat our bodily illness, and its flowers treat our emotions. By accepting the healing qualities of plants, we blend with the inherent balance of Nature. Our greater understanding opens new vistas. Knowledge that has been secret becomes ours in a quest that involves every aspect of life. *Asian Health Secrets* is a gift of love to my many students and clients, and to all those who wish to share in the adventure.

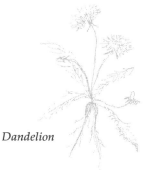

Dandelion

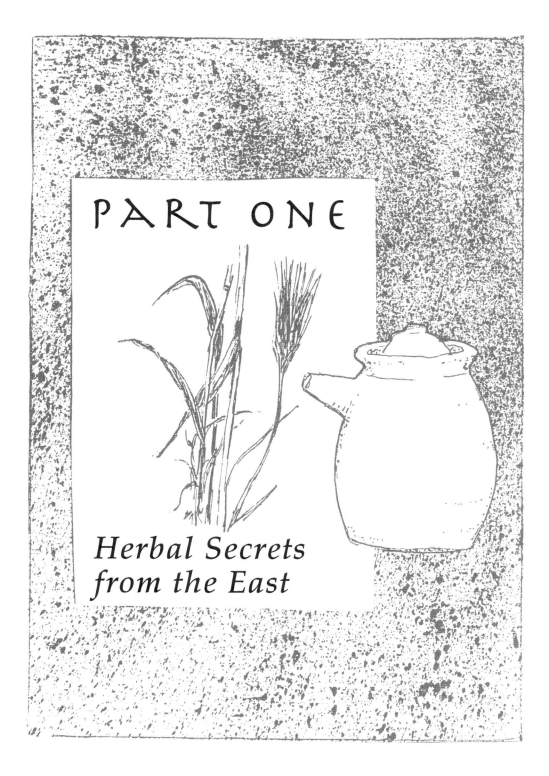

PART ONE

Herbal Secrets from the East

And the woman said unto the serpent, we may eat of the fruit of the trees of the garden; but of the fruit of the tree which is in the midst of the garden, God hath said, Ye shall not eat of it, neither shall ye touch it, lest ye die.

And the serpent said unto the woman, Ye shall not surely die: for God doth know that in the day ye eat thereof, then your eyes shall be opened, and ye shall be as gods, knowing good and evil.

—The Book of Genesis, Chapter 3

Csak egy kislany van a vilagon, as en kedves rozsam galambom.
("There's only one little girl in the world, my sweet rose dove.")
Hungarian love song

1

Granma's Way

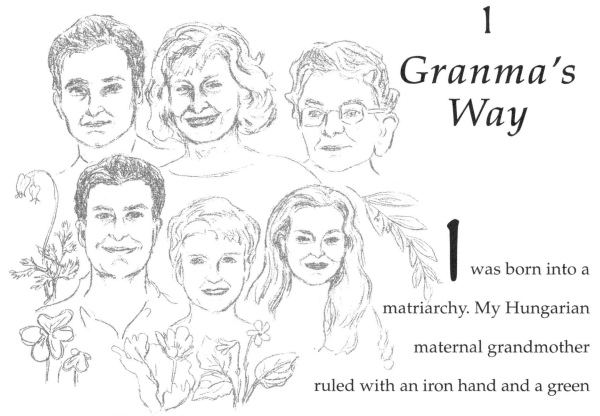

was born into a matriarchy. My Hungarian maternal grandmother ruled with an iron hand and a green thumb. She'd sailed to America in 1904, with a trunk of clothes, a bag of herb seeds, and the family coat of arms. High-spirited and strong-willed, she'd left the Tokay to escape an arranged marriage with a man she did not love. She never learned English or worked at a job, so she lived as if she had never really left Hungary.

In a flowered house dress and babushka, Granma spent her days in her garden. If she got a headache, she tied hot peppers to her forehead with a red bandanna or sniffed a bottle of bad-smelling herbal stuff to clear her sinuses. She always ate bitter salad greens, claiming they cleansed her liver and improved her mood. They may have given her pretty skin, but she had a terrible temper. She chased me with a wooden spoon if I came home late from school, but I usually escaped under a bed.

Once, at eight, I decided to leave home. I was going to live in people's backyards and eat from their gardens. Granma had taught me about edible plants and flowers, but I ended up postponing my travels because it would have made my mother too sad.

As a child, my love of herbs came naturally. I remember at the age of five collecting weeds from the garden to steep a brew for the neighbor kids. The garden's appeal was purely sensory. Its delights were perfumes: tarragon, mint, and dill. I loved the fragrance of marjoram. It gives me pleasure to this day. I didn't know then that marjoram is a vasodilator that can soothe spasms, quiet nerves, and lower blood pressure. The herb created a calm space within me.

My rapport with Asian culture probably began before I was born, like an atavism. Early on, I felt at home breathing in the heady fragrance of incense. I read Lao-tzu and enjoyed Asian music and painting because they were subtle and graceful. Their appeal was immediate, aesthetic.

My introduction to "energetic medicine" (healing methods that affect our energy) came from my beautiful mother. Traditional Asian doctors believe our vital energy is similar to the natural elements of our planet, designated Fire, Earth, Metal, Water, and Wood. I have always felt a certain kinship with Wood, although not for the usual reasons. Born two weeks premature, I required an oxygen tent. None were available, so the doctor, despite my mother's protests, put me into a brown paper bag hooked up to an oxygen hose. Surrounded by a paper cocoon, I wailed for freedom.

Catching a cold, I developed a fever high enough to put me in a coma. The doctors gave me up for dead and asked Mother to leave my room. But she sat by me, she said, sending energy from herself to me. A mother's love cannot be measured scientifically, but it certainly heals. Our energy is powerful, yet invisible. It keeps the heart beating, the breath flowing. Its movement along internal pathways is the focus of Asian medicine.

My formal study of herbs came much later, after a crushing personal loss. In the 1940s, my father worked with Enrico Fermi and other scientists on the first cyclotron at the University of Chicago. Under many feet of concrete in the physics department, two powerful magnets used to split the atom would forever change the way we thought about matter and energy. In addition to building the A-bomb, the scientists hoped to find peaceful uses for atomic power. An attempt was made to isolate nuclear particles in order to shoot them at cancer cells, our first radiation therapy. My father told me that when deuterons were aimed at a man's brain tumor, the cancer was destroyed, but the man's head was blown away.

The scientists who dreamed of harnessing the atom were fueled by the optimism and the postwar economic boom of the 1950s. They wished to control the powers of nature in order to destroy our greatest enemy, disease. But killing germs or sick cells is not enough to prevent illness; we must also strengthen what is weak.

My father, a first-generation American, was temperamentally Hungarian. Intense, fine-featured, he helped design the Saturn rocket that sent men to the moon, and the Sidewinder missile that sped them to their deaths. Despite Dad's top secret work during the 1950s in New Mexico, we were a typical close-knit, emotional Eastern European family. There was usually a Brahms rhapsody playing in the background of our lives.

At age forty my father became seriously ill with periodic fevers and cold sweats. Tiny specks of Teflon, used to coat missile nose cones, had fallen onto his workbench while he rolled his cigarettes. Or perhaps the fevers were related to radiation he had absorbed in testing the cyclotron and weapons at Sandia Laboratory. We will never know for certain, because all his health records were destroyed in a suspicious fire at the Veterans' Hospital. There seem to have been quite a number of such fires at that time.

Then Dad developed symptoms of multiple sclerosis. He became progressively paralyzed. His tall, straight frame sagged. Overnight his hair turned white. He wanted up-to-date medicine, but the doctors offered no help. Mainstream Western medicine recognized no alternatives, so it pronounced him incurable.

Medicine in the sixties was driven by the spirit of the Vietnam War: Search out and destroy the enemy! That mind-set ignored the effects of environmental toxins on the immune system; it aimed to remove the anomaly surgically or kill germs, both useless in my father's case. His condition continued to worsen. For a hobby, Dad made finely crafted, expertly balanced guns. So one day he took one of them, a Colt .45, clicked his heels, and died like a soldier. It was the same day the Saturn rocket he'd helped to perfect lifted the Apollo astronauts to the moon.

I grieved Dad's suicide for years. His diagnosis of "incurable" had become a self-fulfilling prophecy. After his death, I needed to find a new direction for my life. Eventually I realized that out of my despair was born my newfound philosophy about healing and I accepted an approach more sensitive to individual needs. I myself have been diagnosed "incurable" by Western medicine. My own physical and emotional recovery laid the foundation for the years of my health practice. I began to study the human body/mind/spirit as energy, as light-body, as the flow of life itself.

As a rule, Western medicine conceives of illness as a "disease entity," affecting particular areas of the body. According to that view, illness becomes a thing, separate from the interaction of body, mind, and spirit, so that it must be attacked with harsh weapons or be regarded as hopeless. Too often the medical "attack" is worse than the malady it aims to cure: it does not aim at a moving target, but obliterates indiscriminately. We need another way of seeing illness and health, a way that acknowledges change and the flow of energy, a way that does more than seek to destroy.

An Asian approach to human anatomy and physiology stems from a perception of us in a fluid physical and energetic universe. Internal organs and their workings are explained in terms of energy required to make them function. That same view of the material and energetic world was described by the laws of thermodynamics. The first law defined energy within a closed system. The amount of energy within a system—the body, for example—is constant. Energy cannot be destroyed, only changed. The second law postulates entropy, the measure of disorder (change) within a closed system. These axioms laid the foundation for Einstein and others to follow.

Physicists and astronomers have long been accustomed to describing the invisible world of energy by observing its effects. This rationale might well be applied to energetic medicine. Fifty years ago, when we exploded the first atomic bomb, it proved Einstein's theory that energy and matter are interchangeable. That mushroom cloud changed our understanding of physical reality. But why hasn't this heightened awareness pervaded the mainstream practice of medicine? When I've taught at such prestigious institutions as New York Medical College, the oldest such school in the nation, students have been eager to learn how and why energetic medicine works. But for the most part, medical students are still taught that the human heart is an elaborate mechanical pump, neglecting the spark that makes it work. We understand our cars better than we understand our own hearts. We are not cars, but creatures of movement and light as much as flesh.

Not until we investigate the workings of body/mind/spirit with a combined East/West approach can we claim to understand what it is to be human. In Europe and Asia, doctors are required to study in detail both Eastern and Western approaches to medicine, learning the anatomy and physiology of the material body as well as of the energetic body, including acupuncture meridians and the movement of energy along those pathways. This understanding is reflected in diagnosis and treatment in Chinese hospitals where I've worked. Perhaps, in time, we will also accept a healing tradition that goes beyond a material view and even a psychological view, to comprehend our source of life itself, energy.

My father's generation was given the task of splitting apart matter in order to create energy. We must now put our world back together again. My father lived and died by the sword, and my grandmother by the weed. I have chosen Granma's way. It is a nurturing, sustaining approach to life that preserves the connection between nature and myself. It is that approach which has saved my life and brought me to Asia.

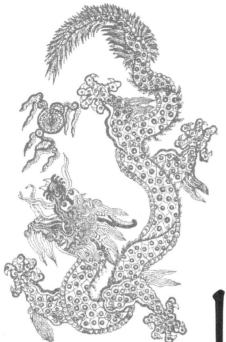

2
A Walk Through Chinatown

I remember the first time I saw New York's Chinatown. It was early morning, just after the stores opened. Sunlight filtered through narrow streets as bundles of bean sprouts were dragged into restaurants by sullen men. The air was filled with bittersweet incense as tiny yellow birds sang in cages high above my head. Chinatown, a huge dragon, yawned and stretched from Broadway toward the East River, scattering worker bees along Canal Street.

I could have been in Seattle, San Francisco, Boston, Toronto, or Hong Kong. In Asian markets throughout the world, the foods and herbs are *the same. What were those fruits carried in baskets by lovely girls? Were they longans? One day I'd buy them in Shanghai's streets. One day in Delhi and Bangkok, I'd find plants for rejuvenation. But I knew nothing of it then. That first day in Chinatown, the dragon watched me from the corner of his eye, knowing I would follow when and where he beckoned. Asia had claimed me.*

By now I've swallowed the Asian herbal tradition whole. I'd rather cook an herbal brew in my own kitchen than see a medical specialist. I'd rather amble through neighborhoods filled with delicious Oriental aromas, sights, and sounds to purchase time-tested medicines than take the most advanced drugs. Visiting Asia in the West is part of the cure for me.

I prefer a cleansing and strengthening approach to health, an approach that the body easily accepts. At home I've used herbs to melt pains, fibroid cysts, and other so-called incurable diseases for myself and others. This has at times left Western doctors stunned and incredulous. Traveling in Asia, I've witnessed a different sort of medicine than we're used to. I've chosen acupuncture doctors in Shanghai and Tibetan doctor monks in Dharamsala for my own illnesses. Besides enjoying the trip, I could better afford the cure there, despite the airfare.

Working alongside doctors in Chinese hospitals, I've occasionally faced antique equipment or primitive sanitary conditions, but I've also observed cures that have made me cry. I've seen people paralyzed with strokes fully recovered in a few months, and others with cancer or mental illness cured with natural medicine. Today, for every four women who die of breast cancer in China, more than twenty-six die in the United States and twenty-nine in the United Kingdom. China has the best survival statistics in the world. How dare we ignore such success? Our Asian communities at home link us to this vast, highly successful store of healing knowledge and experience.

Some of my closest friends work in Chinatown. The merchants and I have a special relationship. We share a respect for their heritage. Herbal medicine is so relevant to everything Chinese that its concepts and vocabulary have provided me a calling card to present to Chinese people here and abroad. This was not always easy. When I first traveled to South China in the mid-1980s, it was barely open to tourism. Twenty-eight dialects were spoken in Yunnan alone, none of them the official Mandarin. Little kids screamed with fright to see my blond hair, never dreaming such creatures existed. I'd be followed by a large, staring crowd when I bought blue worker's clothes or bananas in a market where food was covered with flies. In order to study with acupuncturists in Chinese hospitals, I had to present myself as a patient. When I bought herbs at street markets, I was either ignored or laughed at by merchants unable to imagine that a foreigner could be interested in their medicine. By now student programs for herbs and acupuncture are to be found in Shanghai, Canton, and Beijing, with translations for foreigners.

After returning home from summers abroad, I've conducted educational tours in Asian neighborhoods in New York, Philadelphia, Boston, and Los Angeles. Large communities of Asian Americans live and grow herbs in Oregon, and federally funded clinics, using traditional herbal medicine and acupuncture, exist in Seattle and New York City. Private doctors and acupuncture clinics are found in all major U.S. cities, as well as in Toronto and Vancouver, B.C.

I've become a link between a medicine that does not need an introduction and a captivated public. Now that I've spent years bringing business to Chinatown and Little India, the merchants smile to see me. Several dear friends know that I've chosen to live and thrive with their medicine. If I get sick, I come to them for help. Frank and Susan Lin at Lin Sisters Herb Shop at 4 Bowery Place have concocted herbal brews for me and my health clients for many years. With my suggestions, they have created herbal powders useful for the prevention of breast cancer and the treatment of AIDS. They are among my closest friends in New York. Whenever I teach in Chinatown, the day is not complete until I can take the class to one of my favorite restaurants, Vegetarian Paradise III at 33 Mott Street. There mock ducks, chicken, and fish are made from tofu, gluten, and yams. The healing menu is equaled by the warmth and gracious manner in which we are welcomed.

My tours have varied with the seasons and with the expansion of New York's Asian communities. I always take my students to Do Kham, a Tibetan shop on the northern border of Chinatown, at 51 Prince Street. They sell handmade clothes, jewelry made from silver, turquoise, and red coral, and healing incense. Outside the shop, the flag of free Tibet waves, and inside the sound of monks droning prayers transports you to a higher world. The smiling face of His Holiness Tenzin Gyatso melts all barriers to goodwill and progress. New York City is an island of freedom, money, and power, where enemies can live side by side and engage in commerce.

Chinatowns in America are not all exactly the same. Once I got to see the Chinese New Year, celebrated according to the lunar calendar in February, in both San Francisco and New York. Early morning on Grant Avenue was all California sunshine and smiles. Large floats of dragons and elaborate birds made with flowers lined the parade route, and the costumes and cameras made it look like a movie set. Handsome kung-fu students stood by, casually showing their muscles while drinking orange juice.

A few hours later, in cold New York winter, I watched, crammed into a doorway to escape loud drumming and tough guards who shoved onlookers aside with four-letter New Yorkese to clear a path for the martial-arts boys who carried a dragon's head. When they stopped in front of a store to wish the merchants good luck, the dragon pranced and the fireworks were deafening.

The contrast among Chinatowns is remarkable in other ways, too. In San

Francisco's Chinatown, perhaps America's prettiest, there are lots of tourist shops selling tablecloths, furniture, and clothes, also whole stores devoted to ginseng. There's a wonderful Daoist temple and restaurant, Lotus Garden, on Grant Avenue. In Los Angeles, not far from the wishing well at Meiling Way and Ginling Way, I found the Hong Ning Company on North Broadway, a store that specializes in shark's fins and bones. It's near a Korean community with shops selling ginseng and deer antlers.

New York's no-frills herb stores often have herbal medical doctors for individual consultations, and sell the latest thing from China for stress-related illnesses such as cancer, heart disease, and stroke. In Philadelphia, herb shops are less abundant than private Chinese doctors who sell herbs with a prescription. But as a rule, quite a number of herbal pills are sold in Chinese grocery stores from coast to coast, because Asian people consider herbs necessary as food.

I appreciate the convenience of shopping at big Chinese supermarkets like Kam Man on Canal Street in New York, or Chung May Food Market on Race Street in Philadelphia, or Wild Oats in Santa Fe, but I truly love prying into small side shops. In San Francisco, I found where the fortune cookie was invented during the 1920s. Seven days a week, a tiny nook in Ross Alley has a couple of elderly Chinese women who tear off circles of baked dough from a revolving machine and fill them with sayings they don't understand. It's close to the flower shop where the mother

and aunt in Amy Tan's novel *The Joy Luck Club* worked.

Once in Philadelphia, at Fung Yuan Grocery on North Tenth Street, I found two beautiful sisters aged eight or so. I did business with them because they spoke English, though their kindly grandfather didn't. It's not easy to explain things in any language to kids of that age, and by the time I did, I'd fallen in love. The real fortune in the fortune cookie comes from direct contact with Asia in the West.

Come join me on a walking tour of Chinatown's herbal markets! Certainly you have a favorite restaurant or a shop where you buy silk, gold, or jade, but did you know that all Asian neighborhoods sell powerful medicinal herbs that have been popular for five thousand years? Our markets are miniature versions of those in China. On our walking tour I'll take you behind closed doors to find what few westerners have seen. In Chinatown a casual tourist can get lost. A different logic is at work here from what is found on the straight, broad avenues and cross-streets of the city. You and I will snake through a labyrinth filled with pungent incense and shrill sounds, our entry to an ancient world. By the end of this book, you will be able to apply its secrets to your health and beauty.

We begin our tour in New York City, walking south through Greenwich Village and Soho to the heart of Chinatown, at Canal Street. There always seems to be a crowd in Chinatown. This part of town is booming with new construction. With the influx of Hong Kong wealth, the Chinese borders have extended to include parts of

Little Italy, Chelsea, the Lower East Side, and Brooklyn. Hong Kongers have brought a lot with them: enormous restaurants with ballrooms, streets of chic beauty shops; silk designer clothes line Canal Street. New York has the largest population of Chinese Americans in the country.

The 1960s saw a great period of expansion in American Chinatowns. Many people came from Hong Kong and Canton, one of China's richest provinces and the closest to Western influences. That's why the dialect most often heard here is Cantonese, the language of Chinese opera. Its long, high-pitched diphthongs differ from the short, clipped, guttural sounds of Mandarin.

On Lafayette Street we pass several panhandlers washing car windows, while others sleep in cardboard boxes over the subway gratings. In many years of walking through Chinatown, I've seen only one man asking for money. Begging is not allowed in China, nor is it needed. With socialized medicine and a staggering economic growth rate over the past ten years, China is witnessing a financial boom equaled by no other country. Hong Kong dwarfs New York City in population and visible wealth. We see its influence in bright new buildings everywhere in Chinatown.

The old world is less apparent. As we proceed south toward Canal Street, in the block between Grand and Canal, at 214 Centre Street, is a building with a yellow, iron-grated facade. Passing by this door at 5:00 P.M. on weekdays, we hear a sound like the droning of bees—chanted Chinese prayers, barely audible above the street noise. As we enter, I bow three times in front of a large seated Buddha. Gaudy red, orange, and gold paint and flashing Christmas lights dazzle our eyes as we look up at a hundred carved wooden Buddhas that line the walls. This is a hidden Buddhist temple known only to local residents. No one speaks English here. The master, monks, and nuns who live upstairs hardly venture into the streets.

I've spent quiet evenings here visiting nuns who recite prayers over buckets of birdseed. The next morning at 4:00 A.M., when they spread the seeds on the steps of City Hall, their blessings are carried throughout the city by birds. In Buddhist temples such as the one on Centre Street, ancient Chinese culture has been preserved because there has been less persecution in the West than in mainland China. Tourists are not allowed to participate in ceremonies in China, but are invited to join in here on Sunday mornings.

As we stand near the fat, grinning Buddha, a tiny nun passes, gathering incense for afternoon prayers. She has a shaved head and wears a long gray robe. She smiles a greeting as I bow, hands placed together, and says [*Nee how?*], a Chinese greeting meaning "How are you?" She comes from Shanghai and for a long time was the excellent cook for the temple. When I inquire in Mandarin, she tells me that she's been sick.

I observe her energy and metabolism the way a Chinese doctor would. We'll study this in detail later. Her tongue is red and dry, indicating what traditional Asian doctors call *internal heat*. She does not have a fever, but has dizziness and occasional headaches. Several of the twelve pulses at her radial artery are fast and thin, locating tightness or inflammation inside. She works hard and tends to have high blood pressure. I've seen how, working in the kitchen, she has pushed seventy-pound sacks of rice across the floor. Her wrinkled hands have chopped vegetables for nearly a century.

There are several extremely effective herbal pills that reduce cholesterol and lower blood pressure. One is **Mao Dung Ching,** a capsule form of holly root. Another is **Dan Shen Wan,** a pill made from salvia (red sage), which stimulates blood circulation, and natural camphor. The remedies reduce chest pain by dilating blood vessels near the heart and washing them clean of excess cholesterol by increasing heart action. When I recommend them to her, the nun smiles and answers that her prayers are enough. With her quiet daily rituals, she protects her health by reducing stress. Traditional Chinese doctors would say she protects her *chi,* the vital energy that keeps her alive and well.

The old master of the temple has come in to greet us. He's a very large monk in a bright saffron-colored robe, originally from Beijing. Slowly he sits at a large table covered with Chinese scrolls. He is a famous old monk. During World War II, in the midst of bombing near five sacred mountains at Wu Tai Chan Temple, he recopied a Buddhist text of 600,000 Chinese characters, using his blood for ink while reciting prayers for world peace. Today the master, who is nearly eighty, is very sturdy despite his age. The doctors who kept the monk alive during his devotional rite gave him blood-building herbs: tang kuei, di huang, and others we'll find today in Chinatown.

The old nun is bowing in front of a large standing Buddha of Compassion at the back of the temple. The master is bent over his scrolls with a dipping pen and ink. When I ask the head of the temple if he uses Chinese medicine, he replies in Chinese, "Every morning, hot water and one slice raw ginger in tea." He knows that this oldest of remedies ensures energy and strong digestion. Bidding the ancient world goodbye, we reemerge into sunshine on Centre Street, and direct our steps toward Canal to busy shops full of odd roots, leaves, and berries, strange bottles, and pungent scents. There we'll find some of our oldest friends, Asian spices and teas.

The next stop is Kam Man, a large supermarket located on Canal between Mott and Mulberry streets. On the way we pass by food stands selling hot tofu with sugar sauce, sumptuous shrimp noodles, fried turnip cakes, and pastries made from lotus nuts and sweet black beans. As in much of the world, rice and beans are the staples of an Asian diet, although they're white rice and soybeans. Seasonal vegetables and herbs are sold by people who yell their names in Cantonese. During spring it's fresh leechee and longan fruits, water spinach, foot-long eggplants and green beans, Chinese cabbage and arrowhead, a mild-tasting swamp vegetable; in autumn and winter it's pomegranate, white winter melons to be cooked in soups, and many root vegetables including taro and yams.

You can usually find lotus root year-round. It looks like a thick, light-colored tube with holes running lengthwise inside. When sliced and stir-fried, or used in soups, it's a mild, crunchy vegetable like jicama that reduces phlegm and alleviates diarrhea. There is also bitter melon, which looks like a fat, pale green cucumber with irregular lengthwise grooves. Sautéed or juiced raw, it helps rid the colon of parasites. Considered anti-inflammatory, it's useful for diabetes, chronic fever diseases, and hot flashes. A few vegetable and fish markets on Mulberry and the Bowery label such Oriental vegetables in English for Americans.

At 200 Canal Street, Kam Man looks like a grocery store, but there's lots more to see here than food. Open from 9:00 A.M. to 9:00 P.M. daily, Kam Man is always jammed with people rushing to and fro with baskets of exotic meats, three-foot-long silvery dried eels, fresh noodles, hot pickled vegetables, dried fungus and mushrooms, lotus roots, candied fruits, pottery decorated with gold dragons or blue fishes, and sticks of incense. Walking in the entrance, past a wall of large bottles containing ginseng, shark's fin, and medical herbs, we take the stairs down.

In the stairwell are various herbal sugar substitutes that can relieve dry cough, fever, headache, or blood deficiency. On the ground floor we find spices, dried seaweeds, canned foods, and lovely tableware. A loudspeaker nearby blares in Cantonese as we wander among woks, clay pots, and large Chinese vases. On the main floor are a butcher shop and many frozen foods, as well as packaged slim-

ming teas, medicinal wines, and a collection of dried herbs.

In Chinese supermarkets and meat shops, important seasonal herbs are always displayed so you can't miss them. Often they're near the checkout counter. If you don't know typical herb remedies for seasonal maladies, all you have to do is ask. Everyone Chinese will know. This is because traditionally the basis of family health and happiness comes from eating foods that are in harmony with the season. The custom is basic not only to Chinese medicine but to the Asian lifestyle.

In spring and summer you'll find displayed sweet chrysanthemum flowers for a delicious tea used to prevent headache, eyestrain, and heatstroke, or honeysuckle flowers to cure fever and sore throat. Winter herbs will include warming blood-builders such as tang kuei (also spelled dong guei) and adrenal stimulants.

Year-round you'll find herbs that strengthen immunity against illness and fatigue, such as astragalus, as well as several forms of ginseng for vitality. These are combined with blood and energy tonic herbs sold as soup stocks in all Chinese grocery stores. Simmer a package of mild-tasting soup herbs for about forty-five minutes, then add vegetables or meat. Whoever thought Chinese medicine could taste so good! In Kam Man you can find herbs for soup stocks and sauces on the counter near the ginseng. They are time-tested vegetarian foods, the basis of Chinese health and vitality for over three thousand years.

Premixed soup stocks are instant herbal medicine, because you don't have to combine herbs yourself. The hard part is done for you. In China it's not so easy. There I've browsed in street markets where a Western tourist would not even recognize the herbs. Once, in a small village in Yunnan, I passed an herb seller on a bridge. Looking into his pots, I saw snakes and frogs used for their medicinal value. They are especially appreciated in South China. In Chinatown's supermarkets are a wide variety of quality foods and herbs, but you have to search to find snakes. Powdered turtle shell does turn up in a cooked gelatin, but pills containing dried snakes and insects are sold only at small herb shops.

On the east side of Mulberry Street, past a man selling miniature orange trees, is a fortune-teller who points to drawings of hands, while deciphering the mysteries of the future. Around the corner on Bayard Street, under the shoemaker's yellow umbrella, a barefoot client waits as a new sole is pounded in place. A soprano aria from Chinese opera wafts through the air as the shoemaker works.

One evening I attended the opera in Chengdu (known as "perfect metropolis"), the capital of Szechuan. Szechuan (also spelled Sichuan) is a huge, rich province in western China where, until recently, pandas wandered through dense bamboo forests. Now the bamboo is cut down and pandas doze at the zoo. Chengdu is a busy city, crowded with hundreds of people on bikes, and a main square that boasts a sixty-foot statue of Mao, usually covered with pigeons.

My night at the opera was well worth the few cents' admission. The hot summer

air was drowsy from jasmine blossoms. I had come by rickshaw to a courtyard where many old, bearded men smoked thin, foot-long pipes while sipping tea from tiny cups, either Ch'ing Ch'eng ("Green City") or Meng Ting ("Hidden Peak"), the two best-known green teas from Szechuan. Inside the opera house I was enthralled by acrobats and singers, who could be heard above the rustle of two hundred handheld fans.

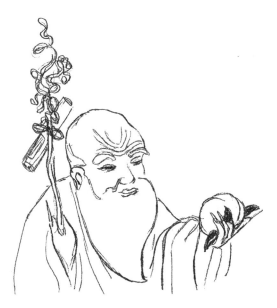

Chinese god of longevity

I also heard opera sung and stories recited by townsfolk near Buddhist temples. There I saw tiny women with bound feet, who must have been a hundred years old. Others told fortunes and sold herbs as water buffalo lounged nearby. In New York's Chinatown, the fortune-tellers congregate near

Columbus Park at Bayard Street. They use Chinese astrology and look at your hand to determine your body type. In a later chapter you'll read more about diagnosis based on constitutional types.

At the junction where Bayard meets Elizabeth Street, we see a dimly lit shop whose window displays large porcelain gods of family, money, and longevity. The Chinese god of longevity is a sage whose bald head resembles the fuzzy peach he holds in his left hand. In his right he carries a walking staff made from a primordial tree. The folds of its twisted shaft hold a Chinese scroll, a medical text. Chinese medicine is based on a tradition that respects longevity born of wisdom. In early times, wisdom was attained by living according to the laws of nature, which involved respecting seasonal changes and using natural remedies to maintain health and happiness.

Once, in an herb shop, the owner told my class to make way for a lady who was over a hundred years old. She had a kindly face. Tibetan and Indian doctors believe the ultimate source of health is love and compassion. Chinese doctors may not agree exactly. They describe diseases coming from outside influences such as wind, cold, and humidity. They use plenty of herbal antibiotics and painkillers. But I've heard from wise old Chinese doctors that when a patient has many illnesses, worries, and complaints, one should treat the heart. I have many heartfelt connections here in Chinatown. No matter what troubles the prevailing winds may bring, I know I'll find friends here in the Asia of the West, among intelligent people dedicated to kindness and good health.

Ending our visit, we pass vendors selling incense, ginkgo nuts, dried mushrooms, and ginseng. It all seems more familiar, but this is only the beginning of your herbal adventures.

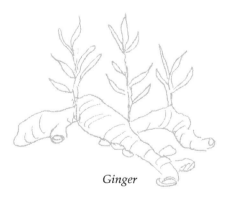

Ginger

陰 陰 陰 陰 陰 陰 陰 陰 陰 陰 陰 陰　陽 陽 陽 陽 陽 陽 陽 陽 陽 陽 陽 陽 陽

Yin: the structive or material aspect　　*Yang: the active or functional aspect of an effective position (e.g., of an internal organ)*

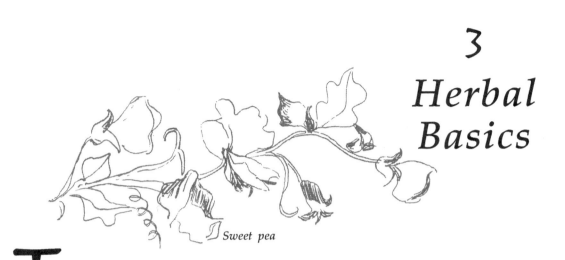

Sweet pea

3
Herbal Basics

The first time I traveled to the jungle, I was afraid of snakes. There is no advantage in such fear; besides, it's unfair. So I bought a baby snake about four inches long and kept him as a pet. He lived in a terrarium with moss and rocks and eventually turned a beautiful green color.

It was when I was attending acupuncture school and living in a tiny room on West Eleventh Street. It was my hut, my nunnery. The entire room was a loft bed. Under it, a window faced a tree. The kitchen filled a closet, and a shared bath was down the hall. The wiring was so old, the walls heated up when I plugged in a fan. Under the loft were plants, books, and acupuncture charts. I *called it my garden. That's where I put Demetri the snake, and the birds in their cage, along with some fish and a toad that honked in the night. My jungle was my home. I lost the fear of snakes when I became Demetri's mother.*

It's time to give up any reservations you may have concerning herbs. It's time to bring Asian herbs home by creating your own herbal pharmacy. You have to live with herbs to understand them, to make them your friends. They can become a part of your life after you trust them. However, we have to start with the basics.

What Is an Asian Herb?

Pearl S. Buck wrote about a Chinese population that was so impoverished they ate anything, even stone soup. Traditional medicines have evolved from such folk cures, but also from the richest and best nostrums, containing pearls and precious gems, used for emperors and kings. In the broadest definition, almost any natural substance can be and probably has been used as an Asian medicinal herb. Oriental doctors have left no stone unturned in an effort to discover medicines.

Standard Chinese herbal *materia medica* texts list more than four hundred herbs, with a collection that contains the unexpected. In Asia, herbs encompass products that are not strictly speaking "herbal." Typical is John Keys's *Chinese Herbs: Their Botany, Chemistry and Pharmacodynamics,* which lists, in addition to plants and fungi, minerals, a variety of animals and their

products, including horn, bone, venom, flying squirrel and bat guano, the discarded shells of beetles, wasp nests, seashells, and even dried, processed human placenta. The rarity of an herb is not as important as its correct use.

People have asked me if Asian herbs are better for treating illness than Western herbs. That depends on the definition of an Asian herb. Does it refer to the herb's origin or type? Do Asian herbs grow in Asia? Are they used by Asians? Cinnamon grows in Asia. Is cinnamon an Asian herb? Not exactly. It grows wherever there is adequate sunshine and humidity. I've seen cinnamon spread out, big sheets of tree bark, drying on rooftops at Canton's Ching Ping market. Next time you order cappuccino, ask the Italian waiter if cinnamon is a Chinese herb. He'll say it's international. Tenren, a Chinese company, grows ginseng in Wisconsin. Does that make it American ginseng? Not at all! American ginseng is an entirely different plant from the Chinese one. They have different Latin names and different effects that we'll study in a later chapter. Neither the origin nor the location of harvest determines an Asian herb.

Is a certain type of herb considered Asian? Asian herbs come in many forms. In shops all over Chinatown, merchants pull dried herbs out of drawers. For generations they've been added to soups and medicinal brews. Prescriptions might include anything from seeds, twigs, and leaves to dried seahorses. If the kind or origin doesn't matter, what is it about an herb that makes it Asian?

A remedy is considered an Asian

medical herb because its use is determined according to Asian medical diagnosis and criteria. It's an Asian herb when used according to traditional Asian medicine. Modern laboratory testing has isolated ingredients and proven the effectiveness of many Asian herbs. As of July 1995, Medline, an international online service that lists medical research abstracts, has 257 entries for ginseng alone. But animal testing is not in keeping with traditional herbal practice. In Asia, *people* have used herbs for thousands of years. The old way is actually easier to understand. We know when herbs work for us, because after using them we look and feel better. Such empirical proof is in keeping with the ancient ways.

HOW DO YOU CHOOSE THE RIGHT HERBS?

Many factors are involved in the effective selection of herbs. The type and source of illness and your age, stress level, and case history are all important. Specific diagnosis includes tongue and pulse readings, observations, questions, and palpation. These determine the herb choice and individualized dosage, which can vary as the treatment progresses in response to changes in your condition.

An appropriate choice for a particular person at a particular time is made from among a wide variety of herb types. For example, it might be a stimulant or a blood-builder, a moistening or drying herb, an anti-inflammatory or antibiotic, or an herb that stimulates circulation. Asian herbs are most often used in combination rather than singly, because their interaction synergistically increases their effectiveness.

HOW DO ASIAN HERBS WORK?

Asian herbs are chosen for their nutritional value as well as for their energetic qualities. Some herbs contain vitamins and minerals, but more often they're used as catalysts for metabolism, circulation, or energy and blood production.

Many plants contain important immunity-building constituents such as flavonoids, like those found in citrus; saponins, used for cancer prevention; or natural steroids that inhibit inflammation. Antibiotic herbs treating local or systemic problems are often combined with cleansing or strengthening herbs in order to facilitate their action and prevent side effects.

Asian medicine accepts a totality of body/mind/spirit. In that view, natural processes are explained not in terms of biochemistry but as changes in the quality, quantity, and directional flow of vital energy.

To understand what is meant by energetic medicine, we have to accept a view of humanness that may be closer to advanced physics than to Western medicine: Vital energy, a component of our being subtler than flesh, bones, and mechanics, is needed to explain what motivates human life. Medicinal herbs influence life's basic elements; they build the "fire" of metabolism, the "water" of blood, saliva, or semen, and "wind," the circulation of nerve impulses throughout the body. Put another way, herbs work by altering vigor, circulation, metabolism, body fluids, hormones, and emotions. Herbs fuel new growth and repair damaged tissue by enhancing nutrition through anabolism and catabolism. Herbs can also kill germs, reduce fever, or do many of the things that medical drugs do.

Because herbs are a part of an elaborate system of Asian medical thought and practice, they are chosen to affect specific parts of the body in particular ways. Herbs can maintain the normal flow of physical processes in organ systems and harmonize emotions in order to reestablish balance. For that reason, they have fewer side effects than Western medicines. To understand how Asian medical herbs work, we must first know a few things about Asian concepts of anatomy and physiology. We must understand that Chinese herbs are chosen according to how they affect *chi*.

What Is Chi?

Imagine for a moment that your body does not have bones, muscles, or blood vessels. Imagine that the internal organs do not have definite shape, but are pulsing with life force. What is it that keeps the heart working, the lungs breathing, or the kidneys filtering blood? Traditional Chinese doctors believe that this force is invisible energy called *chi*. (This word, pronounced "chee," may also be spelled *qi* or *ch'i*.)

Without adequate *chi* circulating through the body, internal organs stop func-

tioning. *Chi*, which fuels all body and mind processes, is augmented by food and oxygen and reduced by illness, toxins, and stress. Chinese anatomy and physiology study the process by which everything in the body/mind/spirit works smoothly, including how *chi* flows through its bodily containers, its channels.

To a traditional Chinese doctor, internal organs and their associated pathways are merely containers of vital energy. Health and happiness depend upon the smooth flow of *chi*, an invisible current somewhat resembling electricity. To study the body by merely dissecting organs would be like trying to research electricity by taking apart a television. You can never see the current because it is like *chi*. We need to observe *chi* in a different way, indirectly.

Westerners tend to be skeptical about *chi*. Because they can't measure it exactly every time, they think it does not exist, that it all sounds strange. And there's no word for *chi* in English. But consider this—we have each of us, without exception, experienced it. Have you ever sat in an airport waiting room and felt "butterflies in the stomach"? That's stuck *chi*. Discomfort is felt because *chi* is not circulating smoothly. If you massaged your stomach, took deep breaths, or imagined a pleasant situation, the stuck *chi* would begin to move more smoothly.

Have you ever wanted to yell at someone, but stopped yourself because the emotions were too strong? Did you feel a lump in the throat? That's stuck *chi*. If the circulation of vital energy is constrained long enough, it might eventually affect the thyroid gland. Chinese doctors believe that many illnesses come from deficient or stuck *chi*. We may even catch a cold because our defenses are low. But this can be reversed with herbs that affect *chi*, because when *chi* is unimpaired, defenses are free to go wherever needed in the body.

There is a healthy direction for the movement of *chi*. In a larger sense, the ley lines of the earth, the directions of winds, the movement of planets, all follow force fields of *chi*. In the human body, *chi* doesn't circulate aimlessly, but in recognizable patterns. This is true for all living beings. Try to pet a cat against the natural direction of his fur, and he'll react with a bite or a scratch. The pathways of *chi* traverse the body like roads. *Chi* moves downward and inward toward internal organs, and also upward and outward to the surface of the skin. When *chi* is adequate and its meridians are balanced, internal organs are held in place, and life's many processes are harmonious.

How do we treat *chi* imbalances? The body always gives us signs. In Part Two of this book you will observe the quantity and quality of your *chi* using traditional diagnosis. Imbalances are indicated by the appearance of the tongue, by facial color, by body language, and in other subtle ways that mark an interruption in the flow of *chi*. After reaching a working diagnosis, we may improve *chi* with herbs that affect specific areas of the body. Depending on the imbalance, it may be necessary to kill

germs, dissolve tumors, remove toxins, and treat a wide variety of chronic complaints. In any case, your metabolism, energy, and mood will improve as the soundness of *chi* is restored. Parts Three, Four, and Five offer you opportunities to determine and regulate the state of your *chi* and blood production so that with herbs the body can begin to heal itself.

Herbs move *chi* through the body's meridians in many ways. Some stimulant herbs lift *chi* toward the head; this is important when treating prolapse problems that come about when energy has become so low that organs literally slip. An example might be chronic diarrhea with extreme weakness. To treat such a condition we might use a stimulant, such as false ginseng (dang shen), along with Chinese wild yam for fatigue and weakness in the legs.

Diaphoretic herbs such as ginger and cinnamon move *chi* from deep inside the body toward the surface, to make us perspire. Such herbs are termed "scattering," and are considered *yang* in that they move energy upward and outward. Ginger and cinnamon are often used to sweat out the early stages of a cold.

Anti-inflammatory herbs cause *chi* to descend from head to feet or move inward toward internal organs. They reduce fever and swelling by taking excess acid wastes and body fluids to the organs of elimination. They move *chi* in a *yin* direction, toward the inside of the body.

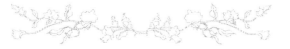

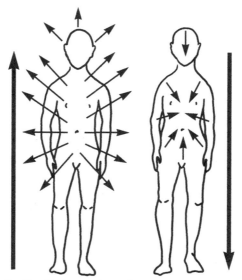

<table>
<tr><th>YANG</th><th>YIN</th></tr>
</table>

YANG

• *Herbs that move* chi *upward and outward toward the surface of the body*

• *Herbs that are stimulant tonics or diaphoretics (cause sweating)*

Examples: herbs that raise blood pressure, speed metabolism, increase inflammation, and treat skin conditions; herbs that lead other herbs to affect various parts of the body

YIN

• *Herbs that move* chi *downward and inward to affect internal organs and body fluids*

• *Herbs that are anti-inflammatory or draining*

Examples: laxatives, diuretics, herbs that lower blood pressure, herbs that reduce congestion or swelling, herbs that increase blood retention of internal organs or generate body fluids, blood-building herbs, sedatives, herbs that slow metabolism

The movement of chi *is described by the terms* yin *and* yang.

Yin *and* Yang

While *chi* represents vital energy, the terms *yin* and *yang* are sometimes used to describe its location, movement, function-ing, or quality. The two words represent many concepts in Chinese medicine, and it is partly the fault of translation that they are inexact in English. Also, *yin, yang,* and *chi* are not precise, absolute terms, but are always relative because they express changing relationships in an ever-evolving body/mind/spirit. In essence, *yin* and *yang* describe a polarity. Herbs are said to have a *yin* or *yang* nature.

One aspect of *yin* and *yang* compares their functions, in which *yin* is passive and *yang* active. The *yin*-producing foods and herbs are moistening, nourishing, and alka-line. They can be sedating or they can slow metabolism. *Yang* herbs, on the other hand,

have an active nature, in that they increase metabolism (seen as increased *chi*) and acidity.

Another aspect of *yin* and *yang* com-pares their location in the body. *Yin* is con-sidered more internal, *yang* more external. In that regard, *yin* refers to deeper acu-puncture meridians and blood and body fluids, whereas *yang* refers to more superfi-cial acupuncture meridians, and to the sur-face of the skin.

How can we use the duality of *yin* and *yang* when choosing herbs? At certain times, because of stress or disease, the body becomes imbalanced. We use herbs of an appropriate nature to bring us back into balance. For example, in fever diseases, dehydration symptoms develop, and moistening is required. Herbs that enhance *yin* (called *yin* tonics) are said to "nourish" or "moisten" the lungs, stomach, liver, or kidneys, which means they can increase blood or fluid retention in those organs. Therefore, when combined with herbs that lead them to affect those areas, *yin* tonics moisten dryness, soften phlegm, and alleviate thirst, dry cough, fever, and night sweats. They treat dehydration diseases such as diabetes, and increase strength and calm the mind. In colloquial English, *yin* tonics prevent burnout by generating fluids.

Yang tonics treat exhaustion and chronic weakness that may result from low adrenal function or irregular metabolism. *Yang* tonic herbs are often stimulants. Traditionally they've been used to reduce timidity, fear of cold weather, cold hands and feet, sore lower back and weak legs, sexual impotence, chronic watery diarrhea, incontinence, and fatigue-related asthma. *Yang* tonics provide the "fire" that drives the endocrine system.

Much of the information in the ancient medical texts that form the core of Asian medicine is metaphorical. For example, natural elements are used to explain body processes because they're easy to visualize. Herbs affect the *chi* of internal organs. Instead of describing how a diuretic herb stimulates the kidneys to remove excess water retention, an herb is said to "remove dampness" from the body. We have all experienced the lethargy similar to fatigue that accompanies humid weather. Whether we believe the body has "dampness" or not, we can still benefit from a diuretic herb that stimulates the *chi* of the kidneys. Digestive herbs such as ginger and pepper increase digestive *chi*, which means they speed digestion.

This gives you an idea why certain herbs are used in many different kinds of herbal remedies: Their energetic function ultimately depends on the role they play in a particular formula. A stimulant herb such as Chinese ginseng (considered *yang*) is often added to nourishing, blood-building herbs (considered *yin*) to ensure their digestion and absorption. Without a stimulant herb to build digestive *chi*, the semisweet fruit or fungus blood-building herbs might cause indigestion. This type of herbal combination parallels and eventually creates healthy digestion. The herbs used are not merely supplements that provide stomach acid or enzymes; they actually ensure the health of digestive organs by stimulating *chi*. Thus, herbs provide both the "food" and the "fire" to cook it.

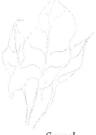

Sorrel

湯藥 湯藥 湯藥 湯藥 湯藥 湯藥 湯藥　湯劑 湯劑 湯劑 湯劑 湯劑 湯劑 湯劑

[tāngyào]　　　　　　　　　　　[tāngjì]

Decoction of medicinal ingredients, a medicine prepared by boiling, to be taken after the dregs are removed

4

How to Use Herbs

In gardens, health-food stores, or herb shops we find leaves, berries, flowers, pods, and other lightweight plant products that can be steeped as tea, called an *infusion*. Twigs, roots, or other heavy, dense

Artichoke

parts of medicinal plants are most often simmered for more than twenty minutes to make a decoction. If you dislike the taste of medicinal herbs, have your herb shop powder them, then fill gelatin capsules (available in health-food stores) with the powder. Some herbs are appreciated for taste as well as effect. Make medicinal liquors by adding digestive herbs, energy tonics, and blood-building elixirs to wine, brandy, or vodka. Add approximately one ounce of dried herbs per pint of liquor. Keep this in an airtight bottle, away from direct sunlight, for three weeks. Gently turn the bottle upside down once or twice a week to mix the ingredients.

The dosage of herbal teas, capsules, or healing brew is always an individual matter based on the diagnosis. Other forms of herbal products include healing baths, massage oils, inhalers, and medicated incense.

This book offers a unique opportunity to participate in an herbal network. Health specialists listed in the Herbal Access appendix are available for questions and individual phone consultations. Herb manufacturers listed can supply mail-order and product information. As your skills in diagnosis improve, you will be able to communicate with them more effectively.

How to Prepare and Cook Herbs

First, clean any herbs you buy. I have found contaminants in the most widely used health food and standard American foods. (I once found a bee in a jar of organic tomato sauce. Another time I saw a chicken bone in a grocery store package of carrots.) Because spices may become moldy or infested, it is good to inspect them. Dried

seaweeds can come with tiny shells or sand; therefore they have to be soaked, and the rinse water changed many times until it's clear. In Asia, herbs are sometimes sun-dried on the ground, and teas can leave a residue of black soil from South China in the bottom of your cup.

I am sometimes asked whether Asian herbs have been sprayed or irradiated. I can't answer precisely, because it depends upon the country of origin. In over ten years of Asian travel through India, Ladakh, Thailand, Tibet, and China, I have walked herb fields. I've watched as Tibetan monks in India's Manali valley picked the year's harvest, spending days chanting and grinding herbs. In the Thai jungle, I've lived with people in huts who had little to eat but herbs. Never were my senses asphyxiated by harsh chemicals.

Most herb-producing countries are too poor to use radiation. One exception is the United States. We are the world's largest producer of hops, used in making beer. Labeling of foods for chemicals and radiation is left to individual states. You may have to call your local health department to find out.

At any rate, herbs should be rinsed before steeping. I usually blanch them with boiling water for a minute, then rinse and prepare them as directed. When you are ready to cook the herbs, use a ceramic-coated or earthenware or glass pot, never Teflon-coated or aluminum. Use pure, fresh water that is free of chemicals and heavy metals.

STEEP LIKE A TEA

Herbs that are delicate
 leaves
 flowers
 grasses
 powdered spices

SIMMER 20 MINUTES OR LONGER

Herbs that are solid
 roots, twigs, bark, pods
 rocks, bones
 fungus, seeds, animal products

There are few hard-and-fast rules governing the preparation of teas. Local custom dominates the use of herbs in China and India, and for better or worse, this has carried over to the West. Chinese herbal doctors call individual potions "teas" or "soups." In Chinatown, doctors prepare individual recipes by spreading dried herbs onto pieces of paper on the shop counter. Often such combinations are so complicated, containing flowers, pods, roots, or fungus, that the ingredients have to be simmered together for several hours in order to blend them. Usually Chinese herbs are cooked a long time, either alone or with meat or soup ingredients.

Ayurvedic physicians sometimes recommend powdered herbs added to warmed milk or rice gruel. Individual differences and food allergies must always be accommodated. Milk is used in India because it is cooling, sweet, and nourishing, and because the cow is sacred. She is loved because she shares her milk with everyone. Because individual digestion and climates can differ, excess phlegm produced by milk may be a problem for people no matter how sacred its source.

Why Asian Herbal Remedies Are Safe

Most of our grandmothers' generation had herb gardens, or used herbs as medicine. Only during this century have herbs come under the scrutiny of government inspection. One reason we must test herbs is economic: Drug companies must show a profit. Roughly one third of all medical drugs come from isolated active plant ingredients. But drug companies can't put a brand name on something that grows like a weed; they have to break down a plant's hundreds of components, testing for years at great expense. Then they can claim to have discovered the active ingredient. However, many times the active ingredient does not work as well as the entire plant. According to tests done in Germany, Saint John's wort, the entire herb, kills the AIDS virus in the test tube, while hypericum, the isolated active ingredient, does not.

Unfortunately, a younger generation seems to have adopted a skeptical attitude concerning the healing properties of herbs because of all the talk about testing. Asian remedies have been tested in the laboratory of life for thousands of years. They are proven safe because people—not rats—have used them for generations without suffering dangerous side effects. Many herbs are even assimilated as foods.

As noted previously, another reason

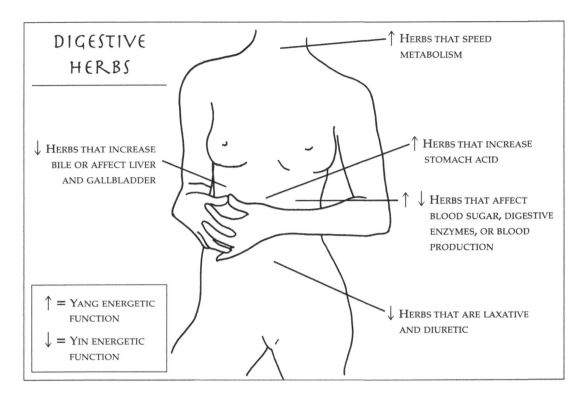

DIGESTIVE HERBS

↑ HERBS THAT SPEED METABOLISM

↓ HERBS THAT INCREASE BILE OR AFFECT LIVER AND GALLBLADDER

↑ HERBS THAT INCREASE STOMACH ACID

↑ ↓ HERBS THAT AFFECT BLOOD SUGAR, DIGESTIVE ENZYMES, OR BLOOD PRODUCTION

↓ HERBS THAT ARE LAXATIVE AND DIURETIC

↑ = YANG ENERGETIC FUNCTION

↓ = YIN ENERGETIC FUNCTION

why Asian herbal cures are safe is that most of them are prepared in *combinations*, not singly. To understand why this is so, consider the body. It is made up of parts working together. The healthy body does more than one thing at a time, and so do herbal combinations. Such natural medicines respect the body's innate need for balance.

The above drawing shows the digestive organs along with the types of herbs that might be used for proper digestion. Digestive herbal combinations are made of such herbs. For example, some may stimulate stomach acids or digestive enzymes, while others may help release bile or reduce water retention in order to smooth digestion. For comfortable, healthy digestion, all

these processes should happen at the same time. This may seem obvious, but it is exactly the reason why many medical drugs have toxic side effects, while herbs do not. Good digestion requires the coordinated functioning of many processes at once, and herbal combinations can do many things at once in order to maintain balance.

Also, the characters of plants and drugs are intrinsically different from each other. There is a built-in safety factor in plants, in that they are made up of many components, sometimes as many as several hundred, that can be isolated into ingredients. A medical drug often uses only one of those chemical ingredients—say, one out of four hundred. Laboratory testing can tell us what effect that drug has on one part of the body. For example, an antacid drug that treats ulcers can inhibit the flow of a particular enzyme. But that same drug also affects other tissues throughout the body. It can cause enzyme activity that is a precursor to a toxin. That is, it can cause a toxic effect in some other part of the body, a bad side effect.

Herbal remedies use more of the plant. Its hundreds of components work together, assuring absorption of the remedy with fewer unpredictable actions. Why? Because the body considers a natural remedy to be a food. The whole herb does not affect cellular activity the way a drug can, because it does not work on the cellular level. Herbs improve nutrition or *chi* production in the way a food does, not in the way an enzyme does.

By using herbal combinations, the remedy's sphere of activity can be guided to the appropriate part of the body, thus avoiding adverse side effects. For example, several medical drugs used to treat high blood pressure coincidentally reduce inflammation throughout the entire body, and have been known to cause sexual impotence, a high price to pay. By contrast, Chinese patent remedies such as **Blood Pressure Repressing Tablets** treat headache and dizziness from hypertension with herbs such as coptis and scutellaria, which affect head symptoms without damaging a person's sex life. Thus the area of treatment becomes more specific with herbal combinations. By combining herbs, we protect ourselves from the weakening effects of any treatment.

Without proper diagnosis, the use of any food or herb might cause temporary unpleasant effects. This happens when innate imbalances are aggravated. For instance, if we had fever and took inflammatory herbs or foods, the fever could rise. If we ate hot peppers for stomachache, or raw salad for diarrhea and cramps, we would feel worse and have bad side effects. By listening to our body, we avoid such mistakes. Often our reaction to poor food choices is enough warning for us to stop. The same kind of instinctive decision is often made with herbs.

Nevertheless, there are times when symptoms become temporarily worse from using natural remedies, such as when the body (or the mind) is fighting to maintain an illness. This is especially true of deep, chronic problems, because bad habits are hard to break, even those that lead to disease. However, discomforts often clear up after only a few doses of herbs, when blocked *chi* is freed. Successful herbal regimens are organized in combinations of herbs that reduce symptoms of withdrawal and discomfort due to cleansing. When in doubt, check with one of the health practitioners listed in the Herbal Access appendix. Often all you will need is reassurance or further directions on dosage or how to take a remedy.

HOW LONG TO USE HERBS

Use herbs while they are effective, then stop or change them as needed. Observing changes in metabolism with Asian tongue diagnosis will be a guide to when to stop a remedy. In general, herbs are not meant to be taken daily, like vitamins. They should be changed with variations in symptoms, lifestyle, stress levels, or seasons.

It is better for beginners not to combine too many remedies at once. Mixing herbs without knowing how they affect each other confuses the body. You may experience temporary dizziness or digestive discomfort. This is a warning to reduce or simplify the remedy. Luckily, there are many time-tested combinations of herbs that are easy to use. In this book we will study many of them to see how they are "built" and how they work.

BUILDING HERBAL COMBINATIONS

Have you ever watched a house being built? First a concrete foundation is laid into a deep hole. This gives the house a solid base. The plumbing pipes are included when laying the foundation, so that pipes on the first floor can connect with others on the second floor. Then the wall framework is constructed on top of the foundation to make the walls. In this way, many rooms can be made.

Building an herbal combination is a bit like building a house. The foundation is the primary energetic function of the combination. Let's look at a real example: **Xiao Yao Wan.** (An alternate spelling is **Hsiao Yao Wan.**) This is a Chinese digestive remedy I often recommend because it accomplishes many important functions at once. **Xiao Yao Wan** is good for digestion, circulation, and blood-building, and treats a number of emotional problems such as nervousness and irritability. It frees *chi* trapped in the digestive center.

How is **Xiao Yao Wan** built? The combination contains paeonia, atractylodes, tang kuei, ginger, mint, bupleurum, licorice root, and poria (fu ling), a fungus. The first four herbs strengthen the functions of stomach, spleen, pancreas, and gallbladder. Mint and bupleurum facilitate the flow of bile downward from the gallbladder to the intestine, and licorice helps with absorption. According to our analogy, all these digestive herbs make up the foundation and walls of the house, making sure digestive energy flows in a healthy direction (from stomach to intestines). In effect, digestive *chi* is strengthened in the center.

If you divided the separate functions of this combination into rooms, you'd have one for blood-building, containing tang kuei and atractylodes; another for smooth digestion, with bupleurum, mint, ginger, and licorice; and one for circulation, with tang kuei and paeonia. Poria, a diuretic, corresponds to the plumbing. It's included because we need a diuretic to remove wastes. By ensuring smooth digestion and circulation, we ease the digestive center. This remedy is safe because it encourages the body to function normally. **Xiao Yao Wan** eliminates low digestive *chi* and poor local circulation that could lead to pain and indigestion.

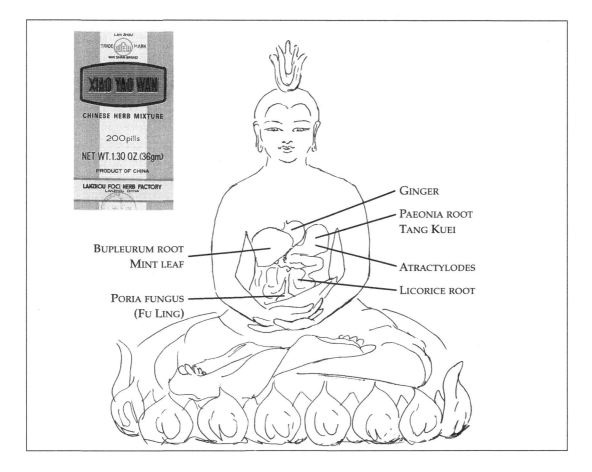

Xiao Yao Wan — Chinese Herb Mixture, 200 pills, Net Wt. 1.30 oz. (36gm), Product of China, Lanzhou Foci Herb Factory

- GINGER
- PAEONIA ROOT
- TANG KUEI
- ATRACTYLODES
- LICORICE ROOT
- BUPLEURUM ROOT
- MINT LEAF
- PORIA FUNGUS (FU LING)

How to Begin a Home Herbal Pharmacy

Your herbal studies will become more meaningful as you directly experience their results. After developing skills in personal diagnosis and a fundamental understanding of herbal energetics with this book, you will be able to treat minor discomforts effectively at home.

Start by setting aside some space in your home for herbs. The area should be free from direct sunlight and extreme heat. Keep your herb collection visible in bottles on a bookshelf or in a cabinet. If the herbs are hidden, you won't learn their names. Label the jars or plastic containers with the names of the herb, their uses, and dates of purchase. Check herbs periodically for freshness. Discard moldy or spoiled herbs.

Section off parts of the shelf for different categories of herbs. See the diagram earlier in this chapter for possible herbs to include. With this book you will study certain qualities of herbs you can put on the labels. For example, digestive herbs such as ginger, cardamom, fennel, and mint can be differentiated by marking which herbs have *heating* and *cooling* properties. Write CARDAMOM—DIGESTION, HEATING on the label, or MINT—COOLING; or a specific function such as DANDELION—LAXATIVE, LIVER CLEANSER. The chapter on culinary medicines will provide you with a large selection of easy-to-use herbs.

Pick one or two major herbs from each category of digestive herbs, stimulants, expectorants, diuretics, and so on. Don't try to complete each group, but pick a wide variety of herbs. Many herbs will be discussed in chapters concerning specific health problems, so that you will get a more refined knowledge of their uses. Study one herb at a time, reading everything you can find from Eastern and Western sources for a few days. After you've studied diagnosis, you may want to cook the herb and use it appropriately for yourself.

When you are ready to start combining herbs, study several Asian patent remedies and traditional combinations in packaged teas. You will notice that they most often combine herbs with different energetic functions, such as stimulant tonics along with blood-builders.

A good way to learn how to combine herbs is by re-creating simple patent remedies at home, using the loose herbs. You might cook **Xiao Yao Wan** from scratch. This book will provide many such recipes. Another fine source is Jake Fratkin's *Chi-*

nese Herbal Patent Formulas. After studying standard patent formulas for a while, you'll be able to make adjustments with ingredients according to specific needs. You will appreciate having the tastes and smells of cooked herbs at home. They create a different energy, foreign but healing, like an aromatherapy trip to China.

If you intend to pursue diagnosing other people, make a commitment to study herbs for several years before you start recommending them. It helps to try out a diversity of herbs on yourself first. Additional home-study courses, herb doctors, teachers, books, and your own experience can be your guide. I've offered some suggestions for further study in the Herbal Access appendix.

Finally, we must acknowledge that although herbal remedies must be individually tailored, some general rules do apply concerning how and when to use herbs most effectively. The following suggestions come with the understanding that there are optimum times to take herbs daily, as well as certain combinations to avoid.

WHEN TO START AND STOP TAKING HERBS

Although blood and energy tonics and herbs that build immune strength can be taken as long-term remedies for chronic weakness, acute maladies should be treated according to their symptoms. This will be covered in detail in later chapters. Always monitor your tongue changes while using herbs (see chapter 11). Also

What Kinds of Herbs to Take, and When

MORNING

Cleansing and laxative teas as needed
Weight-loss, anticholesterol teas as needed
    all day
Herbs for irregular heartbeat (e.g.,
    hawthorn capsules or **Mao Dung
    Ching**) if needed after meals

MEALTIMES

Digestive herbs (containing herbal
    cleansers, antistagnation herbs, and
    blood-building herbs, as well as
    those useful for stomach pain, excess
    bloating, and poor circulation)
Ulcer or antidiarrheal herbal medicines
Blood- and energy-building tonics, along
    with digestive herbs

*BETWEEN MEALS (these do not help
digestion)*

Herbs for sinus, lungs, breathing, and skin
Herbs for the kidneys, adrenal energy,
    back, and legs
Herbs for joint pain, arthritis, hemor-
    rhoids, and injury
Herbs for cold, flu, and fever (may
    increase sweating)
Herbs for the mind

*BEFORE BED (DO NOT MIX WITH
FOODS, ESPECIALLY HOT SPICES)*

Herbs to calm the spirit and the nerves, or
    to increase mental clarity
Sedative herbs for insomnia
Herbs for vision problems
Anti-inflammatory herbs for hot flashes or
    night sweats

monitor digestion. Do you experience pain, diarrhea, or constipation? Add appropriate digestive herbs as needed.

Observe the urine and stools for changes (see chapter 9). You can observe specific imbalances by noting color and consistency.

Women should monitor their menstrual periods. Are they on time? Painful? With PMS or exhaustion? (See the chapters in the Not for Women Only section.)

Complaints may vary according to season as well as internal changes. Thus, herbal formulas must be updated regularly according to individual needs. Check with a knowledgeable herbalist or a traditional Asian doctor periodically to discuss symptoms and results of remedies. The Herbal Access appendix contains the names of herbalists and organizations with referral lists of natural health practitioners.

HERBS AS FOODS AND MEDICINES

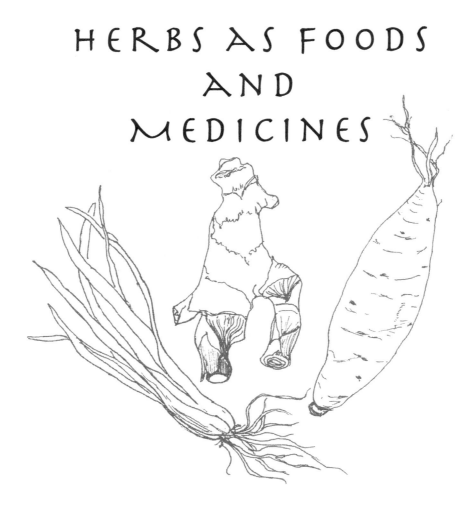

茶茶茶茶茶茶茶茶茶茶茶茶茶　　土方土方土方土方土方土方土方土方

[chá] Medicinal tea, drugs in crude powder or made into small cakes, taken as tea after being infused with boiling water or boiled in water

[tǔfāng] Folk recipe; folk remedy

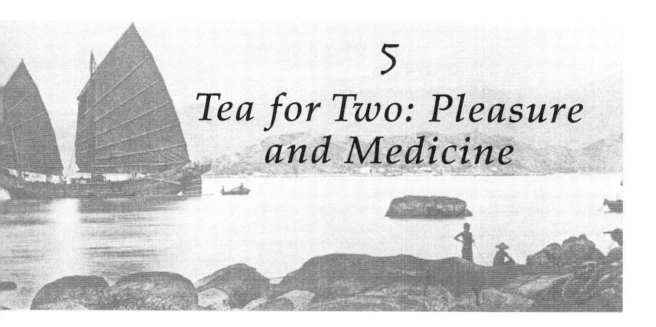

5
Tea for Two: Pleasure and Medicine

If you ever have the mixed pleasure of traveling by train in mainland China, you'll find tea to be the only amenity. Chinese travelers bring along jars of tea leaves that they refresh many times with hot water. There are four classes on Chinese trains. The most basic, called "hard seat," is my specialty, since I travel in summer, when most of the world goes on vacation. The other so-called luxury classes are sold to large tourist groups. "Hard seat" is just like it sounds: a hard seat, metal with no cover. The seats are meant for *two but, in reality, hold both parents, with children sleeping on their laps and underneath the seats, or on top of you. Since they wear open breeches and eat watermelon sold at station stops, the kids provide the train's running water.*

The toilet is always locked, with sick people sitting hopefully outside it. The steaming hot water in a tap at the end of the car is used by all to wash hands, feet, and faces, and to make tea. Everyone is up all night yelling about who's in whose seat. All the men smoke cigarettes in every car, blowing the smoke directly into your face. I rolled along like this for days from Guangzhou through Hunnan into Yunnan's capital, Kunming, where the stench from a cigarette factory permeates the air.

The lovely countryside through Yunnan and Szechuan has many tea fields that wind in concentric circles along steep hillsides. Near Guilin, you pass some of the most spectacular countryside China has to offer. Enormous mountains, once beneath the ocean, are made of limestone. They are so huge, their presence affects the ecology and temperature of the entire planet. During the People's Revolution, this area had collective farms where people worked the fields fourteen to sixteen hours a day. Workers were taken from jobs, university studies, and spouses for up to twenty years in order to ensure zero population growth in China. They were paid a few cents a month and a bag of white rice. Tea was considered medicine or luxury.

Tea was probably the first Asian herb you ever used. It's one of our oldest links to the East, although most westerners are unfamiliar with the wide variety of Chi-

nese teas. Some teas contain caffeine; others don't. Each type has specific medicinal uses: green teas tend to be cooling and cleansing, while red ones are warming and digestive. Teas are easy-to-use, fast-acting medicines. Often their effects are felt after only one or two cups, yet they are mild enough to enjoy all day. Teas as familiar as those sold in grocery stores have figured in Chinese and American history and culture. And their health benefits still play an important role.

In Asia, tea is a highly prized staple of life with considerable health benefits. For example, green tea provides a gentle stimulant for metabolism and the central nervous system, with a negligible amount of caffeine. It contains vitamins A, B_2, C, D, P, and useful flavonoids that increase absorption of vitamin C, thereby strengthening blood capillaries. Recent studies indicate that Chinese green teas reduce cholesterol by lowering blood lipids, so that they reduce the risk of heart disease, stroke, and cancer. They also taste wonderful.

Historically, the emperors had their own private varieties of tea grown for flavor. Thousands of people cared for the young plants growing on hillsides from Yunnan to Fujian. Today we can buy those royal teas together with others from South China, such as oolong and Bohea, the tea that was thrown overboard at the Boston Tea Party.

The New England colonists boiled tea as a beverage, also using the liquid to dye cloth and eating the leaves as a vegetable, with salt and butter. Eventually,

Chinese tea became useful for a number of digestive ailments, including "the gripes," a colorful term for dysentery. If you become an Asian traveler, you may invent your own colorful expressions.

Although practitioners of the traditional medicine of the emperors used rare expensive plants, animals, and precious gems, the medicine of the Chinese countryside has always consisted of foods and teas. There were comparatively few classically trained physicians, not enough to care for the billions of peasants, students, and city dwellers thrown together during the Revolution. Thus a different kind of medicine, using "barefoot doctors," was established, and the remedies employed by them are still used today. Antibiotic teas were widely utilized by "barefoot doctors" for fevers and infectious diseases. Their training also included simple first-aid and folk remedies designed to get workers back to the fields as soon as possible. Some tea remedies are powerful and unpleasant tasting; others prevent chronic problems related to indigestion, and are great for everyday use.

Classifications of Chinese Teas

Chinese teas are classified according to taste, color, and energetic effects. For example, Tuocha is considered a bitter green tea that has mildly sedative and anticholesterol properties. When tea is used as medicine, its most important aspect is its energetic effect.

THE ENERGETIC EFFECTS OF TEA: DIGESTIVE AND STIMULANT

When we speak of a tea's energetic effects, we are referring to how it affects *chi*. Tea stimulates "digestive *chi*" or metabolism. Chinese teas are slightly laxative, or help clear phlegm without irritating the nervous system. Coffee can make you nervous, but tea clears your head while it stimulates digestion. Which teas are best for you depends on your needs. Tea has two main features: taste and medicinal effect.

THE COLORS AND TASTES OF TEAS

For those who think that tea grows in bags or that they're no more exciting than the usual brands, Chinese teas offer a delightful change. Teas in China are white, green, black, or red in color. The white and green teas are the least fermented and contain the least caffeine. They are refreshing and range from very mild in flavor to slightly bitter, whereas the red and black teas are more bracing. Many of the following popular teas are easily found in Chinese grocery stores.

White teas

White teas are the most pale when brewed and mildest in flavor because they are sun-dried and receive little processing. Of all the varieties, white tea tastes the most like freshly picked tea leaves. For example,

Sow Mee ("Old Man's Eyebrows") has a light fragrance and shiny silver leaves.

White teas are sometimes combined with cleansing herbs that reduce cholesterol. For example, Bojenmi is the brand name of a famous weight-loss tea made from white tea leaves combined with slimming herbs (see chapter 15).

Green teas

Green teas are more bitter in flavor than white teas. The leaves are dark green and the effect is slightly laxative. So much research has been done on the health benefits of green tea that its fame has reached the West, where *The New York Times* has reported its cancer-preventing properties. In addition to reducing cholesterol, green teas' flavonoids help absorption of vitamin C, which boosts immune strength.

Green teas can be bracing teas like the type called "gunpowder," or milder ones like Lung Ching. It's good to start the day with a bitter green tea that eliminates poorly digested food. Green tea acts as a stimulant because it clears phlegm. Do you awaken feeling foggy? It's probably digestive phlegm. Not all teas cleanse in the same way. Jasmine tea, often classified as green tea, is made by adding jasmine flowers to teas. It may not be the best tea for first thing in the morning, because jasmine flowers are considered *cooling* (anti-inflammatory) and moistening. They may create phlegm in some persons. The rule of thumb is that the tea that works well, feels refreshing, energizing, and cleansing is the best morning tea for you.

Differences between white and green teas

How can you differentiate between a white tea and a green one? Green teas have dark green leaves that are sometimes curled, and a stronger aroma and taste. White teas are rarer, with flat, sliced, silvery leaves. Many green teas are named for their sources, such as Shih Feng ("Lion's Peak"), Pai Yun ("White Cloud"), Pao Yun ("Jeweled Cloud"), Tz'e-sun ("Purple Sprout"), Hsieh Tou ("Snow Gorge"), and Jin Chu ("Sun-Poured" or "Sun-Fused"), which originate from Zhejiang province, near Fujian in the southeast.

All about oolong

Oolong is a gem of teas that is actually semifermented and lies somewhere between green and black tea. It has less caffeine than either black tea or coffee. It also has been touted in China as a cancer preventative because of its acids and flavonoids. Oolong, like many other green teas, hails from Fujian, the part of mainland China closest to Taiwan. Fujian shares Taiwan's humid climate, but that's where the comparison stops. Taiwan is one of the richest countries in the world, with more gold bullion and foreign exchange saved than any other. It is modern, powerful, and traditionally Buddhist. Fujian, one of China's poorest provinces, is often closed to tourists.

Oolong is digestive, stimulant, and delicious. It lifts the spirits. With green or oolong tea, we are satisfied by the flavor without suffering any draining effects. Coffee may be a stimulant and laxative, but long-term use weakens both digestion and the heart by overstimulation.

The names of Chinese teas often reflect their qualities; for example, one oolong tea is delicate enough to be called Hsien Shui ("Water Nymph"). Another famous brand is Ti Kuan Yin ("Iron Goddess of Mercy"), named after Kuan Yin, the Chinese Bodhisattva of Compassion. Another variety, Tit Koon Yum (Kuan Yin's name in Cantonese), comes from Hong Kong. A wake-up tea, it packs a stronger punch than other oolongs.

We often see porcelain statues of Kuan Yin, a beautiful female deity, in Chinatown stores, dressed in a long white gown, carrying a golden vase containing the nectar of compassion. She is loved by her devotees, who celebrate her with a special day in Taiwan because whenever asked for happiness, health, or children, she always responds by showering them with her nectar of compassion. The cleansing effects of oolong, not to mention the blessings from Kuan Yin, seem a better deal than the usual morning "mud-in-yer-eye."

The most prized tea quality is called "first picked" because it comes from the early spring tea harvest. One delicious example among the green teas is Lung Ching ("Dragon Well"), produced in Zhejiang province near Hangzhou's West Lake. The tea grows on several peaks of the T'ieh Mu mountain range, the choicest variety coming from Lion's Peak. The fragrance of this tea is so delicate that connoisseurs recommend storing it in airtight containers: exposure to air would ruin the flavor and aroma. Brewed, Lung Ching has a subtle bouquet that is best enjoyed without interference from stronger tastes of meat or cheese. A tea worthy of enjoyment all by itself during a moment's contemplation, Lung Ching is more expensive than other green teas, and worth it.

Red and black teas

There is some confusion about whether some teas are considered black or red. This may be because their hues blend with steeping. For example, one called Tsui Yang Fei ("Drunken Concubine Yang") is described by John Blofeld in his book *The Chinese Art of Tea:*

When processed, the tea becomes black, but with a reddish tinge suggestive of a beauty's cherry lips, making "people feel drunk with joy!" However, it is rare and its taste not particularly good.

Chinese black teas contain the most caffeine. They are strong stimulants without some of the damaging effects of coffee. They may have potent flavors like Chinese "brick tea," Lok On, orange pekoe, or Yingteh. They may be perfumed with rose petals or essential oils. When smoked, black tea becomes Lapsang Souchong. British dignitaries admired this delicious tea sweetened with milk for late-afternoon sipping. (True Chinese tea aficionados would cringe at the thought of milk or sugar.)

Red tea, the most fermented type, contains no more caffeine than green tea, but has a full-bodied taste. Some red teas are also classified as "black," but their effect is more important than their color. Chinese red tea, like Japanese bancha twig, is digestive. Teas that increase digestion are called carminative. For persons troubled by slow, painful digestion, a digestive tea can actually be a stimulant because it increases digestive *chi*. The body has better vital energy and circulation because it is not struggling to digest.

Pu-Erh is a well-known carminative tea, grown at Nam Nor mountain in Yunnan province. The red color of the tea matches the red soil of the region. Pu-Erh is mildly sweet, with a flavor reminiscent of autumn leaves.

Pu-Erh is a good tea for those who eat unwisely. It reduces digestive phlegm so that it cures indigestion from an overly rich diet of meat or creamy or fried food. In China it has other uses. The diet in South China's ricefields is meager and not always clean. Human fertilizer is used to raise crops, and this makes it necessary to cook everything thoroughly. Also, oily and sweet foods can lead to excess phlegm. The result is often parasites. Pu-Erh tea is a folk remedy for dysentery because it reduces digestive phlegm, the playground for parasites.

Pu-Erh is also popular for hangovers. The Chinese seem to have quite a few such household remedies. (Also see American ginseng tea, chapter 32.) Pu-Erh tea clears head and palate at the same time. Fancy dim sum parlors have been known to serve this digestive red-colored tea, but you'll have to ask for it. Restaurateurs most often

serve jasmine tea because they think it's the only Chinese tea we know, while the staff is probably drinking a lesser-known red tea in the backroom. It'll likely be a digestive such as Pu-Erh or Po Nee. Their rich flavors are well suited to dim sum delights. Just ask for [*hong cha*], which means "red tea." (Do you want the long version? [*Ching wen! Gay wah suma hong cha.*] "Please give me some red tea.")

Long-term Benefits of Tea

Some have claimed that tea makes you beautiful, others that it makes you smart. The greatest benefit is that tea is digestive, and that's no small thing. Asians know that excess weight and cholesterol, along with stress and sedentary lifestyle, can lead to serious problems. Obesity is not a problem in China. For one thing, people travel everywhere on bicycles. They have less heart disease than we do. Many people attribute this to diet, but it's not as simple as that. Let's consider for a moment the relationship of heart disease to cholesterol.

CHOLESTEROL, HEART PROBLEMS, AND TEA

Many experts say that a low-fat diet is helpful in preventing excess cholesterol. Chinese doctors say digestion requires "digestive *chi*," the energy of metabolism. When the body labors to digest a rich, fatty meal, less *chi* is available for breathing, thinking, and maintaining a steady heartbeat. Poor digestion increases stress, and vice versa. Plaque is made up of fat, cholesterol, calcium, clotting factor, and cellular waste. This is what can eventually clog blood vessels, choking off circulation.

According to Chinese medicine, diets high in fat and cholesterol not only increase body weight but also create poor circulation. Oily or fat foods also encourage what Chinese doctors call *she,* a term used to describe digestive wastes, precursors to fat, cellulite, and tumors.

What is it that makes Chinese people more healthy? They have a lot working against them. *The New York Times* reported six-year studies done by Western universities that have shown the reduced protein intake of the typical Chinese diet to be effective in reducing arthritis and heart disease. Although this is true, such studies, done near Beijing, do not take into account the diet of the near-starving populations in the southern countryside, where problems of poverty and poor sanitation have witnessed a rise in hepatitis and plague.

The everyday diet in rural China is white rice, white flour, sugar, and grease from pork, with practically no fruits and vegetables. Breakfast in Yunnan is a bowl of oily liquid with white noodles. Workers eat this while squatting in their blue uniforms in early-morning street markets. No one looks up to smile. To this phlegm-producing diet is added pollution from burning coal and cigarette smoke, and the combination produces two of South China's major health problems: asthma and stroke.

Aside from diet and pollution, external stress is another contributing factor to health. Left over from the People's Revolution is an elaborate hierarchy of local authorities. This cadre controls the economic, social, and personal maneuvering of the majority of Chinese people. No one can open a business, get permission to marry, or have a child without the cadre's consent. They oversee the quotas.

You'd think that stress-related hypertension would be difficult to control in China, but this is not the case. When I asked Dr. Xiao Wu, an acupuncturist in Chengdu, a historically important medical center, how successfully he treated stroke, he said that symptoms of paralysis and aphasia were often totally reversed with acupuncture and herbs within two months, when the patient received early treatment. Like most other Chinese doctors, he also recommended a wise diet and several teas for prevention of excess cholesterol.

For prevention and treatment of hypertension and stroke, traditional Chinese medicine (abbreviated TCM) recommends a diet low in both fats and sweets. This is because fats, nuts, and fried foods inhibit the functioning of liver and gallbladder, while sweets slow the functioning of spleen and pancreas. Put another way, hard-to-digest foods reduce digestive *chi.* We can find remedies for these problems in all Chinese grocery stores, in the form of delicious anticholesterol teas.

Chinese anticholesterol teas

One tea famous for reducing cholesterol is Tuocha. It's a relaxing tea. Although it's available packaged loose or in bags, my favorite form is a rock-hard cone that comes from Yunnan. You have to dig at it with a knife to get a spoonful for your teapot. Served hot, its perfume transports you to ricefields after a rain, where the air is dank and heavy, yet refreshing.

Other Chinese anticholesterol teas include Temple of Heaven gunpowder tea, a bitter green tea. Despite its name, it contains very little caffeine. Many weight-loss teas, including Bojenmi and The Well-Known Tea, contain hawthorn, which reduces cholesterol. (See Part Four on weight loss and raw tienchi ginseng.)

ADDITIONS TO TEA: SPICES AND SWEETENERS

For added flavor and special benefits, try adding pungent cooking spices to teas. A pinch of turmeric powder increases cleansing. It's a natural antibiotic that improves intestinal flora, which helps absorption. Cardamom stimulates the heart and increases digestive *chi*. It lifts energy and mood. Add just a pinch of these strong flavors. Fennel seeds provide digestive energy as well as a mild, sweet taste. Fennel settles the stomach. Anise is sweet and increases appetite.

I have a favorite candied ginger from Chinatown made with ginger, sugar, salt, and licorice, but a slice of raw ginger in tea enhances digestion as well. Bitter green tea with pungent ginger or turmeric is especially good for digestion, cleansing, and weight loss.

In Tibet and Mongolia, countries of high altitudes and cold climates, tea drinkers add salt and butter to black tea, amplifying its warming, sedating effects. The milk is so rich it tastes like a meal in itself. Tibetan butter tea, made from the churned milk of a *dri* (the female yak), tastes rich as British creamed tea and has a hue that the explorer Alexandra David-Neel described as "the color of faded roses."

I like adding strong curative herbs to morning tea. Sometimes that's the only time I have for them. I might steep a handful of crushed dried gardenia pods (in Latin, *Gardenia jasminoidis fructus*; in Chinese, *zhi zi*) in green tea. They're anti-inflammatory for headaches, irritability, and bloodshot eyes. Gardenia pods clear phlegm that's thick and yellowish. At other times I might add dried citrus peel (chen pi) to clear the head.

At times I've been known to throw food-combining rules to the winds. Normally it's best not to mix fruit with either protein or starch, or to mix beer with rice; it causes indigestion. But there is always an herbal remedy for indiscretions. I might drink green tea, adding homeopathic nux vomica (30c potency) or Pu-Erh tea with a pinch of nutmeg. Pu-Erh soothes after a hearty meal. The little pinch of nutmeg is a carminative that quiets the ever-active cosmopolitan mind.

Tea sweeteners

Most westerners sweeten tea, which changes its energetic effects. For green tea to act as a laxative, it should remain bitter.

But for those who indulge, some sweeteners are better than others.

Many people regard honey as a healthy sweetener. But it requires a warning: it must be used carefully, never heated, which makes it hard to digest and destroys most of its value as a medicine. Even its energetic effects can be a problem. Honey is considered "scattering," according to Chinese doctors, which means it moves *chi* outward, causing perspiration. This might be beneficial, especially for chronic bronchitis, but honey's diaphoretic action also sends digestive acids to irritate joints. This means honey not only slows digestion but can aggravate inflammatory arthritis for some people. Tea sweetened with raw honey is best enjoyed between meals.

In Chinatown you will find a number of Chinese teas packaged as instant cubes or granules that are easy-to-use sugar substitutes. The following four instant drinks are available in Chinese grocery stores around the world. They can also be ordered by mail from addresses provided at the back of this book. Some contain medicinal herbs along with cane sugar or dates. Others use sweet-tasting herbs. They are so sweet I use them instead of sugar.

One delicious sweetener is **She She Cao Instant Beverage** made from two herbs native to Guangzhou (Canton). There it is enjoyed daily by those who wish to prevent blemishes. Traditionally, one of the ingredients, bai hua she she cao (in Latin, *oldenlandia*), has been combined with other herbs to treat cancer in head, neck, and breast, and to cleanse the skin of what Chinese doctors call "toxic swellings," i.e.,

boils and congested lymph glands. According to researchers, it's said to have the ability to "activate the reticuloendothelial system and increase phagocytosis by lymphocytes." This makes it effective against many infectious diseases. Huang qin (in Latin, *scutellaria*; in English, skullcap), an anti-inflammatory, reduces fever, thirst, headache, red eyes, and a bitter taste in the mouth. Used together in **She She Cao** tea, these two herbs provide the liver-cleansing and antibiotic properties necessary to clear troubled skin.

Lo Han Kuo Instant Beverage, recommended for dry throat and cough, is a favorite of smokers and singers for its soothing effects. It is made of 95 percent powdered lo han kuo, an empty pod about the size of a tennis ball, and 5 percent cane sugar. Conveniently packaged as a cube, it can be added to tea or coffee. I have also found cubes called **Lo Han Kuo Hawthorn Beverage,** which combine those two herbs, one for cooling lung inflammation, the other for strengthening digestion and the heart. They seem the perfect addition to balance the heating and weakening effects of coffee.

I use these cube or granule sweeteners when cooking vegetables or pies, or in anything to which I might add sugar. I add one half to one cube sweetener per pot of tea or one cube for each quarter cup sugar in recipes, but tastes vary.

Ling zhi, the famous reishi mushroom, is not known for its sweet flavor so much as for its cleansing, anticancer effects. Although the mushroom itself is not sweet, the instant cube is. Ling zhi (in

Latin, *ganoderma*) is valued as a treasure that ensures longevity. I add one cube of **Instant Ling Zhi** per pot of bitter tea.

Another herbal sugar substitute is **Essence of Tienchi Flowers.** Tienchi, a form of ginseng that greatly increases blood circulation, is sometimes an ingredient in Chinese remedies for injury and bruises. The flowers, which make up this sugar substitute, work in another way. This sweet powder is anti-inflammatory. Recommended for liverish headaches, pimples, high blood pressure, irritability, and grinding of teeth during sleep, it can help reduce doctor and dental bills.

The Tea Ceremony

I am sometimes asked if there is a Chinese tea ceremony. I've never seen it in mainland China, probably because it's traditionally associated with Buddhism. But a simple form is practiced in Taiwan, where many Buddhist rituals are still observed.

Originally, as in Japan, tea was made by whipping powdered leaves in hot water with a bamboo brush. Later, during the Ming Dynasty, tea was steeped in pots for the first time. A complete tea service from that time includes a tiny clay pot and thimble-size cups, a bowl for disposing of used tea or water, and a pitcher for boiling water.

My instructor for the tea ceremony was a Taiwanese Buddhist friend I met in a Chinese restaurant. James came to America as a tourist and fell in love with this country. After selling his factory in Taipei, he took a "slave" job as a waiter in New York, working twelve-hour shifts, sharing a company cell at night with ten other men. Eventually he bought his own restaurant, a pizza parlor!

A lover of Chinese opera and antiques, he had a fine sense of style. "The perfume of oolong," he said, "is enhanced when made in a *yixing* clay pot and steeped no longer than one minute. You must fill the pot at least three quarters full with tea." This miniature clay pot fits into the palm of your hand. The cups are Lilliputian, a small amount of the powerful brew being as satisfying as a pot. The special clay *yixing* teapot was developed to enhance the rich flavor and reddish color of oolong.

First, the pot and cups are placed in a small bowl. The pot is filled with loose oolong tea. The tea is washed once by pouring boiling water over it, then immediately emptying the pot of water. Then enough boiling water is poured into the pot to make the tea, and more is poured over the closed pot and little cups to keep them warm. The warmed cups are removed from the water and placed onto the platter. After the tea has steeped, all the tiny cups are filled. Then, according to James, you must first admire the tea, sniffing the aroma, tasting just a sip, and finally drinking all the cups, one after another. This is best done in early morning while listening to the music of an *yi wu*, a two-stringed violin, or reading famous classical poems dedicated to the art of tea, such as the following by Chiao-Jen of the T'ang Dynasty:

TYPES OF CHINESE TEAS

COLOR/TYPE	EXAMPLES	FLAVOR	CAFFEINE	BENEFITS
white	Sow Mee	very mild	none	refreshing
	Bojenmi	"	"	slimming
green	jasmine	fragrant	slight	*cooling*
	gunpowder	bitter	"	anticancer, anticholesterol
	Loong Tseng	strongly bitter	"	stimulant
	Lung Ching	delicate	"	refreshing
	Tit Koon Yum	bitter	"	stimulant
oolong	Ti Kuan Yin	bitter	moderate	*cooling*, laxative
	Shui Hsien	"	"	"
red	Pu-Erh	rich, pungent	"	digestive
black	Ying Teh	rich, bitter	strong	stimulant
	Keemun	"	"	"
	Bohea	"	"	"
	Lapsang Souchong*	smoky	"	"

Note: All teas contain tannic acid, which makes them digestive.

A friend from Yueh presented me
With tender leaves of Yen-Hsi tea,
For which I chose a kettle
Of ivory-mounted gold,
A mixing-bowl of snow-white earth.
With its clear bright froth and fragrance,
It was like the nectar of Immortals.
The first bowl washed the cobwebs from my
    mind—
The whole world seemed to sparkle.

A second cleaned my spirit
Like purifying showers of rain.
A third and I was one with the Immortals—
What need now for austerities
To purge our human sorrows?
Worldly people, by going in for wine,
Sadly deceive themselves.
For now I know the Way of Tea is real.
Who but Tan Ch'iu [an immortal] could
    find it?

6
The Taste and Energy of Foods

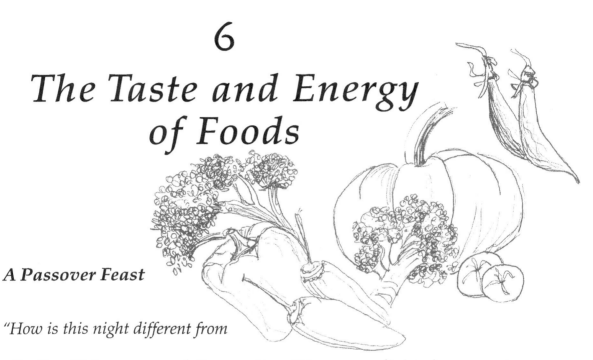

A Passover Feast

"How is this night different from all others?" Someone read the question. We were reclining in a sumptuous Lower Manhattan loft filled with Asian antiques, Swedish glass sculptures, huge oil paintings, and potted trees. As I looked up through the leaves to the balcony, thirteen carved wooden Lo Han monks lined the hall bookcase leading to the music room and its Tibetan thangkas. I have worshiped in this temple of art many times. Peter and Billy have long been my favorite New York couple. As a kid newly arrived in the city, I attended their Sunday teas once a month,

where I'd meet actors, singers, directors, budding boys, and Brahmins alike, all mingled in an atmosphere of love. While I studied voice with Peter, his instruction included urging me to put on weight. He laughed when I called him my Jewish mother. Billy invariably said something or touched my shoulder in a certain way to give me food for thought. Their love and encouragement has never had limits. That's part of why Pesach has become special for me.

We'd read the Haggadah around a circle that included a rabbi in blue jeans and me, the only shiksa. We sampled the traditional tastes: bitter, salty, sour, hot, and sweet. For bitter we had hyssop, a digestive herb tea used since biblical times. Peter dipped a boiled egg into salt water to symbolize the tears of an oppressed people, and chewed a twist of lemon. This was followed by a bite of sharp radish. Personally, I preferred the sweet apple and nuts of the charoses.

The overall effect of dinner was bittersweet. Our ranks varied slightly year to year, a place being set not for Isaiah, but for "The Epidemic" (AIDS). I'd sit like "the stupid son," listening to the music of droned Hebrew, reflecting upon the personal stories about freedom told by the guests. I think freedom comes in learning how to survive, how to prevent oppression and illness, and in realizing that your family are the friends at home in your heart.

Most people don't think of Jewish cooking as Oriental, but the ancient Hebrew tribes had Eastern roots. The five tastes of the Passover feast are the same as those found in Asian herbal tradition. Bitter, sweet, hot, salty, and sour are universal flavors, transcending limits of time and place.

The most important advice I can give you in this chapter is that if you want to be healthy and happy, eat all five flavors with each meal. Try not to eat too much of any one, but balance them all. Each of the flavors affects different internal organs, and illness comes from stressing the body by relying too heavily on a particular taste. In this chapter you will learn how each taste affects your *chi*, so that you'll be able to successfully use more or less of it.

The Energetic Actions of Herbs

We've already learned that *chi* is not as simple as the Western concept of "energy." For one thing, there are different types: "digestive *chi*" refers to metabolism; "protective *chi*" describes resistance to illness; and "original *chi*" represents our inherited strengths and weaknesses, the genetic codes found in DNA.

Sometimes *chi* refers to the strength or weakness of particular internal organs. For example, a Chinese doctor may say an herb "builds the *chi*" of a particular organ system. Ginger stimulates the *chi* of the stomach, which means it increases or strengthens its actions.

Here is my translation of the energetic effects of the five flavors: The hot or pungent flavor is stimulating and diaphoretic; that is, it may cause sweating. Sour is astringent or cleansing. Sweet, bland, or oily tastes slow digestion, affect blood sugar, and quiet the nerves. Bitter is a stimulant and sometimes a laxative. The salty taste can be stimulating and digestive, and can influence water retention. In each case the flavor's energetic effects are more important than the taste. Later in this chapter we will study more about the relation of tastes to the Five Elements.

HERBS: TASTE, TEMPERATURE, AND TYPE

If we were to examine medicinal herbs the way a traditional doctor does in China, we'd consider an herb's taste because it affects *chi,* which involves all body and mind functions. We would also consider the herb's temperature—whether it has *heating* (inflammatory) or *cooling* (anti-inflammatory) properties. We would pay attention to which acupuncture meridians the herb affects, and any other specific actions—for instance, how it affects digestion, circulation, or breathing. That is considered the herb's type.

Are there general rules? For example, do *all* bitter herbs or *all* heating herbs work the same way? Sorry, but studying herbology is like meeting several hundred new friends. It will take a few years to know them well. But they will have similarities.

It's interesting to note that some Western-trained herbalists also categorize herbs according to the energetic effects, although they might take this information for granted. I once met Sabinita, a wise herbal woman in Truchas, a tiny eagle's nest high in the mountains of northern

New Mexico. Her Chicano background embraced a great respect for herbs with Anglo as well as American Indian names, but she used the same *type* of herbs to treat a cold that I would. She said, "We use this herb to sweat out a cold," exactly the way a Chinese doctor would use a diaphoretic herb. That is because she understood the *energetic effects* of herbs. Western and Asian herbalists use many of the same categories when describing an herb's energy. Herbs that stimulate and speed metabolism are called "stimulants" or "tonics." Herbs that reduce inflammation or fever are designated "anti-inflammatory" or "antipyretic." Drying herbs are called "astringent." They clear the sinuses, are digestive, or treat diarrhea. Herbs that increase perspiration are "diaphoretic," while "diuretic" herbs increase urination.

Unfortunately, most Western-trained herbalists do not consider all the energetic aspects of herbs. That can lead to problems. One striking example is what an Oriental herbalist calls the *temperature* of herbs. We will examine this concept in detail later, but for now, here is an example: A pungent antibiotic such as garlic or echinacea is considered *heating* (even hotter than *warming*) not only because it tastes hot but because it increases inflammation or dehydration symptoms. A Western-trained herbalist might recommend such an herb, regardless of its *heating* effects, because of its conventional use as an antibiotic. But this ignores the herb's *temperature.* It also completely ignores the patient. Such a denial of individual needs can magnify inflammation symptoms such as fever, nervousness, hot flashes, or night sweats. Chronic fever diseases, including AIDS, require anti-inflammatory herbal antibiotics such as honeysuckle flower and wild indigo (isatis), not *heating* ones such as echinacea.

Many Western-trained herbalists and medical doctors treat the disease entity, not the person. To use herbal medicines effectively, you must choose them based upon individual diagnosis, not on case studies. I cannot stress this enough. During the last century, much research was done on herbs by medical doctors who did not consider the energetic effects of herbs, but only their biochemical ingredients. They also ignored the taste and temperature of an herb. In other words, they did not study what Chinese doctors describe as *chi.* That's why herbs in America are too often found on spice racks and in specialty shops, not in hospitals, as they are in China.

This is partly due to miscommunication or prejudice. Western doctors have not taken the time and trouble to investigate the energetic system of anatomy and physiology native to Asian medicine.

Asian doctors do not describe internal organs as we do in the West. Their explanation of anatomy is energetic, not material, because internal organs encompass associated pathways of energy sometimes called channels or meridians. Some have described this anatomical construct (an organ and its associated meridian) as an "organ system." These systems make up human anatomy according to Chinese medicine. Other Asian traditions also describe channels of energy (called *srotas* in Sanskrit). Here is an analogy. A Western understanding of an internal organ would be: "The capital of Vermont is Montpelier," whereas an Asian view would be: "The capital of Vermont is Montpelier, along with all the roads leading to and from it."

Vital energy that flows along channels carries out the organ system's physiological functions. Since the channels run through the body like a road map of energy, they affect areas that are distant from the internal organ. Perhaps this corresponds most closely to what we describe in the West as the lymph system or neural pathways. But it is difficult to make direct connections between Eastern and Western views of anatomy. The functions of organ systems, as you will see, are affected by the energetic properties of the five tastes.

The Five Elements and the Five Tastes

There are various schools of thought throughout Asia concerning exactly what elements make up the body. Indian and Tibetan doctors describe five elements: Ether (space), Air, Fire, Water, and Earth. Dr. Vasant Lad, in his book *Ayurveda: The Science of Self-Healing,* summarizes the creation of the Five Elements in this way:

> *From a state of unified consciousness, the subtle vibrations of the cosmic soundless sound* aum *manifested. From that vibration there first appeared the Ether element. When this ethereal element began to move, it created Air, which is Ether in action. With friction heat was generated. Particles of heat-energy combined to form*

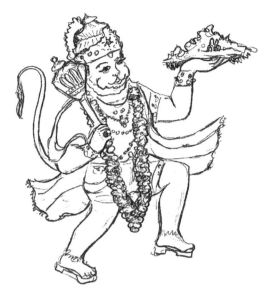

The East Indian monkey god Hanumen. In the Ramayana he brings a mountain of herbs to help Rama.

intense light and from this light the Fire element manifested. Through the heat of the Fire certain ethereal elements dissolved and liquified manifesting the Water element and then solidified to form the molecules of Earth. In this way, Ether manifested into the four elements of Air, Fire, Water and Earth.

Chinese doctors describe this process of creation in another way and acknowledge five different elements, designated Fire, Earth, Metal, Water, and Wood. Let's look more closely at the Chinese Five Elements in order to see how foods and herbs affect energy. By understanding this relationship, we can make better use of the five flavors.

FIRE: THE BITTER TASTE

fire

Fire cooks our food and protects us from danger. Without the light and comfort of fire, civilization would not be possible. There is also an aspect of fire in our metabolism. It is what keeps us warm, sends our blood circulating through blood vessels, and helps us digest and assimilate food. In the human body, the Fire element is said to maintain the heart and pericardium, which allow the "smooth rhythm of bodily functions, maintaining circulation and emotional balance." The small intestine, also part of the Fire element, assimilates useful food and sends waste to the large intestine. A related meridian, the Triple Heater, helps maintain balance of body temperature and metabolism.

Many factors affect the functioning of internal organs. Those energized by Fire are temporarily stimulated by the bitter taste. For example, our morning coffee or tea speeds the heart and stirs digestive and nervous systems. Overuse of a bitter stimulant "hardens the pulse," according to Chinese doctors, so that circulation becomes no longer smooth. Many bitter tastes are laxative, affecting the small intestine. Overuse of bitter foods dehydrates, or "withers the skin." If you wish to avoid wrinkles, eliminate coffee, black tea, and cigarettes.

To reverse the bitter taste's dehydrating effects, combine it with hot, sweet, or salty tastes. For example, add cardamom (hot and sweet) to coffee and ginger (hot) to tea. Bitter green vegetables cooked with fresh ginger, pepper, salt, and a natural sweetener will even taste better.

EARTH: THE SWEET TASTE

earth

We are nourished by the generosity of the earth. She sustains life with rich soil and a temperate climate. The Earth element in the body corresponds to the stomach and spleen/pancreas, seen as one organ function. The stomach is said to ripen food, while "the spleen makes blood and gives pleasing shape to the body." Treatment of cellulite and blood sugar imbalances often include herbs that enhance the functioning of spleen/pancreas.

Western nutritionists agree with Chinese doctors that "the spleen makes blood," although it is explained indirectly. The pancreas releases enzymes that digest B vitamins. A healthy Earth element provides the rich soil to nourish growth.

The sweet taste affects the Earth element in several ways. Many nourishing, blood-building herbs are actually sweet fruits (plums, berries, peaches) or fungus such as tang kuei (Latin: *Angelica sinensis*), which strengthens "spleen" function. However, persons troubled by blood sugar imbalances and obesity are warned against eating sweet foods. (See chapter 16.)

Chinese doctors say a slightly sweet taste such as the herb licorice "harmonizes" digestion, because it reduces cramps. But concentrated sweets and acid-producing foods, such as refined sugar, or phlegm-producing foods such as pasta, cheese, and nuts can disturb energy and digestion, causing bloating from indigestion and "aching in the bones." Certain pains are made worse from phlegm-producing foods so that Chinese herbal formulas for rheumatoid arthritis as well as sinus congestion often contain barley, an antiphlegm food.

Balance sedating, phlegm-producing (sweet) foods with stimulants that are bitter, hot, sour, and drying. Add radish, bitter greens, pungent sauces, caraway seeds, pepper, ginger, and seaweeds to pastas. Bitter, sour, hot, and drying tastes reverse the sedating and congesting effects of sweet by stimulating digestive *chi*. Another example, hawthorn berries (bitter and sour), are recommended in Chinese slimming teas such as Bojenmi or The Well-Known Tea. Or steep a handful of hawthorn berries in a bottle of wine or vodka for three weeks to make a pleasant after-dinner digestive.

METAL: THE PUNGENT TASTE

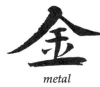
metal

The richness of the earth also makes possible the production of energy, oxygen, precious metals, and gems. Diamonds are formed from decaying waste compressed under pressure. The transformation of oxygen and waste is the domain of the Metal element. The associated organ systems are lung, large intestine, and skin.

Dianne Connelly, in her beautiful book *Traditional Acupuncture: The Law of the Five Elements*, writes,

> *If we think of the vast network of the human body, the structure of being able to take in food and air, to assimilate and utilize the fuel, then to let go of the unnecessary things, these are some life-sustaining aspects of the element of Metal.*

The lungs exchange oxygen and waste while gathering energy for the cells. The large intestine passes waste through elimination; the skin is also a vital organ of breathing and elimination.

Spice creates an acidic environment by increasing digestive *chi* so that we eliminate toxins and absorb minerals. Pungent foods reduce waste by stimulating sweating or elimination. Many are diaphoretic or laxative. However, excess use of hot foods and spices burns internal tissue or causes skin blemishes. Pungent spices are important additions to our diet when we need to create more appetite and speed digestion, while extreme temperatures, either very cold or hot, cause spasms. As you will learn later, hot spices can increase menstrual pain, colitis, headaches, and nervous tics.

Hot is balanced by bitter and sour. To hot, spicy foods add green vegetables and bitter, cleansing herbs, dandelion, parsley, mint, or red clover tea. Cooking spices such as cumin and coriander reduce the burn of hot foods. Lemon juice counteracts the drying effects of hot flavors.

WATER: THE SALTY TASTE

water

When life on earth began from combining gases such as ammonia and carbon dioxide, it was sustained by water. In the womb, we too were nourished by a liquid similar to seawater. The Water element in the body is represented by the bladder and kidney organ systems. The "kidney," in Chinese medicine, also comprises the adrenal glands and hormonal functions. The Water element maintains adequate moisture throughout the body, as well as normal hormone secretions. When the kidney, adrenal glands, and hormonal functions are not healthy, we experience wide-ranging physical and emotional problems. These might include kidney and bladder problems per se, but also irregularities of fertility, sexual strength or desire, poor immunity against illness, and extremes in mood.

Internal moisture ensures blood, saliva, sexual fluids, and hormone balance. Skin and hair have luster; bones are strong and well formed; teeth, fingernails, and nerves are healthy. Adequate moisture engenders rest and calm, allowing emotions to become more profound.

Sodium-rich foods such as celery promote cleansing, but overuse of salty stimulants, even miso and tamari, causes problems. Extreme use of hot, dry, or salty foods can drive us to excess speed, paranoia, or maniacal expressions of willpower. Energetically, such overstimulation is experienced as *heating* and *drying*: It creates thirst, hunger, and anxiety. One example of this is the unpleasant jolt we feel after eating a popular Japanese cure for exhaustion: one raw egg mixed with a dash of soy sauce. The egg transports the fermented soy (a hot, salty, drying stimulant) to the brain and nerves. Your heart pounds as you break into a sweat.

The Water element contains what the Chinese call *jing,* described as the original *chi* we inherited. Modern scientists might call it genetic programming. In any case, vitality and life force are protected by the Water element. That is why it is said that damaging the Water element reduces resistance to illness and our ability to heal. With weakened adrenals, we make fewer white blood cells.

According to traditional Chinese doctors, excess stimulation from drugs, jet flights, late nights, stress, fatigue, and excessive sexual activity shortens our lives. A little salt in our foods creates good appetite and digestion; too much leads to constriction of blood vessels and high blood pressure in some persons. Prolonged illness, as well as high doses of anti-inflammatory drugs and chemotherapy, weaken adrenal energy, blood, and bone marrow. The results of such therapies can be weakness and depression for years afterward.

In a later chapter we'll study nourishing foods and moistening herbs that rebuild blood and sexual fluid. Other "kidney remedies" repair exhaustion and the effects of aging. They profoundly influence energy, circulation, emotions, and our capacity to create and maintain life.

WOOD: THE SOUR TASTE

wood

With rich soil, adequate sun, moisture, and oxygen, the earth sends forth life in the form of plants. Each spring the process begins again. We rejoice in the force of nature and her offspring, the flowers and trees. The Wood element becomes most active at this time.

The Wood element is associated with the liver and gallbladder organ systems. According to the *Nei Ching,* an ancient medical text, these affect not only digestion but also the health of nerves, muscles, tendons, and joints, as well as the soul and its outlet, the eyes. Indirectly, the Wood element affects muscle strength, since an important function of the liver is the absorption of calcium, which strengthens muscle fiber and quickens muscle response. The Wood element, therefore, affects smooth circulation and heart function.

Overstimulation of the liver and gall-

Bitter: stimulant, laxative, reduces sweet cravings
Sweet and oily: sedative, can be fattening
Pungent: stimulates energy, digestion, appetite, nervousness
Salt: heating and drying, can be a stimulant
Sour: cleanses liver, reduces fat and cravings for sweets

A QUICK REFERENCE
1

TASTE	BALANCE WITH
BITTER	pungent, sweet, salty (also sedating)
SWEET	bitter, pungent, sour (also *drying*)
PUNGENT	bitter, sour, sweet (*cooling,* sedating)
SALTY	sour and bitter (*cooling* and moistening), also sweet and oily (sedating)
SOUR	pungent

2

TASTE	EXAMPLE	IMBALANCE IN THE BODY	POSSIBLE REMEDY
BITTER	coffee	weakens digestion and heart (exhaustion, depression)	cardamom
	green tea	laxative, *cooling*	ginger
	chocolate	stimulant/depressant	cardamom
	tobacco	dehydrating	almonds, oatmeal
SWEET	milk	creates *phlegm* (lethargy)	cardamom, pepper
	pasta	creates *phlegm*	pungent spices
	ice cream	*phlegm*, fatigue	clove
	white sugar	irritates nervous system	bee pollen, maple syrup
	legumes	flatulence	pepper, garlic, ginger
PUNGENT	chili pepper	burns, dehydrates	cumin
	garlic	anger, inflammation, pimples	coriander, mint
	yogurt	*phlegm*	cucumber, cumin
SALTY	watermelon	water retention	the seeds (a diuretic tea)
	miso	water retention (anxiety)	cucumber
	salt	water retention	parsley, juniper berry
SOUR	lemon	draining	honey, maple syrup, ginger

HOW MUCH OF EACH DO YOU CONSUME DAILY?

BITTER	SWEET	HOT/PUNGENT	SALTY	SOUR
Laxative/ Stimulant	*Sedative*	*Stimulant/ Digestive*	Drying	*Cleansing*
coffee	sugar	pepper, cayenne	salt	lemon
tea	pastry	onion	miso	grapefruit
cigarettes	breads	garlic	soy sauce	apple
salad	sweet fruits:	hot sauce	watermelon	pickles
dandelion	peach, apricot,	ginger	green olives	sauerkraut
chicory	cantaloupe,	radish	pickles	vinegar
Chinese	banana	turmeric	ripe olives	lecithin
slimming teas	cheese	clove	cheddar cheese	
bitter and sour	nuts		chips	
herbal minerals:	pasta		seaweeds:	
alfalfa, nettle,	licorice		(stimulants)	
spirulina,	beef		dulse, kelp,	
dandelion,	pork		laminaria	
kelp, parsley,				
hijiki				

bladder with excessive hot, spicy foods encourages muscle spasms, headaches, aching joints, and some allergic reactions. Our eyes become dry or painful from inadequate moisture and blood circulation. We might become nervous or aggressive. We thus lose the flexibility of tender green wood to become brittle and tyrannical.

When the Wood element is congested from a rich diet, it cannot absorb adequate calcium to produce a steady heartbeat. Emotional problems can thereby ensue.

Sour tastes drain the Wood element; pungent tastes stimulate it. When used together, they cleanse and normalize its function. Hot water and lemon juice after a rich meal help us process fats.

The liver manufactures enzymes, cholesterol, proteins, vitamin A (from carotene), blood coagulation factor, and bile. Smooth digestion depends on adequate production of bile, which is bitter and sour, alkaline and laxative. As a laxative, it cleanses excess acids from the intestines. Homeopathic natrum sulphate (sodium sulphate) also has a draining effect because it eliminates toxic liquid from the cells and stimulates the flow of bile. Natrum sulphate is recommended for nausea, constipation, and lethargy from slow digestion. This is an important consideration for those who wish to eat healthfully and live longer.

In order to prepare healthful and delicious meals, the caring cook serves all five tastes each day, preferably in the same meal.

In Quick Reference 1 you'll find a summary of the five tastes along with their balancing tastes. Table 2 shows examples of the tastes and the effects of their imbalance in the body and mind, along with herbs that might be used to create balance. Do you consume one taste more than others?

At this point you have not learned enough about Asian medicine for it to have changed your point of view. You may still be thinking in Western medical categories. The following advice will help destroy old habits so that you can better observe your energy.

Observe Yourself and Understand Yourself

In every chapter of this book I shall repeat that herb use must be individual, but you cannot fully understand what that means until you've mastered the skills of adequately observing yourself.

Step One: Accept a new mind-set that reads like this: The choice and optimum dosage of herbs and foods varies according to your needs at a given time. Some considerations that determine dosage include your age, weight, symptoms, stress level, emotional needs, and other factors. This means that all the standard dosages found on labels of health-food store or other herb bottles are inappropriate for more than half of the people who buy them. Later, using Asian diagnostic techniques, you can determine your exact dosage.

Step Two: The following questions will point you in the right direction:

෴ The bitter flavor tends to be a heart stimulant or laxative. Do you use coffee or cigarettes to wake you up? Do you really need a heart stimulant or laxative? Does your heart often feel slow and weak? Do you have excess cholesterol or chest pain? Do you need more peristalsis of the colon? Or do you need less bitter? If so, you may have chronic diarrhea or be too thin, nervous, irritable, or weak. Or do you need to reduce your craving for sweets? (See chapters 14, 15, and 16.)

෴ The sweet and oily flavors tend to be sedative. Do you feel tired after eating a rich meal? Do you eat too many sedating foods such as oils, avocados, cabbage, turnips, grains, sweets, pastries, dairy products, or alcohol? They put on weight. Or do you need sedatives to quiet your nerves? (See chapters 33 and 35.)

෴ Hot and pungent flavors are *heating*, and stimulate energy, digestion, and appetite. Do you use too many? If so, you may be too hungry too often, or have dry, itchy skin, irritated eyes, excessive thirst, cough, nervousness, or insomnia. Or do you need more *heating* foods because you have a poor appetite, indigestion, shortness of breath, chills, and weakness?

෴ The salty flavor is *heating, drying,* and a stimulant. Do you use too much salt? If so, you may become hungry and thirsty after eating salty food, your mouth may feel dry, or you may become irritable or develop headaches. Does your body retain water or feel puffy? Or do you need more strength and appetite?

ᡭᢙ The sour flavor is digestive. It helps release bile, which is laxative. Do you need more sour foods? If so, you may get constipated and irritable, or feel congested or tender in the rib cage area after eating fat or hot foods, or you may crave too many fat foods or alcohol.

Such questions as those listed above can help determine your problem areas and possible solutions. By the end of this book, you will be able to generate your own questions and begin to balance digestive and other energetic problems by blending the five flavors. This is as ordinary as making a salad. Vegetables of many colors offer a variety of flavors as well as many vitamins and minerals.

Most salad greens are bitter, sour, and pungent stimulants. (Parsley stimulates the kidneys to reduce water retention; carrots feed and stimulate the liver; onions and garlic are potent heating sexual stimulants.) Dressing oil is sweet in nature and fattening, because it's sedating. A dash of salt, mustard, or black pepper is digestive, while vinegar and lemon are cleansing.

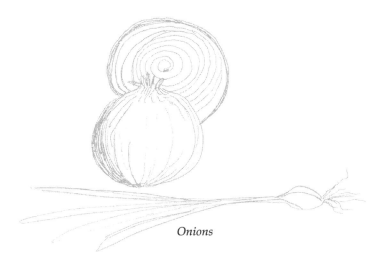

Onions

四氣 四氣 四氣 四氣 四氣 四氣 四氣　　四性 四性 四性 四性 四性 四性 四性
[sìqì]　　　　　　　　　　　　*[sìxìng]*

The four properties of drugs: cold, hot, warm, and cool, classified according to their therapeutic effects

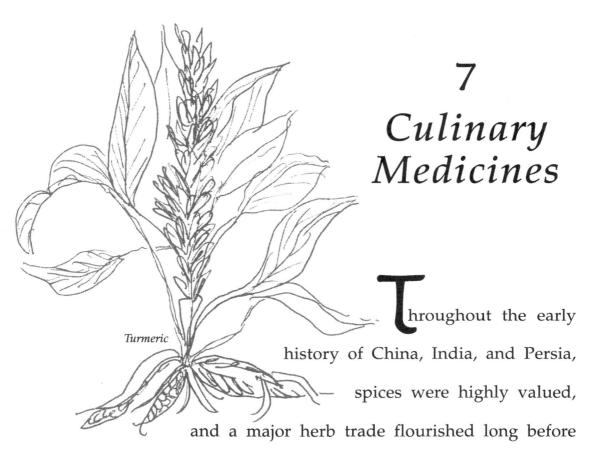

Turmeric

7
Culinary Medicines

Throughout the early history of China, India, and Persia, spices were highly valued, and a major herb trade flourished long before there were separate countries. The Crusades were carried on to win herbs and spices used for medicine and food preservation. In 1492, Columbus set sail for the Spice Islands in search of nutmeg, a well-known narcotic, and a sea route in order to carry on the extremely lucrative spice trade.

Most people use spices, never questioning which ones are healthy for them. We think taste is all that matters. But taste, temperature, and energy of culinary herbs and spices profoundly affect well-being. Good health begins with good digestion. You can eat the most nourishing and expensive health foods, but if digestive *chi* is weak, it turns to waste.

How can we determine whether or not digestion is faulty? Simple observation. If we feel stuffed or experience burping, nausea, or fatigue after eating, our foods are too rich or fat. Then we can add pungent and bitter digestive herbs and spices that stimulate digestion.

Digestive capacity varies greatly with stress and fatigue because we need adequate *chi* to maintain breathing, blood circulation, and muscle strength. When tired or upset, or after eating too many oily and sweet foods, we have less available energy. Heavy foods slow digestion and vitality. But digestive herbs and spices work as stimulants to help us overcome the harmful effects of rich cooking in order to build health.

Today, only traditional Asian doctors know how spices can be used as medicines, because they are used to evaluating the energy potential of herbs. Like medicines, culinary spices can be stimulants, sedatives, diuretics, laxatives, or antibiotics. Their flavors are also involved. For example, *heating* pungent herbs such as citrus peel, ginger, pepper, and cardamom are sometimes used in herbal formulas to improve the digestion of other herbs.

Chinese "patent remedies" (herbal combinations patented centuries ago) may contain cinnamon to stimulate blood circulation, clove to increase sexual potency, turmeric to help dissolve tumors, or ginger to cure indigestion.

Since we have this pharmacopoeia in the kitchen, all we need are some guidelines to unlock the energy potential latent in Chinese medicine. A later section will cover personal diagnosis. But for now we can examine your home stock of remedies, useful throughout the rest of the book. Is your kitchen well furnished with spices for energy and health? The following chart will help you decide. It shows many commonly used culinary herbs and spices along with their medicinal uses.

The culinary remedies in this chart can be added to foods or brewed as teas when needed. Their choice and amounts will vary according to individual usage, based on Asian tongue diagnosis. You may wish to add stimulant digestive spices to rich dishes, or make a spicy afternoon tea to stir energy and enthusiasm.

At what age can we start using herbs and spices? In Asia, it's very young. Chinese mothers give their babies **Xiaoer Qixing Cha** as their last bottle of the day. These instant granules, available in Chinese groceries, combine powdered barley sprouts with herbs that facilitate digestion and prevent colic. I'm convinced that it works, because I've never seen a crabby Chinese baby. Napping in a sling tied to Mother's back, they're a picture of contentment.

SPICE REMEDIES

Digestives (all carminative for indigestion)

WARMING (stimulates digestion)	COOLING (anti-inflammatory)	ADDITIONAL USES
ALLSPICE		stimulant
ANISE		sweetener
ASAFOETIDA		stimulant, antispasm
BASIL		increases sweating, i.e., diaphoretic
BAY LEAF		laxative
CARAWAY		reduces phlegm
CARDAMOM		heart stimulant
CAYENNE		increases circulation
	CHICORY	blood cleanser
CINNAMON		circulation, diaphoretic for arthritis, colds, and flu
CLOVES		adrenal stimulant for asthma, impotence
	CORIANDER	diuretic
	CUMIN	cools ulcer pain
	DANDELION	diuretic, laxative, lymph cleanser
	DILL	expectorant
	FENNEL	diuretic
FENUGREEK		sexual stimulant
GARLIC		liver stimulant, antibiotic
GINGER		diaphoretic
HAWTHORN BERRIES		reduces cholesterol, heart stimulant
JUNIPER BERRIES		diuretic
KELP		minerals
	LEMON	vitamin C, expectorant
	LEMONGRASS	diaphoretic

SPICE REMEDIES *(cont.)*

WARMING (stimulates digestion)	*COOLING* (anti-inflammatory)	ADDITIONAL USES
	LICORICE	demulcent, laxative, source of estrogen
MACE		antispasm, expectorant
MARJORAM		calming, antispasm
MUSTARD SEEDS		stimulant, expectorant
NUTMEG		sedative
ONION		blood cleanser, tonic
ORANGE PEEL		dries phlegm, stimulant
OREGANO		stimulant, diaphoretic
PAPRIKA		stimulant
PARSLEY		blood cleanser; diuretic; increases menstruation, i.e., emmenagogue
	PEPPERMINT	diaphoretic
	POMEGRANATE	dries phlegm
ROSEMARY		strong stimulant
SAFFLOWER		increases circulation
	SAFFRON	liver cleanser, emmenagogue
SAGE		stimulant, expectorant, stops excessive sweating
SAVORY		stimulant
SESAME SEEDS		nerve tonic, rejuvenator
	SPEARMINT	diaphoretic, diuretic
TARRAGON		emmenagogue, diuretic, antiseptic, liver stimulant
THYME		antispasmodic, dries phlegm, increases breath
TURMERIC		stimulant, antibacterial, increases circulation and intestinal flora, antitumor

The Yin *and* Yang *of Chinese Cooking*

Yin and *yang* are broad concepts we'll examine in many different contexts. The terms describe a number of interrelationships in Chinese medicine, which differ from their use in macrobiotic cooking. When describing energetic actions of foods, *yin*-increasing foods moisturize because they contain water. They are also alkaline in nature, like cabbage. Some reduce stomach acid in a number of ways, for example, because they're laxative or diuretic in effect. Green vegetables and lettuce are considered *yin* for this reason. *Yin*-increasing foods can also augment body fluids or water retention when they slow metabolism.

On the other hand, *yang*-increasing foods are often hot spices that speed digestion and metabolism. In the simplest terms, *yin*-increasing foods are nourishing and sedative, and *yang*-increasing foods are stimulants.

In order to achieve balance, we would blend *yin* and *yang* in the following way: Green vegetables (*yin*) slow digestion by diluting stomach acid. So cooking them with hot spices, pepper, and ginger (*yang*) speeds digestion. Hot spices balance alkaline foods by creating stomach acid. Further, spices affect energy. Traditional Asian medicine shows us that many pungent spices increase *digestive energy*. Digestive energy (what Chinese doctors call digestive *chi*) is the result of acids and enzymes produced by healthy digestive organs. Asian doctors do not improve digestion with supplements of digestive acids, enzymes, or glandular extracts; instead, they stimulate the *functioning* of digestive organs with herbs and spices. By stimulating metabolism with spices, we prevent digestion from becoming lazy.

This is the basis of herbal energetic medicine: We choose an herb according to its effect upon *chi*.

CULINARY REMEDIES AND *CHI*

Chi is found everywhere in the body, so spices can do more than heal indigestion. The *chi* of an herb can be observed through its taste, temperature, and effects. For example, herbal stimulants can cure insufficient *chi*, resulting in such problems as menstrual irregularity, depression, or overweight.

Herbs that increase circulation treat stuck *chi*, leading to pain or bruises. Anti-inflammatory herbs can reduce fever, pain, or other signs of inflammation due to illness or injury. Those types of remedies will be covered throughout this book.

Now we can explore their temperature, focusing on *warming* and *cooling* herbs and spices in cooking.

COOKING WITH HERBS

Cooking can transform your life because herbs protect us against illness, fatigue, and depression. When you understand how herbs and spices affect *chi*, you can enhance health, beauty, and longevity. Let's approach the concepts of *internal heat* and *internal cold* by examining some remedies used to balance them.

How to balance an imbalance

If you wanted to put out a fire, would you add more wood? The answer seems obvious. But I have met many people who are hot-tempered and have reddish skin rashes, bloodshot eyes, chronic thirst, hunger, and insomnia, who love to eat rich, spicy foods. This increases internal inflammation. To treat an energetic imbalance, we must add the opposite: Balance *internal heat* symptoms with *cooling* herbs, and *internal cold* symptoms with *warming* herbs.

What kinds of herbs are warming *and* cooling?

Warming herbs and spices are the most common ones in the kitchen; we've used them since before the Crusades. Ginger and black pepper are stimulant digestives. Some hot spices can even increase blood production or energy, affecting *chi* in a variety of ways. Ginger makes us feel warmer, but it also increases digestive *chi* by encouraging the production of stomach acid to warm digestion. Increased digestive *chi* heightens appetite, reduces wastes, improves breathing, and builds protection against weakness.

A *warming* herb or spice is considered *heating* when it creates or increases inflammatory symptoms. Its use can aggravate preexisting disharmony, pain, fever, irritability, or other signs of *internal heat*. Ginger stimulates appetite and energy for most people. But if you suffer from stomach ulcers, it can cause pain from excess acidity. To a certain extent, an herb's energetic effects depend upon the health of the user. At the same time, an herb must be considered independently. Some herbal medicines are considered to be very *heating*—we have already mentioned echinacea. You will learn to use the temperature of herbs correctly as you study diagnosis.

Many *cooling* herbs are laxatives, diuretics, or blood cleansers that rid the body of excess acid or toxins that create inflammation. The cleansing of inflammatory acid makes an herb *cooling* in its effects. Some *cooling* herbs also include antibiotics or kill parasites. (The latter type is called a *vermifuge.*) Some reduce blood pressure or blood sugar. Others slow metabolism by increasing water retention or body fluids. Clearly, *warming* and *cooling,* when used in classifying herbs, refers to more than the regulation of body temperature.

Warming *herbs and spices*

Warming herbs speed metabolism and all body processes. They are stimulants and energy tonics. They can be used to increase circulation or raise blood pressure, improve appetite, or stimulate brain, heart, or adrenal glands to enhance mental capacities and improve memory. When we are weak, *warming* stimulant herbs make things happen faster. When we're exhausted or nervous, *warming* sedatives can quiet the nerves to help us rest. But not all *warming* herbs work the same way.

We all know what it means to eat something hot and spicy. Mexican, Arabic, African, Indian, and Thai cuisines all use a rich variety of pungent spices with a satisfying hot flavor. Some spices even make us perspire. But does perspiring make us feel warmer? Actually, it normalizes body temperature. The pungent flavor alone does not stimulate perspiration; it is the diaphoretic action of the herb that induces sweating.

Looking at the Spice Remedies chart earlier in this chapter, we find a number of *warming* stimulants. For example, anise, asafoetida, cardamom, cayenne, garlic, ginger, hawthorn berries, and paprika stimulate stomach acid to warm digestive *chi*. Other *warming* spices are *drying* to remove excess digestive phlegm, which indirectly enhances digestive *chi*. These include orange peel and caraway.

Some *warming* spices stimulate specific internal organs. Cloves, fenugreek, juniper berries, and parsley are stimulants that build the *chi* of the kidneys or adrenal glands. Rosemary stimulates both adrenals and heart. Thyme increases the *chi* of the lungs to strengthen breathing.

Some *warming* herbs affect the body in a global manner, acting on more than one internal organ or function at a time. For example, sage stimulates the functioning of all the Five Elements at once.

Cooling *herbs and spices*

A *cooling* herb or food reduces heat and inflammation in the body either by increasing sweating or by reducing acid through its laxative or diuretic qualities. (*Cooling* diuretics cause acids or inflammatory wastes to be excreted in urine.) *Cooling* herbs reduce fever, pain, and inflammation. Some can eventually slow metabolism and circulation.

The Spice Remedies chart provides a number of examples from among *cooling* remedies, including *cooling* digestive herbs that reduce stomach acid, such as cumin, dill, and dandelion. They are useful for ulcers because they do not slow digestion, but remove excess stomach acid. *Cooling* diuretics include coriander seed and leaf, dandelion, and spearmint. Several herbs, such as chicory, dandelion, and saffron, cleanse the liver of toxins and acids. They are either laxative or relax spasms by reducing excess acid through increased urination.

HERB AND SPICE COMBINING

Chinese herbal patent remedies often employ *warming* and *cooling* herbs together to move stuck *chi*. *Warming* herbs can move *chi* that is stuck from weakness, while *cooling* herbs reduce wastes. A good combination of spices would be similar to **Xiao Yao Wan,** the pill remedy we studied in detail in chapter 4. We can substitute the kitchen spices ginger, mint, tarragon, and parsley for several of the Chinese herbs in **Xiao Yao Wan.**

The choice of an herb according to taste, temperature, and function requires practice in guided observation. The Diagnostic Questionnaire in the next chapter will help clear up many questions you may still have.

PART TWO

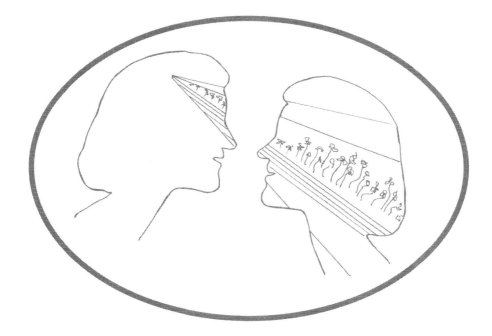

Diagnosis and Diet

Diagnosis is a way of looking and listening, where all methods have the value of bringing us closer to understanding what we are. Become more sensitive; it will enhance your ability to heal.

得神 得神 得神 得神 得神 得神 得神 得神 得神 得神 得神 得神 得神 得神

*[déshén] Being full of spirit. A patient full of spirit is apt to recover from his illness
and usually has a good prognosis.*

8

"Here's Looking at You . . ."

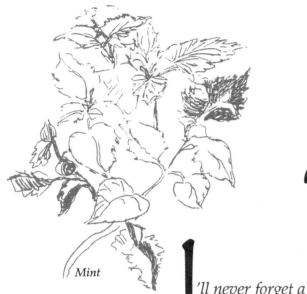

Mint

I'll never forget a medical doctor who once was a student in my Saturday class. He'd brought his whole family to explore Chinese herb markets. His bright little boy was studying Mandarin, and they all beamed with enthusiasm. After the class was over, the doctor told me emotionally, "We are moving to China. I'm going to study acupuncture in Beijing. I was an anesthesiologist for twelve years, and I'm sick of seeing people die on the operating table!"

Few doctors are willing to start over with their studies, or even to admit that there might be a better way. Western medical school costs too much time, effort, and money. Also, I think giving up a Western approach completely would

73

be mistaken. After all, medical tests and monitoring devices do provide sensitive data, useful to all kinds of health practitioners.

What the doctor and I agree upon is that diagnosis and treatment must be individualized. Only then can medicine be exact. What we seek with diagnosis determines, in part, what we perceive and the tools we choose to effect a cure. If we try to cure an illness instead of a person, using the same type of treatment or the same dosage of medicine for all, many people will surely die. But even more will never be seen, understood, or helped. That is because the aim of any good treatment is to bring the person back into balance, which involves much more than curing the disease at hand.

A Layered Approach

The next five chapters analyze your particular needs according to Asian medicine, then Part Three, Bringing You into Balance, helps you apply what you've learned. Diagnosis and Diet also offers a layered approach to herbal study. If you want the simplest approach to herb choice, skip ahead now to chapter 11, Your Tongue and You. Asian tongue diagnosis is fast, easy, and convenient. It will help you to recognize the type and location of many health problems.

Otherwise, if you desire a more in-depth approach, a chance to increase self-awareness and learn how to choose Asian herbs, read all the chapters in Part Two. The herbal remedies discussed in this book are made using the principles of health and balance found in these chapters.

Taken as a whole, Part Two provides an experience in self-observation similar to what you might expect when consulting an Asian health practitioner. Also, by using many sorts of observations from traditional Asian diagnosis and several detailed questionnaires, we finally approach the heart of the matter: Why do imbalances occur?

☞ NOW: SKIP TO CHAPTER 11, OR CONTINUE READING CHAPTERS 8 TO 12

Before we can understand *chi,* even before we begin to observe others, we need to observe ourselves. Since Asian diagnosis is as easy as noticing a particular tone of voice, change of complexion, or physical sensation that occurs during stress, we can easily use it to become more sensitive to our own well-being.

The next few chapters give us the opportunity to consider some basic concepts. They include *internal heat* and *internal cold,* which do not indicate body temperature but, among other things, refer to the speed and ease of metabolism. We will also cover what Chinese doctors call *dampness.* (The original word is *she,* but the concept exists in all other Asian medical disciplines. It is at times translated as "phlegm" or its equivalent in Sanskrit or Tibetan.)

Another subject covered is *stagnant chi,* also called "stuck energy" or *stagnation.* I introduced the concept of *chi* in the Herbal Basics chapter as the engine that drives all vital functions. In this one we learn about discomforts that occur when energy becomes either too agitated or too low. *Stagnation* leads to poorly functioning internal organs and a variety of physical and emotional complaints.

Finally we'll look at the Correspondences, constitutional types, and Asian tongue diagnosis. The best possible examples for diagnosis will come from you. The chapters in the diagnostic section serve as an introduction to your unique blend of body, mind, and spirit. In later chapters you won't have to go through every step as I have laid them out here, but will apply your personal observations to the study of particular ailments. By the end of this book, you will have learned many ways to observe your total health.

Studying Asian medical concepts is like counting the growth rings of a tree. It takes time. The rings appear to look alike but are somehow different. When you finally get to the core, it's still the same tree, but you can see much deeper. The word *chi*

will be used many times in this book, and each time you study its forms and movements, you will gain a better understanding of its importance.

Please complete the questionnaire below in order to observe your energy in a new way. Don't hesitate over the answers, but note down your first impression. Then total the number of checks at the end of each section. We will use the responses later both as a basis for personal analysis and as examples.

Remember, this questionnaire is not intended to diagnose illness but to illustrate concepts of energy. Any condition that is affected by the flow of *chi* is by nature temporary. Don't worry if you mark something that seems to be a problem. It can improve with herbs.

You ought to answer this questionnaire periodically, because responses vary slightly with the change of seasons or if you have a cold. You may also want to use the questionnaire to judge the effects of stress upon your *chi.*

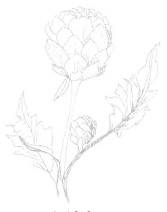

Artichoke

Diagnostic Questionnaire

I. Heat

1. FIRE

____ I have a fast or irregular heartbeat.
____ I often have nightmares or anxiety attacks that awaken me.
____ I'm anxious or emotional about a lot of things.
____ I tend to have a reddish face, or often blush.
____ I talk and laugh a lot.
____ Sometimes I get diarrhea with yellow mucus or blood.

2. EARTH

_✓_ I'm hungry all the time.
____ I crave sweets.
_✓_ I have ulcers or heartburn.
_✓_ I can't sleep from too much thinking.
_✓_ I think, move, talk, and eat fast.
_✓_ At times I think so quickly, I almost feel I'm out of my body.

3. METAL

____ I have a dry cough or yellow mucus.
____ I'm often thirsty. I keep water by the bed at night.
____ I have an itchy red skin rash or very dry skin.
____ I smoke cigarettes or take stimulant drugs.
____ I have colitis or painful intestinal spasms.

____ When I get angry, I'm as tough as steel.

4. WATER

____ I'm a very sexual person. I crave sex often.
____ My urine tends to be sparse or concentrated.
____ I have tightness in my back or behind the knees.
____ I usually know what's best for me and everyone else.
____ I tend toward extremes in work and play.
____ I've been very thin or very heavy.
____ I have a thick white, yellow, or pink discharge from the vagina.

5. WOOD

____ My eyes are dry and red. I have blurry vision or am nearsighted.
____ I can really get impatient or get so mad I yell.
____ My nervousness can become extreme.
____ I get headaches, spasms, or allergies under stress.
____ I stay up very late and can't wake up the next morning.
____ I'm a perfectionist. I get upset when things don't work.
____ I have painful joints.

_5_ Total number of checks in this section. Which element(s) had more checks?

II. Cold

1. FIRE

_____ I often have low energy and a slow heartbeat.

_____ I reach for coffee or tea to speed me up.

_____ I'm losing my memory.

_____ I can't sort things out clearly.

_____ My face is pale, and I feel listless.

_____ I have really stiff shoulders and enjoy warming massages.

2. EARTH

_____ I'm queasy and have lots of saliva, especially in the morning.

_____ I want to be alone when I'm tired. People drain me.

_____ I'm not very hungry. I often get indigestion and bloating.

_____ I get diarrhea with undigested food in the stools.

_____ I tend to obsess or complain.

_____ I reach for sweets or creamy foods to comfort me.

3. METAL

_____ I have lots of watery phlegm and congestion.

_____ I find it hard to breathe when I'm tired. I'm weak climbing stairs.

_____ I'm depressed. I feel heavy in the chest and closed in.

_____ I sigh from fatigue or I wheeze when breathing.

_____ Smoking cigarettes helps me to wake up and focus.

_____ I feel or look very pale.

4. WATER

_____ I have frequent urination that's like clear water.

_____ I have low sexual energy.

_____ I catch every cold and flu that goes around.

_____ I have poor concentration and memory, especially when tired.

_____ I groan from fatigue, and sleep a lot.

_____ I'm most tired during late afternoon.

_____ I feel I lack self-confidence.

5. WOOD

_____ It's hard for me to make up my mind; I'm indecisive.

_____ My muscle tone and strength are poor.

_____ Nothing interesting goes on in my life.

_____ I'm not very enthusiastic about sex.

_____ I crave rich foods and alcohol but don't tolerate them well.

_____ My skin is sallow or greenish.

_____ Total number of checks in this section. Which element(s) had more checks?

Diagnostic Questionnaire (cont.)

III. Stagnation

1. FIRE

_____ I get confused and perplexed when I'm stressed.

_____ I forget what I'm saying in the middle of a sentence.

_____ I stammer when I'm tired or nervous.

_____ I feel pressure in my chest.

_____ Sometimes my hands or arms go numb.

_____ When it comes to lovemaking, I'd rather read a novel.

2. EARTH

_____ I have pain in my stomach, and I can't think clearly after I eat.

_____ I worry, worry, worry.

_____ I burp a lot.

_____ I feel spacey when I don't eat.

_____ I don't feel grounded in my home or work or relationships.

_____ I have a large waistline.

_____ I have very irregular eating habits and poor digestion.

3. METAL

_____ When I start coughing, I can't stop.

_____ I seem to hold all my emotions in my chest.

_____ I often sneeze or get hiccups.

_____ My joints hurt with a dull, heavy ache in cold damp weather.

_____ My problems seem hopeless.

_____ I have chronic sinusitis, swollen lymph glands, or bronchitis.

4. WATER

_____ I have stiffness that comes and goes during cold weather.

_____ I have amenorrhea (no menstrual period) or am infertile.

_____ I seem to have lost my capacity for sex.

_____ I have prostate trouble.

_____ My bones are weak and break easily.

_____ I've lost my hair or it's turned white.

_____ I have chronic urinary tract infections.

5. WOOD

_____ I have spasms or seizures.

_____ I have pains that shoot through my body like the wind.

_____ My chest is tight.

_____ It's hard to swallow.

_____ I have poor circulation.

_____ Lately my life is very frustrating.

_____ I often have to control my rage.

FOR NUMBERS 1–5 OF STAGNATION

_____ I've had chemotherapy, radiation, or large doses of antibiotics.

_____ I take antidepressant or other psychiatric drugs.

_____ I'm addicted to street drugs.

____ I drink more than an occasional glass of wine or beer.

____ I take birth control pills.

____ Total number of checks in this section. Which element(s) had more checks?

My totals for these sections are:

_5_ I. Heat

_8_ II. Cold

_4_ III. Stagnation

The totals in detail are:

	HEAT	COLD	STAGNATION
Fire	0	3	0
Earth	5	3	1
Metal	0	1	1
Water	0	1	0
Wood	0	0	1

For the record:

During what season have you filled out this questionnaire?

_✓_ Spring

____ Summer

____ Indian summer (early autumn or between autumn and winter)

____ Fall

____ Winter

Do you have a cold or flu?

What changes in lifestyle are happening at this time? (For example, moving, changing jobs, loss of a loved one, fallen in love, living in a different climate, etc.)

EVALUATING YOUR RESPONSES

The questionnaire above is not meant to be a test in the ordinary sense. No answer should be considered right or wrong; they can be used to indicate your energetic tendencies right now. These will change as your diet and lifestyle change. You might have quite a mixture of check marks in each of the Heat, Cold, and Stagnation sections. We are rarely just one or another of these types. If you had many responses in only one section, your temporary imbalance would be rather extreme.

Each of the sections has subheadings labeled Fire, Earth, Metal, Water, and Wood,

which refer to the Five Elements you studied in chapter 6. This questionnaire gives you a succinct profile of metabolism and the functioning of the endocrine system, according to traditional Chinese medicine.

If you checked many items in the first section, labeled Heat, you have what Asian doctors call *internal heat* symptoms. Those discomforts could result from dehydration, inflammation, or a hyperactive state of metabolism. In each case the symptoms are described according to TCM, and do not indicate diseases described by Western medicine. For example, under subhead 3, "I have a dry cough" refers to dryness in the lungs or throat. In another example, "I talk and laugh a lot," under subhead 1, shows hyperactivity in the Fire element. As such, it could refer to either the heart or the pericardium.

Note that "heat" doesn't imply a weather condition. It can be used to describe fever, inflammation, and the balance of moisture and dryness of internal tissue. "Heat" symptoms may be due to illness, long-term stress, a spicy diet, or habits that are considered heating and drying, such as smoking cigarettes.

If you checked items under Cold, you have *internal cold* symptoms. These could be the result of a hypoactive (slow) metabolism, the opposite of inflammation. The symptoms might be the result of fatigue, weakness, undernourishment, depression, or a diet of extremely cold raw foods.

Items checked under Stagnation refer to *stagnant chi.* It results when long-term stress from inflammation or exhaustion has made internal organs function in an irregular manner. *Stagnation* can result from either extreme *internal heat* or *internal cold* symptoms. Perhaps the body's energy is "stuck" because a spasm or pain is blocking the flow of *chi. Stagnation* symptoms result in irregular heartbeat, pain, or indigestion from physical or emotional stress.

In the following sections of this chapter we'll explore Asian diagnosis using the information from your questionnaire responses, in order to see how signs of *internal heat* or *internal cold* affect the Five Elements. First, however, we need to better understand what is meant by *heat* and *cold* when referring to metabolism, the functioning of the nervous system, and anything else that is controlled by *chi.*

Is It Hot or Not?

To use the Diagnostic Questionnaire successfully, you'll need to look more closely at the fact that all Asian medical systems use the concepts of *hot* and *cold* symptoms. We've already learned that *internal heat* is a condition of inflammation, dehydration, or hyperactivity of metabolism. Conversely, *internal cold* symptoms arise from hypoactivity, or underfunctioning metabolism. How we can correct such imbalances with herbs is the subject of the rest of this book.

In chapter 4, we stated that to fully understand Asian energetic medicine, we have to consider herbs according to taste, temperature, and type. The questionnaire indicates your current imbalances among the Five Elements, according to their type and temperature. For example, you may find that you need to use *warming* digestive herbs or *cooling* diuretic herbs at present. You can learn this by noting the frequency of your responses in the Heat, Cold, and Stagnation sections.

HOW DO YOU KNOW IF YOU NEED A *WARMING* OR *COOLING* HERB?

Look back at your responses to the Diagnostic Questionnaire. In the first section under Heat, we see *internal heat* symptoms as they affect the Fire element. The associated organ systems for the Fire element are heart, pericardium, Triple Heater, and small intestine. Since heat symptoms include discomfort that is inflammatory in nature, we see overstimulation of the heart with fast or irregular heartbeat, anxiety, nightmares, reddish face, and hyperexcitability. However, we don't always know the origin of these conditions. Perhaps they result from temporary stress or prolonged problems such as excess cholesterol, side effects from medication, or addictions. When dealing with heart irregularities, it pays to use additional methods of diagnosis, possibly even Western medical testing for cholesterol or high blood pressure. Then we can choose herbs that do not simply sedate the heart, but get to the root of the problem.

Another example: It is easy to understand clear-cut problems relating to inflammation in subhead 2, Earth, of the Heat section. The associated organ systems are stomach and spleen/pancreas. Excess stomach acid from *internal heat* causes hunger and burning. You may have ulcers, heartburn, or symptoms related to hyperactivity of spleen/pancreas (obsessive thinking or craving sweets, according to Chinese doctors), because these are considered to be part of the same energetic system: the Earth element. You need to avoid creating more stomach acid by eating cooling alkaline foods and herbs such as bitter greens.

Now go through the questionnaire, noting the number of your responses for each element. If you have three or more checks in the sections pertaining to Heat for an element, you may need some *cooling* herbs and spices, which balance that organ system. If you checked three or more items in the Cold section of a given element, *warming* herbs and spices, are appropriate

for you. You may need both *heating* and *cooling* herbs among various elements. We will study specific needs later, using several methods of observation. For now, we can generalize in the following way:

HEAT

Indicates inflammation or dehydration and requires *cooling* (anti-inflammatory or moistening) herbs.

- In the Fire element, might require heart-moderating, anticholesterol, or weight-loss herbs, *cooling* laxatives, or sedatives for anxiety.
- In the Earth element, might require *cooling* digestive herbs for indigestion or ulcers.
- In the Metal element, might require *cooling* herbs for cough, thick mucus, colds, flu, skin allergies, or rashes.
- In the Water element, might require *cooling* diuretic herbs.
- In the Wood element, might require *cooling* herbs that treat liver and gallbladder problems leading to indigestion, headaches, allergies, eye problems, or arthritis.

COLD

Indicates internal weakness or slow metabolism and requires herbal stimulants or tonics.

- In the Fire element, might require heart-moderating or anticholesterol herbs.
- In the Earth element, might require *warming* stimulant herbs, affecting

digestion, blood-building, or hypo-glycemia.

𝕾 In the Metal element, might require *warming* stimulant herbs for fatigue, shortness of breath, or depression.

𝕾 In the Water element, might require *warming* stimulants for fatigue or sexual weakness.

𝕾 In the Wood element, might require *warming* digestive herbs or herbs that affect circulation.

STAGNATION

This will require combinations of both *warming* and *cooling* herbs that might treat pain, periodic symptoms (those that come and go), or emotional balance.

The following will help you understand how *cooling, heating,* and *antistagnation* herbs work.

COOLING HERBS AND SPICES

Cooling spices are anti-inflammatory because they eliminate *internal heat* symptoms in a variety of ways, depending upon their location. (Also see chapter 4.) In describing the actions of *cooling* herbs, I shall refer to sections of the Diagnostic Questionnaire so you can see which kinds apply to you.

Cooling *digestive herbs*

Some people need herbs for indigestion, but can't tolerate spices because they create stomach acid (subhead 2, Earth, of Heat section). For burning pain of ulcers or excess acid inflammation, use a *cooling* digestive herb—for example, cumin, dill, or mint—and highly alkaline foods such as cabbage.

Cooling digestive spices tend to be bitter. For that reason many are laxative. Some are diuretic, which means they stimulate urination. This helps eliminate acid that causes the overly hot condition. Digestive acid is best eliminated in the stools, not through sweating. Diaphoretic (perspiration-inducing) herbs can spread excess acid through the body to aggravate inflammatory joint pain or skin rash.

Cooling *laxatives*

The following herbs are useful for balancing symptoms of *internal heat* (subhead 2, Earth, of Heat section, affecting stomach and spleen/pancreas; or subhead 3, Metal, affecting lung and large intestine). Generally what we eat affects not only digestive organs, but also lungs, large intestine, and skin. Traditional Chinese anatomy links all of these. Excess inflammation in these areas can lead to ulcer pains, excess hunger, thirst, dry skin, or irritable bowel symptoms. In each case, to soothe inflammation we use *cooling* alkaline-producing herbs such as aloe.

Aloe vera is highly alkaline, slightly bitter, and an excellent source of natural vitamin E. It heals the burn of ulcers, cools the digestive tract, and detoxifies liver and spleen. The gel (or juice), available in health-food stores, helps clear blemishes and bad breath. It is slightly laxative. You can drink aloe vera gel in water, tea, or apple juice.

If you scored high in subheads 2, Earth, and 5, Wood, of the Heat section, you will need anti-inflammatory herbs that affect not only digestion but also joints. Rhubarb is an effective laxative food that helps eliminate toxins from the digestive tract and uric acid from the joints. If cooked rhubarb tastes too bitter and sour, you might add some fennel seeds as a sweetener. Do not use honey, which is *warming.*

Blood cleansers

Cooling bitter herbs can be used as blood cleansers to detoxify the liver and blood so that we have less inflammation, irritability, and skin rash. They apply to subhead 5, Wood, of the Heat section. Saffron is used for painful and enlarged liver. Dandelion and burdock eliminate constipation and pimples. Bitter *cooling* herbs such as dandelion or aloe vera cleanse toxins because they are laxatives as well as liver cleansers.

Cooling *diuretics*

Internal heat can cause sparse concentrated urine or frequent urges to urinate. (See subhead 4, Water, of Heat section.) Excess tension energy in the acupuncture meridian related to the bladder can be experienced as tightness or spasms in the back and legs. It can pull a person straight upward to stand tall and strut, or it can make movement painful. Notice the psychological equivalent of strutting from plentiful *chi* in the bladder meridian: "I usually

know what's best for me and everyone else." When back spasm is accompanied by dark urine, a *cooling* diuretic can ease discomfort from *internal heat.*

Coriander seed and leaf cilantro are *cooling* and diuretic to combat burning urination and urinary infections.

Cooling diuretics are sometimes used to lower blood sugar in diabetes. For example, cornsilk tea is used for weight loss and diabetes. Just boil the cornsilk along with the corn, and drink the cooking water like tea.

Cooling *digestive herbs that affect absorption*

Cooling digestive herbs help absorption of nutrients when they increase the flow of bile. For example, gentian is used traditionally for ulcers in the stomach and small intestine. Fever, jaundice, hepatitis, enlarged liver, acne, diabetes, and cancer have also been treated with this *cooling* herb. Most often used for chronic diarrhea, poor absorption, shortness of breath, and depression, gentian is widely used in popular after-dinner liquors. Gentian is useful for persons who checked responses in the Earth, Metal, and Wood sections of the Diagnostic Questionnaire.

Warming *digestive spices*

Warming spices facilitate absorption by stimulating the production of acids and enzymes while drying excess moisture in the intestines. They are useful for people who checked responses in subhead 2, Earth, of the Cold section for *internal cold* symptoms that apply to the Earth element. Those people tend to have slow digestion, are tired after eating, or have indigestion and bloating. When digestion is slow, the body has difficulty transforming food into energy and blood. At the same time, the elimination of toxins is impaired. Poorly digested food turns into cholesterol, cellulite, asthmatic phlegm, tumors, or any number of other problems. By adding certain pungent spices to foods, we speed their processing because we increase energy and appetite while increasing stomach acid.

Our individual needs for *warming* digestive spices will vary according to age, stress level, and speed of metabolism. Usage of *warming* spices must be adequate to digest meals without creating excess acidity. Overuse of hot spices causes burning or nervousness.

Some *heating* digestive spices are ginger, pepper, clove, anise, nutmeg, turmeric, caraway, allspice, cardamom, cinnamon, and combinations such as those found in pumpkin pie spice and Chinese Five Spice powder. Most people know that these delicious spices are used in pastries, without knowing they are so *heating* they provide an energy boost.

Rosemary stimulates the adrenal glands and heart, and is useful for subhead 4, Water, and subhead 1, Fire, of Cold. Sage curbs excessive sweating from weakness. Enjoy rosemary or sage as teas by using only a small pinch of the herb for each cup. Since they are extremely *heating*, rosemary and sage are best enjoyed by persons with *internal cold* symptoms.

The caring cook will use *warming*

digestive spices to create more appetite. Spices create not only appetite for food but appetite for life. They are stimulants creating extroverted high energy that gets you out of your chair. They are fine for most people in the morning, but could cause sleepless nights when eaten too late in the evening. As we shall see later, however, persons with chronic *internal heat* symptoms should not use *heating* spices at all. Long-term imbalances affecting all aspects of metabolism can occur with the misuse of foods. We see the effects of these imbalances in symptoms that traditional Chinese doctors describe as *stagnation* or *stagnant chi.*

Internal heat *or* cold *symptoms and* stagnant chi

In real life, many different kinds of responses happen simultaneously. For example, a person might experience inflammatory arthritis along with weak digestion. In that case, the choice of herbs becomes more complicated. Such problems result from *stagnant* or stuck *chi.*

Stagnation

The flow of vital energy or *chi* can become stuck anywhere in the body. When this occurs in the upper body due to rich diet, poor heart function, physical trauma, or emotional blocks, we feel pressure and tightness in the chest. An irregular heartbeat can create other symptoms. Subhead 1, Fire, of Stagnation refers to stagnant energy affecting the Fire element.

Often stagnant *chi* is trapped in the

shoulders, chest, or digestive area. Moving the stuck *chi* with stimulant herbs breaks up congested energy in the entire body, not just where we feel it most. Then we feel more relaxed and have more energy. Both indigestion and emotional blocks improve when we free *chi* stuck in our center.

Herbs that "move stuck *chi*" can be *warming, cooling,* or what the Chinese call *scattering. Scattering* herbs can cause sweating while increasing circulation. For example, two remedies, **Xiao Yao Wan** and **Shu Gan Wan,** are widely used to ease digestive and emotional discomfort related to stuck *chi.* These remedies increase blood circulation and digestion while helping rid the body of accumulated wastes. See chapter 4 for information on how **Xiao Yao Wan** and other such herbal combinations are "built."

Now that you know about the five tastes and the energetic effects of *warming* and *cooling* herbs, you can better understand how a combination like **Xiao Yao Wan** works. That formula is considered effective for treating stagnant digestive *chi.* Its pungent, stimulant herbs increase digestion and blood production, while its bitter, cleansing herbs facilitate the flow of *chi.*

The herbal remedies you will ultimately use depend on more-refined methods of diagnosis we shall learn in the following chapters. The harmonious workings of body/mind/spirit are more complicated than information on the general or traditional uses of herbs found in books, or the questions found in a questionnaire. We can use questionnaires such as the one at the beginning of this chapter only to gather information along the way to greater understanding.

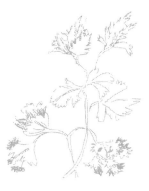

Parsley

9

Informal Asian Health Diagnosis

To learn without thinking is fatal.
But to think without learning is very dangerous.

—Confucius

Confucius

The learning process referred to by Confucius means understanding the teachings of the ancients. In the *I Ching* we are advised to study the laws of the universe in order to better understand ourselves. We're told that "the great [person] gains wisdom by understanding how the invisible [energy] affects the visible [matter]." *Chi* is invisible to the naked eye like a stream of electrons, so that we must study its effects in order to perceive it. Asian diagnosis gives us a framework by which to observe *chi*.

Most herbals ask us to learn without thinking because they

offer no individualized advice, only general information on herbs. Western medical books demand thinking without ancient learning. They lack the wisdom of experience; their insights are splintered into specialties. We need a different approach.

In the previous chapter we learned what is meant by *internal heat, internal cold,* and *stagnation.* Now we can refine our perception with another concept, the notion of Correspondences. My laboratory is often the supermarket.

Have you ever looked closely at the foods people buy, then observed their appearance and behavior? You can learn important things by looking and listening. Traditional Asian doctors collect lots of information that way. They analyze details most people wouldn't notice at all. Then, with inductive reasoning, they make a working diagnosis based on Asian medical theories, and choose the appropriate herbs and therapies. These can vary during the course of treatment, according to subtle changes noticed by the doctor.

For example, at a checkout counter I watched an old New York couple. She, in a bright green sweater, was scolding him, in a maroon shirt. They had probably fought together for forty years. Looking to the crowd for approval, they each made their points loudly. He had a tic—a twitch in his lips—and an overly red face. She had gnarled hands with joints that resembled pincers. Both were browned with liver spots and had thin gray hair. His voice was high-pitched, hers a whine. Most people wouldn't consider these to be symptoms of illness, but with training in Asian

diagnosis, I always remark imbalances in appearance and behavior.

In their shopping cart I saw red meat, processed cheese, white bread, potato chips, coffee, jelly doughnuts, and a packaged cake. "Dangerous fats, sweets, salt, and irritants leading to excess acid, inflammation, poor circulation, and *phlegm,*" I thought. With a diet like that, I could predict high cholesterol, circulation problems, impaired vision, sciatica, eventually heart problems, arthritis, and, more likely than not, cancer. Perhaps the woman's gnarled, painful joints were encouraged by an overly acid and fatty diet of sugar and red meat. That diet would be too *heating,* causing congestion of *chi* circulation. We cannot know exactly how representative these foods are of this couple's diet, but we can make a good guess by looking closely at them.

The foods we choose most often indicate our health tendencies, while those we eat under stress indicate our addictions. These are the foods we choose to comfort us or drive us faster. In either case, we suffer their consequences.

Asian health practitioners usually do not follow their patients into the grocery store. They may inquire about diet, but most often they notice the *effects* of imbalance resulting from years of dietary abuse. Observation of the body is as important in diagnosis as asking questions, taking a medical history, or observing the patient's tongue and pulse.

For example, facial color can indicate the state of blood circulation or blood production. A reddish hue noticed around nose and mouth can indicate the presence of acids leading to broken capillaries or blemishes. A high cholesterol count can also lead to an overly red face. A ruddy complexion is generally considered a sign of *internal heat* affecting the circulatory or digestive system.

Pallid, greenish, or sallow complexion can indicate blood deficiency or poor circulation, generally resulting from *internal cold* conditions. *Stagnation* from weakness or poor circulation can be present in either case. It is often observed as purplish lips. These types of indications are used only to form a working diagnosis.

This diagnosis is further confirmed by observing the tongue and pulse and by asking questions such as: Are the woman's joints painful? Does cold weather (which constricts blood circulation) make the pain worse? Do certain foods make the pain worse? Other questions will arise from what we notice in the observation of tongue and pulse.

The Correspondences

These corresponding factors are not random, but are part of a cohesive diagnostic method used in Chinese medicine, called "Correspondences." It is a means of explaining the origins and manifestations of *chi*, a way of observing life through a specialized vision. The ancients thought all sights, sounds, smells, directions of wind currents, and everything else were expressions of *chi:* The laws of heaven were observed in movements of energy on earth. In medical terms, anything that affects the functioning of internal organs can be observed through the Correspondences. In that view, we can see what's happening inside by viewing the outside.

This concept is not at all foreign to Western holistic medicine, especially herbalism. I have several books on desert herbs by Mexican *curanderos* that feature such herbs as boldo, used to treat "coppery-colored facial tone, anger, and violent behavior due to biliousness of the liver." We determine the choice and effectiveness of herbs by observing changing signs and symptoms.

CORRESPONDING TASTES

According to Asian diet theories, five tastes affect associated internal organs. The tastes can either stimulate or drain each of the Five Elements. When used in diagnosis, a corresponding taste shows us a problem in the element. We experience a "sour" taste in the mouth with indigestion from liver problems. The sour taste corresponds to a problem in the Wood element. When sick, we can also crave the associated taste because an imbalance strives to perpetuate itself. We will examine this further when we address the problem of addictions.

Many other Correspondences are also associated with the Five Elements. For example, each element is more or less active or full of energy during different times of the year. Certain climates threaten the health and balance of each element. The body has a predictable odor, the complexion an associated color, and the voice a characteristic timbre when an element is out of balance. I have summarized some of the Correspondences in the following chart.

Although the chart may not look immediately useful, when we understand the relationships represented, it becomes quite interesting. Take, for example, our quarrelsome couple in the supermarket. She has poor circulation and arthritis, with damaged joints and liver spots. These strongly indicate problems in the Wood element. According to TCM, the Wood element is responsible for the smooth flow of *chi* affecting joints, muscles, tendons, and circulation in the chest, neck, and eyes.

Looking at the chart under the Wood element, we find green color, sour taste, rancid smell, shouting voice, and problems with the ligaments. The woman is wearing a green sweater. This may be meaningful if she wears it very often. Perhaps, without knowing it, she is wearing the color like a badge that reads, "Wood: I have liverish problems." But perhaps green is this year's fashion. I am more interested to know if her urine, stools, phlegm, the coating on her tongue, or her skin color is greenish. These may indicate internal problems with Wood (liver/gallbladder function), especially the production and circulation of bile.

If I were close enough and she had an *internal heat* condition, she'd have a slightly rancid odor. The liver is an important organ of detoxification. If it suffers, impurities mount, leading to such symptoms.

Another more obvious indication is her tone of voice. Various sounds, such as shouting and whining, correspond to imbalances in the elements. The woman in the supermarket shouts when arguing, but if her voice sounded like a shout even when she spoke normally, it would indicate prob-

FIVE ELEMENT CORRESPONDENCES

ELEMENT	WOOD	FIRE	EARTH	METAL	WATER
SEASON	spring	summer	late summer	autumn	winter
CLIMATE	wind	heat	humidity	dryness	cold
ORGAN	liver/ gallbladder	heart/small intestine	spleen/ stomach	lung/large intestine	kidney/ bladder
COLOR	green	red	yellow	white	black
FLAVOR	sour	bitter	sweet	pungent	salt
ODOR	rancid	scorched	fragrant	rotten	putrid
SOUND	shout	laugh	sing	weep	groan
EMOTION	anger	joy	sympathy	grief	fear
ORIFICE	eyes	ears	nose	mouth	urinary
HELPFUL GRAINS	wheat	glutinous-millet	millet	rice	beans peas

lems in Wood. A whine indicates trouble in Earth; a sigh, weakness in Metal; and a groan, weakness in the Water element. Most people have problems in more than one element at a time, but the corresponding voice, complexion, and so forth can indicate the more important imbalances.

Why is a shouting voice associated with Wood problems? Tightness in the neck and jaws gives the voice a shouting sound. People with stiff neck and jaw often suffer from tight muscles in the chest and the sides, resulting from poor circulation (*stagnant chi*) affecting the Wood Element.

The woman's appearance, odor, voice quality, and difficulty of movement are indicative of problems in Wood, which originate from *internal heat* and *stagnation*. There are other factors involved, but these symptoms alone are enough to indicate Wood.

The man in the maroon shirt has a twitch at the mouth. This muscle spasm may be a habit, or it may be related to high blood pressure or repressed anger. Certainly the man has other signs pointing to *internal heat*. What I noticed most was his red face. This might only be temporary. If not, however, it could be an indication of *internal heat* affecting the heart. He would be advised to check his cholesterol and blood pressure. His high-pitched voice could be from strain or fatigue. If chronic, it could also indicate a problem of *heat* and *stagnation* in the Fire element.

The Correspondences are only guideposts for further analysis; they are not themselves the answer. If we saw a man in the supermarket with a red face who often laughed, we couldn't know, beyond a doubt, that he had a heart problem. Perhaps he was embarrassed or had just seen a Buster Keaton movie. The Correspondences give us things to look for, but such signs and symptoms of illness must be confirmed with tongue and pulse diagnosis and sometimes with Western medical reports.

The advantage of Asian medical diagnosis is that it takes into account things that escape the attention of Western medical diagnosis. These are the little complaints that seem annoying but unimportant, that make a Western doctor throw up his hands and say, "Forget it. You're just growing older," or "See a psychotherapist."

Asian medical diagnosis is based on an ancient view of humanity that links body, mind, and spirit, where subtle indications from any part of our vital energy speak for the whole. In this way, Asian diagnosis is a most valuable tool for predicting and preventing future illness. By understanding the present, we can look into the future. This awareness stems from an ancient wisdom that links the invisible (mind) with the visible (body).

OBSERVATION OF DATA

At this point, you know enough Asian diagnosis to be confused. The first few years I studied acupuncture, it seemed like peeling the layers of an onion. You have to go over the same concepts many times in different ways. *Chi* is always *chi*, but our comprehension grows from experience. That lends meaning to what Lao-tzu wrote during the fourth century B.C. in his *Tao Te Ching:*

To be great is to go forward,
To go forward is to travel far,
To travel far is to return.

As you refine your skills in observation, people will seem different. Your understanding of them will be deeper, your intuitions more true. After studying your constitutional type and tongue in the next couple of chapters, you'll begin to have a reasonable grasp of what is happening with your *chi*. Then you can apply what you've learned to others.

The Eight Principles

Traditional Chinese doctors use a specific method of analysis called the Eight Principles. Briefly, they are a series of questions: Are the symptoms excess or deficient, hot or cold, *yin* or *yang*, internal or external? These determine the nature, location, and origin of symptoms. They are not easy concepts. The difference between a good herbalist and someone who chooses herbs according to general knowledge (from laboratory studies or traditional custom), speculation, or magic is their use of the Eight Principles.

Without going into exhaustive detail, we can say that the nature of symptoms can be excess (more *chi* than normal, or congested *chi*)—for example, swelling, sinus congestion, severe pain, and throbbing. Or they can be deficient (*chi* or blood), leading to weakness, paleness, fatigue, or wounds that don't heal.

Their nature can also be considered hot (for example, fever, ruddiness, or dehydrated body fluids) or cold (lots of liquid discharge, such as watery urine, runny mucus, or diarrhea).

The location of symptoms can be deep, affecting the *yin* parts of the body such as internal organs or blood. Or they can be more superficial, affecting the *yang* (the muscles, the surface of the skin).

The origin or source of the problem can be external, resulting from the climate, germs, or pollution. Or it can be internal from imbalance, weakness, stress, or emotions. Understanding how these factors work to create illness will determine the choice of herbs. Of course, they overlap. It becomes evident when we address the emotions. We are more susceptible to illness when we are weak, tired, or upset.

Emotions and the Five Elements

Our emotions are the combined product of body and energy. As such, they can be influenced by herbs.

Each of the Five Elements is said to contain a spirit that provides an emotion. Happiness comes from the heart, anger from the liver, obsession from the spleen, anxiety from the lungs, and fear from the kidneys. When an element is troubled, its associated emotion can surface to announce an imbalance. Nuances are possible. For example, indecision can be seen as an *internal cold* symptom affecting Wood.

Emotions are perceived indirectly. We can hear anger in a harsh voice or con-

The Correspondences Applied to You

Let's observe you in the way an Asian health practitioner would. Please mark the items that apply to you.

I often have problems with:

WOOD

____ liver or gallbladder
____ chronic headaches, allergies
____ hepatitis or herpes
____ muscle spasms, seizures, epilepsy
____ blood pressure
____ nearsightedness
____ arthritis
____ menstrual pain and PMS

FIRE

____ heart trouble
____ rheumatic heart disease
____ high cholesterol
____ poor circulation
____ anxiety or depression
____ numbness of limbs

EARTH

____ spleen or stomach
____ digestive disturbances
____ emotional ungroundedness
____ diabetes or hypoglycemia
____ addictions to sugar or alcohol
____ edema or cellulite
____ chronic diarrhea
____ bruises

METAL

____ cough
____ asthma, emphysema
____ shortness of breath
____ diarrhea or constipation
____ chronic fatigue
____ depression
____ skin rashes

WATER

____ kidney or bladder function
____ poor concentration or memory
____ lower back pain
____ fragile bones, sprains, fractures
____ urinary incontinence or infections
____ sexual problems
____ infertility
____ hair loss, premature white hair
____ low immune strength

Totals ___ Wood, ___ Fire, ___ Earth, ___ Metal, ___ Water

My facial color shows this hue (observe in adequate lighting, not direct sunlight; notice the entire face, then the areas around the nose and mouth and under the eyes):

____ greenish   ___ white
____ reddish   ___ dark
____ yellow or brown

My urine tends to be (observe the urine when you have not taken vitamins that would affect its color):

____ greenish
____ reddish
____ deep yellow or brown
____ clear or bluish
____ cloudy
____ grainy or with sediment
____ oily
____ streaked with red

My stools are:

____ runny, watery
____ long, thin
____ dry
____ contain undigested food
____ light or yellowish
____ greenish
____ orange
____ streaked with blood
____ streaked with phlegm
____ black

In foods and drinks I crave:

____ sour
____ bitter
____ sweet, bland
____ hot, pungent
____ salty

Lately I've been:

____ angry, emotional, demanding
____ exhibitionist or anxious
____ whining, clingy
____ sad
____ fearful, distrustful

I have:

____ dry, red eyes
____ watery eyes
____ a red nose, broken capillaries
____ bleeding gums
____ bad breath
____ difficulty hearing
____ oversensitivity to noise

INTERPRETATION:

Internal cold symptoms tend to be pale skin; watery, runny, and clear body fluids; emotional depression or dependency; low *chi* with possible difficulties in concentration and hearing.

Internal heat tends to be characterized by reddish skin. Urine is dark yellow, reddish, oily, or streaked with blood. Stools are dry or dark, or streaked with phlegm or blood. Emotions are hot, such as anger or exuberance. Other heat symptoms can be red eyes and broken capillaries.

Stagnation (or *stagnant chi*) underlies all chronic problems, and is often related to poor circulation and pain.

tentment in laughter. The Correspondences take all such observations into account, everything from tone of voice to facial hue or body odor. It is by observing the Correspondences that the basic aspects of life—spirit, blood, and *chi*—become apparent. But for the present, let's consider only what we've observed in the two previous questionnaires, the nature and location of symptoms.

First, notice where you marked the most responses in questionnaires on pages 76 and 92. One or more sections will stand out as important for you. Compare your responses in the element sections of both questionnaires. If you marked many items for one or more of the Five Elements, it indicates areas for further investigation. Usually, the larger the number of responses, the more troubled the element. Although the responses may be influenced by having a cold or by emotional or seasonal considerations, if the problems have been chronic, it's a good indication that the element is out of balance.

People react to stress differently. Perhaps you get a headache, an allergy, or a rash, or perhaps you get angry. All these responses situate your problems in the Wood element. If you treat a headache with an aspirin, you miss the benefits of bringing the element back into balance. Many other uncomfortable symptoms would persist.

By taking herbs that cool *internal heat* problems of Wood, we can reduce headaches, muscle spasms, skin rashes, nervousness, allergies, hypertension, inflammatory arthritis, and certain eye problems. The forms that our symptoms take mirror imbal-

ances in our energy, and their location depends upon the health of the Five Elements.

The Five Element Correspondences and Their Hot and Cold Symptoms

Please look back at the chart of Five Element Correspondences as we study how each of the elements has its related *internal heat* and *internal cold* symptoms.

THE WOOD ELEMENT

Nature Hot: pain, spasm, fever, anger
Cold: weakness, paleness, indecision
Location liver, gallbladder, muscles, nerves, eyes, emotions
Origin internal and external *wind*, frustration
Color green
Taste sour

wood

In TCM it is said that the liver "contains the blood," which nourishes muscles and eyes. We can better understand what that means by looking at the symptoms of *internal heat*.

Wood and internal heat

Internal heat symptoms affecting Wood often yield sharp pains or muscle spasms. The Wood element influences the smooth circulation of *chi*, and also the health of nerves, muscles, tendons, and eyesight. When the Wood element flourishes, there are no spasms or tremors because we have a better chance of adequate calcium absorption for strong muscles, smooth circulation, and good vision.

Internal heat symptoms for the Wood element, as listed in The Correspondences Applied to You, include chronic headaches and allergies, hepatitis, herpes, muscle spasms and seizures, high blood pressure, inflammatory arthritis, and sharp menstrual pain.

Wood and internal cold

Internal cold affecting the Wood element is usually part of a bigger picture of general weakness or exhaustion. Deficiency or *internal cold* symptoms of Wood could lead to poor muscle tone and weak, ridged fingernails because enzyme activity and calcium absorption are impaired. *Internal cold* affecting Wood weakens muscle strength anywhere in the body. It can affect heart rhythm and blood circulation. Muscle tone is also important for healthy vision. Nearsightedness is often indicative of problems in Wood.

I have listed fewer *internal cold* symptoms than *internal heat* symptoms for Wood in the questionnaire because they are seen less frequently in practice. Aside from anemia and certain vision problems, we most often see weak muscle tone. In most cases, herbal doctors treat liver weakness with *warming* remedies that treat *stagnation* to stimulate the functioning of the liver organ

system, clearing congestion. This ensures the smooth flow of *chi*.

The origin of imbalance in Wood goes beyond poor nutrition. Taking calcium pills is not enough to ensure a healthy liver. The Chinese medical explanation of many imbalances in Wood is found in the concept of *wind*.

Wood and wind

According to the Correspondences, the weather condition that most threatens the Wood element is *wind*. But "wind" has two separate meanings. The origin of wind as a weather condition is external. It's the wind that blows on windy days. However another sense of *wind* is as an internal imbalance. To complicate matters, the effects of external wind can become internal. As we shall see, its method of entry and location will determine how *wind* is treated.

The most frequent example of illness caused by external wind is the common cold. Because the symptoms indicate an excess condition (stiffness and chills) with an external origin (wind from outside the body), the correct herbal treatment for the first stage of a cold is diaphoretic: sweating out cold air trapped in muscles gets rid of the problem by reversing the symptoms, sending what should be outside out again.

In a modern understanding of the term, "evil wind" can also carry infectious disease. In that case, many internal imbalances such as fever, jaundice, and aches occur. The correct treatment would not be with diaphoretic herbs (as though it were merely an external problem), but with antibiotic and anti-inflammatory herbs, treating it as an internal imbalance.

Internal *wind* in the body is said to be created by inflammation. *Heat* originating from the liver rises up to the head, causing pain, dizziness, or blurry vision. The result can be a sick headache. Or the *wind* can go elsewhere, to congest circulation in the muscles, joints, or skin. In many cases, *cooling* herbs are useful. But *warming* herbs can also "ground the wind." For example, valerian, a nerve sedative, is useful for migraines and dizziness. I take capsules of valerian during long flights to Asia to "ground" me and clear up in-flight headaches caused by stale air and excess nerve stimulation.

When "rising liver *wind*" symptoms such as dizziness or headache come from poor digestion, herbal blood cleansers such as aloe vera are necessary; when they result from excessive nerve stimulation, a nervine (nerve sedative) is useful. These are important distinctions because we use different types of herbs to treat pain depending upon its origin.

Wood and foods

A chronic sour taste in the mouth can result from poor digestion from stuck *chi*. Excess oily and sweet foods interfere with both Wood and Earth elements, resulting in excess cholesterol or stones. A sour taste or a green-brown coating on the tongue, along with other bilious symptoms (nausea and constipation), can be alleviated with liver-cleansing herbs—for example, ginger and lemon tea.

According to the Correspondences, wheat is associated with the Wood element because it quiets the nerves and soothes an addled spirit. It's a warming, grounding grain. It creates phlegm, a balm for mucous membranes. The Wood person runs on nervous energy, which makes great demands on nerves, stamina, and muscle strength. Wheat can relax and recharge a tired Wood person.

THE FIRE ELEMENT

Nature   Hot: tachycardia, anxiety, insomnia
Cold: weakness, numb extremities, depression
Location heart, chest, face, emotions, small intestine, abdomen, shoulders
Origin   heat, stress, poor digestion
Color   red
Taste   bitter

fire

Fire creates heat. In the body, the Fire element warms us with a glow of health by circulating blood through blood vessels. The small intestine separates food from waste. The workings of any one of the Five Elements also affects the others. When Wood is sufficient, the heart can be strong enough to warm us. With enough bile, the small intestine can absorb nutrients, and calcium can create a smooth, steady heartbeat. It's beautiful how it all works together.

Fire and internal heat

Internal heat in the Fire element can be provoked by hot weather, spicy foods, or inflammatory emotions such as anxiety, rage, or jealousy. That is why Chinese doctors say, "Heat damages Fire." Inflammation symptoms of the heart can include spasms, chest pain, or irregular heartbeat. *Internal heat* affecting the small intestine can lead to spasms and diarrhea with blood or yellow mucus. Chinese doctors treat the Triple Heater acupuncture meridian for certain illnesses increased by *internal heat* and dryness—for example, diabetes and epilepsy.

Red is the color associated with illness in the Fire element. According to the Correspondences, *heat* in the heart results in a reddish facial color. Reddish purple indicates *stagnant chi.* We may see this in people with high cholesterol or chest pains.

The Correspondences offer observations that may seem old-fashioned, but can be very useful. The odors associated with imbalances are a case in point. The scorched smell of fever or high blood pressure can sometimes be a not-so-subtle indication that the Fire element is overheated. I once walked into my room and perceived the unpleasant odor of fever. My parakeet smelled like burnt bird. He was thrashing aimlessly, suffering from a sudden attack of *internal heat.* Parakeets are known to die of fits. Quickly I gave him a tiny pill of homeopathic ferrum phosphate (iron) and saved his life.

Other signs of *internal heat* affecting Fire are less evident—for example, excessive laughter. Laughter and joy are wonderful things except when they become extreme in mania, a sign of *internal heat.* Conversely, we can think of depression as a lack of joy, a disease of weakness and *stagnation.* Several Chinese patent formulas (such as **Cerebral Tonic Pills**) treat mania, lack of mental clarity, and poor memory by regulating heart rhythm and cholesterol, thus easing circulation in the chest and brain.

How much laughter is healthy? I've heard wise old Chinese doctors say that worry injures the heart. Certainly it obstructs *chi* circulation. I like to remember a story I once heard about a man who said he was spontaneously cured of cancer when he watched Charlie Chaplin movies all day for a few months. That seems like the right amount of laughter.

In general, signs of *internal heat* affecting the heart are inflammatory: fast heartbeat, red skin, a scorched odor, and manic behavior. Symptoms indicating *internal heat* from the Correspondence questionnaire are heart trouble and anxiety.

Fire and internal cold

Internal cold signs affecting the heart and pericardium include lethargy, lack of joy, pallor, and poor circulation. These are also signs of weakness, often treated with herbal tonics for energy and longevity. Signs of *cold* in the Fire element listed in the questionnaire include depression and numbness of limbs. These are also signs of *stagnant chi.*

Stagnant energy is the inevitable result of heart weakness (*internal cold* affecting the heart). It can result from age, illness, or exhaustion, leading to weak muscles and undernourishment. *Stagnant chi* affecting the heart can lead to heart pain, poor concentration, or chronic heart failure.

Fire and foods

Bitter stimulants and laxatives activate the Fire element. But the taste can also be a warning signal. A chronic bitter taste in the mouth indicates poor digestion and stuck bile. This usually leads to chest discomfort and increased cholesterol. Bad breath may accompany constipation.

Digestive herbs are helpful for the heart. So is hawthorn, a bitter, hot, sour herb used to stimulate and strengthen a weak heart. A strong, steady heartbeat eventually helps control stress, fatigue, and cholesterol levels.

Millet is suggested for both Fire and Earth elements because, being a seed, not a grain, it's more easily digested and results in less phlegm.

THE EARTH ELEMENT

Nature Hot: ulcer pain, halitosis, blemishes, mania
Cold: nausea, excessive saliva, depression, obsession
Location stomach, spleen, flesh, blood, emotions
Origin humidity (food and climate), worry

Color yellow or brown
Taste sweet

earth

Symptoms troubling Earth involve indigestion, anemia, low energy, poor concentration, blood sugar irregularities, over- or underweight, menstrual irregularities, and mood swings. When Earth is troubled, we feel removed from our center, vulnerable, ungrounded. Life seems uncertain. We imagine that illness comes out of nowhere, for no reason, because we cannot see the results of our actions.

Earth and internal heat

Internal heat symptoms include pain and burning of ulcers, or excessive hunger. They can result from excess acid and stress. At times, stomach irritation can become so intense it leads to hyperactivity and insomnia. Chinese medicine links hyperthyroid mania with *internal heat* affecting Earth. In China, acupuncture treatments of stomach meridian points are used to reduce mania and hallucinations so that patients regain their center.

Items from the Correspondences questionnaire pertaining to *heat* in Earth include diabetes and sugar cravings.

Earth and internal cold

Internal cold symptoms result from a diet that is too often raw or cold in nature or from chronic illness. The resulting blood sugar irregularities tend toward hypoglycemia. Slow metabolism, excess weight, fatigue, pallor, and blood deficiency all result from slow digestion due to an *internal cold* condition.

Internal cold affecting the spleen leads to chronic diarrhea, malnourishment, thinness, blood deficiency, and poor concentration. The person tends to feel spacey, obsess, worry, and crave sweets. Symptoms from the Correspondences questionnaire concerning *internal cold* in Earth are digestive disturbances, emotional ungroundedness, hypoglycemia, addictions, edema and cellulite, chronic diarrhea, and bruises. Bruises and fragile capillaries can be related to poor absorption.

We observe the nose as an indication of the health of the Earth element. Excess mucus indicates a problem. Some Chinese doctors say the color and texture of the skin on the nose indicates general health. Many alcoholic persons have red noses with broken capillaries. The blood vessels are weak, and the body's ability to make blood is lessened when the spleen and pancreas are damaged.

Earth and emotional woes

A singing sound in the voice and the symptom of sympathy show imbalances in the Earth element that pertain to *internal cold* affecting the emotions. After years as a health practitioner, I can recognize the person with a spleen imbalance, whose voice may be songlike but does not sound grounded on earth, and whose constant demand for help is a nasal cry for sympathy.

These symptoms are not bad in themselves. Persons who savor their feelings can become adept at processing life's ups and downs; they are often very successful in artistic or spiritual work. Many people with an important spleen dynamic become health professionals, counselors, or clergy, devoting their lives not only to listening and feeling others' pain but helping to alleviate it.

But at times, the splenic person can fall in love with suffering. What to us may seem self-indulgence, for the person with "weak spleen" becomes the joy of self-analysis. This joy can go over the edge into schizophrenia, in which case we need to strengthen the spleen with herbs such as gentian, which tends to normalize blood sugar and improve mental clarity.

Dampness

Earth is said to be damaged by humidity (called *dampness* by TCM). *Dampness,* like *wind,* has two sources, one internal, the other external. Humid weather tends to slow digestive *chi,* making us feel hazy, lazy, and phlegmy.

Mucus-producing foods such as sweets, oils, and dairy foods slow digestion. They require digestive acids and enzymes for a longer period than simple sugars. Slowing digestion can be very useful in certain cases. For example, complex carbohydrates lower blood sugar because they are slow to digest, leaving us satisfied longer. They are useful for diabetes.

Conversely, too much cheese, pasta, nuts, and sweets causes bloating, indigestion pain, phlegm, and fatigue: that's *dampness*. Troubles arise when a phlegm-producing diet leads to overweight, cellulite, chronic phlegm conditions, and problems with mental clarity. *Dampness* can be hot or cold. Think of it as hot phlegm (thick and yellow) or cold phlegm (watery, runny, thin, and white). *Dampness* plays a big part in all the body's discharges, from sinuses to vagina.

Earth and foods

The sweet taste and fragrance are signs of imbalance in Earth. People with problems in Earth crave sweets. The diabetic person's body odor and urine smell sweet. These people should avoid all sweets, even beets and carrots. In Chinese medicine, diabetes is controlled with moisturizing, *cooling* herbs that lower blood sugar (such as cornsilk tea) and anti-inflammatory acupuncture treatments affecting lungs, stomach, and spleen, which ease excess thirst, hunger, and craving of sweets.

Hypoglycemia, a *deficiency* or *internal cold* problem, is treated accordingly with *warming* tonic herb combinations such as **Xiao Yao Wan**. Millet, a drying seed, not a grain, dries the excess *dampness* of spleen.

THE METAL ELEMENT

Nature Hot: cough, thirst, blemishes, anxiety
Cold: wheezing, fatigue, depression, diarrhea
Location lungs, large intestine, skin, emotions

Origin dryness (diet and climate)
Color white
Taste pungent

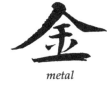
metal

According to Chinese anatomy, the lungs and large intestine are linked by the same meridian system. This means that cold or hot air penetrates easily from the most superficial organ, the lungs, to one of the deepest, the large intestine. For us to remain healthy, the lungs must be a barrier to extremes in weather. Otherwise we may develop cough and colds.

The large intestine assimilates important nutrients and passes wastes from the body. It is affected by hot and cold temperatures of foods and spice. Imbalances in the large intestine can result in pain, spasm, diarrhea, constipation, or chronic illness such as colitis, a problem usually resulting from weakness and *dampness.*

Metal and internal heat

Internal heat affecting the lungs creates spasm (coughing fits that do not stop), pain, and difficult breathing, panting, fever, thirst from dehydration, night sweats, and thick yellow or green mucus. Overheating the lungs can cause fatigue and blood deficiency. Shortness of breath and accompanying depression give the voice a weeping quality.

Inflammation in the Metal element can result from infection or from *heating* and *drying* substances. Internal imbalance can also be involved. For example, menopausal symptoms such as hot flashes and night sweats can be somewhat reduced with herbs that cool lung inflammation and build blood.

Dry cough, shortness of breath, chronic fatigue, and asthma (could be either *internal heat* or *cold*), emphysema, TB, and skin rashes apply more to the lungs than the large intestine and need further clarification with diagnosis. Large intestine *internal heat* results in spasm, urgency, and pain with bowel movements, possibly containing blood or thick mucus.

Signs of imbalance in Metal show up in the mouth. The mouth, especially when we include the tongue, is one of those areas of the body where we can view the health or imbalance of the entire person. If the mouth is dry, it could mean lungs and throat need moisturizing herbs. Bleeding gums, another sign of inflammation, are associated with excess heat in the large intestine organ system.

Inflammation makes body odors pronounced. The so-called rotten odor, an indication of imbalance in Metal, can apply to body odor but also to smoker's breath. Smoking is heating and drying enough to damage the lungs. Herbal bad-breath remedies such as aloe vera refresh the throat, lungs, and stomach.

Metal and internal cold

Internal cold symptoms for Metal would include all those involving watery phlegm, oozing sores, heavy congestion, fatigue from shortness of breath, and related depression. Those discomforts apply mostly to the lungs, but *internal cold* can also affect the large intestine, resulting in watery diarrhea and weakness.

Grief is an important sign of *internal cold* affecting lungs and adrenal glands. It is the associated emotion indicating trouble in the Metal element. Another way of looking at it is that grief makes it harder for us to breathe. Grief is what we "hold in" our chest or gut. Certain natural remedies that dry thick phlegm, such as homeopathic ignatia amara, 30c, also have a beneficial effect upon worry and grief.

The white color is associated with problems in Metal because very white skin or phlegm is a sign of weakness from *internal cold* or deficiency. Racial heritage does not matter with Asian diagnosis. People with darker skin tones will also experience paleness as one of the signs of extreme imbalance in Metal.

Metal and dryness

Dryness is said to damage the Metal element, although a reasonable amount is healthy. *Dryness* can be external or internal. One cure for asthma used to be moving to Arizona. But that worked best for people with *internal cold* affecting the lungs. Hot and dry is not always better.

Prudent use of pungent (*heating* and *drying*) foods and spices stimulates digestion and detoxification while clearing phlegm, whereas an excessively spicy diet and cigarettes are damaging. *Dryness*, for persons who are already dry, damages sensitive lung tissue so that we absorb less oxygen with each breath. *Dryness* of the large intestine is often a chronic problem for older people, leading to constipation or bloating. The appropriate remedy would be strengthening and moistening herbs, such as a tea made by boiling apricot kernels.

Metal and foods

A dry cough shows *heat,* whereas a wet, wheezing cough is symptomatic of *internal cold.* To correct *dryness,* rice, a moistening, *cooling* grain, is recommended. For excess phlegm, a *drying* grain such as barley is useful. Herbal remedies for breathing problems and excess phlegm will be covered in chapter 30.

THE WATER ELEMENT

Nature Hot: hyperkinetic energy and sexual drive, urinary urgency, paranoia
Cold: weakness, impotence, low immune strength, poor memory
Location kidney, bladder, back, legs, hormones, brain
Origin *cold,* stress, illness, stimulants, jet lag, drugs
Color blue or black
Taste salty

water

The Water element is made up of a complex organ system including the kidney, urinary bladder, and adrenal glands and those aspects of our nervous system affected by them, the pituitary and certain brain functions such as hormone balance, memory, and concentration. Here is an area where further study by Western medicine could show how brain chemicals affecting emotions and body are related. A few Western doctors who research communication in the cells are finally admitting that mind and body are somehow linked mysteriously by way of emotions.

According to TCM, the deepest, most fundamental source of *chi* and immune strength is the Water element. When, in later chapters, we study fatigue, mental clarity, depression, and immune-threatening disease, it will be useful to remember that the vital energy as well as both *yin* and *yang* (fluids and functioning) of the Water element affects the entire body.

The Chinese classic texts say *cold* damages the kidneys. Cold weather or excessive intake of cold or raw foods reduces *chi.* Mental and physical exhaustion, jet lag, or overuse of stimulants also damages the Water element. Stimulants, including coffee and cocaine, can be temporarily *heating,* but become so draining that they leave us utterly spent and feeling cold. Chinese medicine also considers excessive or unwise sexual activity exhausting. The ancients recommended special sexual practices and herbs to overcome fatigue and weakness. We will cover them in a later chapter.

Water and internal heat

An *internal heat* condition affecting the kidneys leads to sparse, dark-colored urine and urinary urgency. But few people complain of it. Neither do they complain of *internal heat* affecting the adrenal glands, with excess sexual excitement and insomnia. The most frequently discussed Water element problems concern *internal cold*.

Water and internal cold

Symptoms of low *chi* or *internal cold* of the kidneys are not only urinary, with frequent urination, but can be as diverse as fatigue, poor memory, premature senility, lumbago, and low sexual energy and drive, as well as poor immune strength. That is because the "kidneys," as defined by Chinese medicine, comprise a complex organ system including the adrenal glands and brain.

According to the law of Correspondences, black is the color most associated with weakness in Water. Accordingly, facial symptoms of *internal cold* or *stagnation* are dark circles under the eyes and a grayish tone to the skin. Groaning is the sound we make when we feel dead tired. Some people with chronic adrenal fatigue drink lots of coffee and speak in groans and whispers.

The symptoms of illness that I included in the Correspondences chart are all those of *internal cold:* mental exhaustion, poor concentration and memory, lower-back pain, fragile bones, fractures, urinary incontinence and infections, sexual weakness, infertility, and hair loss, to name a few.

Water and foods

Peas and beans were recommended in ancient times to treat weakness in Water, probably because they physically resemble kidneys. Doctors then thought that foods found in nature that looked like internal organs should be used to cure them. It was called the "doctrine of signatures." We now know beans are a good source of protein, fat, and starch. Good nourishment and rest are necessary, as much as herbs, to heal the Water element.

The Generation Cycle

The Generation Cycle is a metaphoric explanation used by the ancients wherein the Five Elements are connected, with each strengthening the next: Wood builds Fire, which strengthens Earth, which strengthens Metal, which strengthens Water, which strengthens Wood. When one part of the body is weakened, the rest suffers.

There is a fine-tuned balance, like a dance, in the workings of body/mind/spirit. Some early Chinese anatomy charts place the Earth element in the center, with the others arrayed around it in a circle. In order for chi to be adequate and smooth-flowing, in order for blood production to be adequate, our Five Elements turn around each other in a circle, each lending energy to the next. Try the following exercise to visualize your balance.

A Meditation to Balance the Five Elements

Sit in a relaxed manner, breathing deeply and slowly. Imagine a slow dance revolving in your center: Your chest is relaxed, then your left side, your left lung, and the left side of the intestine relax. Then relax the lower abdomen, the right side, the right side of the intestine, and the right lung. Relax all the way through to the back. Breathe slowly and deeply, making no noise. Put your hands at the navel and relax there. Send your breath downward from your head to your feet. Imagine the elements joining hands and turning in the circle while you relax.

Is there an area of resistance? Of pain or tension? Are there emotions coming to the surface as you pass by an area? The areas of *internal heat* will feel tight or sharp; the areas of *internal cold* will feel heavy or empty. *Stagnant chi* will feel stuck.

When you experience your imbalance, you can dissolve it with foods, herbs, or meditation. To become more aware of *heat*, *cold*, and *stagnation*, ask yourself the types of questions found in the Five Elements questionnaire. Using the Correspondences, try to see, hear, and smell stuck *chi*, areas of blockage or resistance. Or try to sense *internal heat* and *cold* more directly with sensory meditation, as we did above. It all works.

Do not be misled: Modern diagnosis may be exact, but it is not always better. Ancient methods have great value because they bring us into a communion of all aspects of body and mind, from the coarsest to the most subtle. Correct use of herbs based on self-knowledge is more effective than knowing how herbs are used traditionally or in laboratory studies. For one thing, a scientific approach describes a process that can always be repeated. Can the phenomenon of you, yourself, in this instant of time and place, be forever repeated?

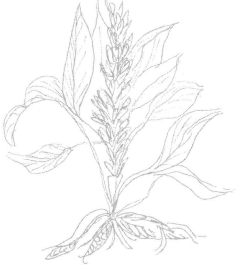

Turmeric

10
Diagnostic Shorthand Methods

You may not wish to go through a complicated rigmarole to begin observing your *chi*, so I'll offer a couple of shorthand methods to get you started. They require no special skill, and can be fun to use.

These observations have another application as well: Since the following techniques are based on the Correspondences and Five Element theory, they elaborate energetic tendencies, i.e., our usual reactions. As such, they have predictive power. It is generally accepted by Asian medicine that a good doctor prevents future disease. If we could really predict the future, we'd be able to forecast our soundness with the accuracy of a Wall Street average. But the tendencies of our energy are actually easier to find, and are a more certain indicator of our future health than any statistical probabilities based on random samples. That is because by now we know our usual reactions to stress. The shorthand methods covered in this chapter only help to make sense of them.

Physical Karma

When I meet someone for the first time professionally, he or she arrives loaded with health complaints. I have to decide which one to treat first. A glance at the person's hands, facial hue, or figure can give me an indication of the kinds of problems that might be considered "constitutional," that is, according to their inherited type. Often this becomes background information I use intuitively to reach a diagnosis. Such observations, culled from the Correspondences, cannot give me specific information on a person's illness, but more an understanding of their health tendencies or of what I call Physical Karma.

Physical Karma illuminates a person's present health circumstances and possible future illnesses. It involves no moral judgment, such as "good" or "bad" karma, but is the sum of health tendencies stemming from our inherited energy. For example, under stress, do you tend to get angry, nervous, sentimental, or afraid? Do you get diarrhea, a headache, a rash? Do you reach for a cigarette, drugs, or sweets? These tendencies can be ex-

plained and, to some extent, predicted according to our physical and energetic makeup, our Physical Karma. Furthermore, they can be interpreted when seen through the filter of the Correspondences and the Five Elements.

Observing Physical Karma is intuitive, but is based upon traditional Asian diagnosis and experience I have developed during my healing practice. I will explain the method briefly so that you can begin to observe yourself and protect your future good health.

CONSTITUTIONAL TYPES

All traditional Asian medical theories describe constitutional types, indicating possible predispositions toward physical and emotional states. One organizing principle for determining a type is the Five Elements, in which possible types include Fire, Earth, Metal, Water, and Wood. For example, a Fire-type person would be expected to have more problems involving the Fire element.

Another way of looking at Physical Karma is with the concept of *humors*, in which the possibilities are *wind*, *bile*, and *phlegm* types. I introduced these *humors* in the preceding chapter, but they will be illustrated in greater detail here. When Asian doctors refer to a person's body type, it's only part of what is considered their constitution, because our energetic tendencies involve more than our body. Some people believe it is ultimately our energy that gives shape to the body. You can use the following shorthand methods to observe your energy. Choose whichever one resonates best with your interests.

CONSTITUTIONAL TYPES ACCORDING TO THE FIVE ELEMENTS

I call this method a "shorthand" approach because some Asian doctors observe the hands in order to perceive certain health problems. Its origin is the notion of Correspondences. The idea is that a part of the body (usually the hands, nose, ears, or tongue) can represent a microcosm of the whole body. A Chinese herbalist may, for example, inspect your fingernails. They feel that a healthy pink color under the nails indicates adequate blood production and circulation. If the nail has crosswise grooves or ridges, the Chinese doctor may suspect you have weak nails from liver problems leading to poor absorption of calcium. Blood deficiency and poor calcium absorption indicate problems with the Wood element. With this information, the herbalist would continue to clarify the observations, using other methods of diagnosis, and finally make a prescription of herbs to correct the imbalance.

Another variation comes from the work of Dr. Yves Requena, a French endocrinologist, trained in traditional Chinese medicine and ancient palmistry. According to this theory, physical tendencies and personality are given shape by each of the Five Elements. We can determine the constitutional type by observing the shape and markings of hands and fingernails. I modify that approach somewhat, depending upon circumstances; for example, nail polish and false fingernails interfere with the interpretation. I mainly rely on the shape, coloring, and skin texture of the hands.

The shape of the hand is its most outstanding feature. That determines its element. Descriptions and examples are provided for each element.

Internal heat makes the hand feel warm and look dry, red, and scaly. *Internal cold* makes the hand cold and pale. *Dampness* makes the hand feel clammy. And *stagnation* makes the hand look purplish.

When reviewing my drawings, keep in mind that the person with a Fire hand would be expected to have more Fire-related symptoms, the Wood person to have Wood symptoms, and so on. See the questionnaire on Correspondences and the Diagnostic Questionnaire for examples.

A person often comprises more than one constitutional type, according to the Five Elements. We might, for example, have a hand that shows both Earth and Metal elements. It takes some practice to become adept at this form of diagnosis, and it should be combined with other methods. Here are some things I've learned from looking at hands for years.

THE FIRE PERSON

Those people who have a Fire hand tend to have their *chi* centered higher in their body than normal. Their heart and chest

THE FIRE HAND

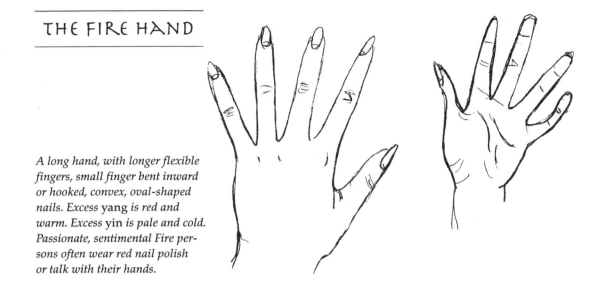

A long hand, with longer flexible fingers, small finger bent inward or hooked, convex, oval-shaped nails. Excess yang *is red and warm. Excess* yin *is pale and cold. Passionate, sentimental Fire persons often wear red nail polish or talk with their hands.*

symptoms (and emotions!) are important. For that reason they can often be hyperactive, anxious, insomniac, or emotionally unstable. Feeling "out of sync" can become their karmic issue. They tend to be very sensitive to their surroundings and relationships; sentimental, they come from the heart. Life can be very painful for them when *chi* becomes stuck in the chest, resulting in chest pains from emotional issues, stimulants, exhaustion, drugs, or medications.

If you are a Fire person, respect your need for rest and recovery from stress. Try to avoid the emotional sabotage caused by others who may ask a great deal from you. Avoid the use of stimulants such as caffeine and overwork. Too much of either of these can make you feel out of touch with yourself or with everybody else. (See chapters 31 and 35.)

THE METAL PERSON

The person with the Metal hand is vulnerable in the lung and large intestine areas. *Chi* can become a problem when it is deficient or stuck. Possible emotional issues for the Metal person are related to breathing and elimination. They may have trouble taking in enough air to feel strong. Some smoke to feel calm or to "put up a smoke screen." Addictions are said to be more common for this type of person than for others. A Metal person's issues involve distance to or from others: Such a person may keep you waiting for a phone call, but react with surprise if you accuse him or her of coldness.

Sometimes Metal persons feel quite at ease when isolated from others. Solitude protects their energy, inspiration, and calm, allowing them to do the spiritual or artistic

THE METAL HAND

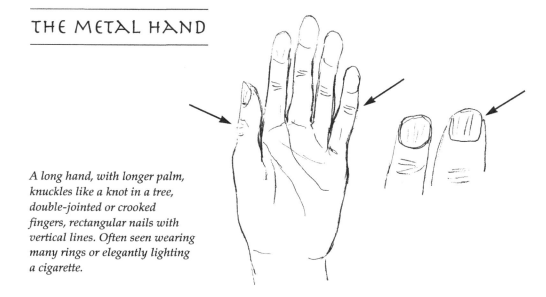

A long hand, with longer palm, knuckles like a knot in a tree, double-jointed or crooked fingers, rectangular nails with vertical lines. Often seen wearing many rings or elegantly lighting a cigarette.

work they love. It's as though they want to take in just enough of the outside, but not too much. Other, less fortunate Metal types may feel the sting of isolation and become antisocial.

Metal types with a large-intestine imbalance will have problems regarding elimination or letting go of the past. Cleansing or weight-loss teas help with constipation. Otherwise, for the Metal person who suffers from stress-related diarrhea, a few drops of gentian extract, taken with water, will often do the trick.

THE EARTH PERSON

Persons with the Earth hand require adequate *chi* in their digestive center. Since their digestive organs, especially stomach, spleen, and pancreas, as well as their blood-sugar balance, are at issue, they may crave

sweets and feel woozy from hunger. They'll reach for sweets or rich foods for comfort, grounding, or energy. Earth and Metal types are those most prone to food addictions. When depressed, they gorge on ice cream or cheese, which can lead to overweight and phlegm, resulting in difficult breathing and tumors. Without a healthy diet and exercise routine, low energy and poor digestion lead the Earth person to heart trouble, diabetes, or hypoglycemia.

Earth types need to feel comfort in their emotional center. This includes home, relationships, and work. They like everything to be smooth and friendly. At their best, they are peacemakers. Untiring, they struggle to bring forth an idea or make a group cohere. At worst, they eat to satisfy the unsatisfiable. Emotional issues for the Earth person involve incorporation. If they love you, they can "eat you up." They crave stability and warmth. They

THE EARTH HAND

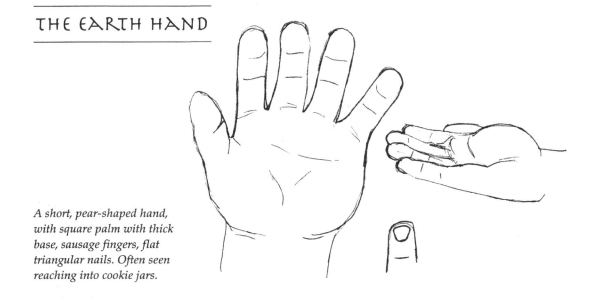

A short, pear-shaped hand, with square palm with thick base, sausage fingers, flat triangular nails. Often seen reaching into cookie jars.

love having congenial family around, especially at feasts. Their karmic issue is rumination. Do they process, worry, and digest their ideas ad nauseam? Or do they get something done?

If you are an Earth type, you should exercise, bend in the middle with sit-ups. I once heard how a Tibetan doctor told a friend of mine to do one thousand prostrations before an image of the Buddha. He slowly went down onto his knees and bowed gently while exhaling until his head reached his meditation pillow. He did this twenty times twice daily, in front of a beautiful painting he'd bought in Asia. By the time he had finished the required number of prostrations, he had lost his stomachaches and extra weight. Exercise will help balance your blood sugar and lift your spirits. It will help bring you into your cen-

ter of balance and well-being. (See chapters 15, 16, and 31.)

THE WOOD PERSON

The person with the Wood hand has many lines on the inside of the fingers and palm. This is not only from dry skin but possibly from poor circulation, and could result in problems with joints or headaches. The *chi* of the Wood person tends to be focused in the liver and gallbladder organ systems, located on the right side of the ribs and in the chest and neck. Allergies, high blood pressure, and headaches are tendencies for Wood with *internal heat*. Poor muscle tone, vision problems, and indecision can indicate *internal cold*. The Wood element motivates movement; with strong muscles and

THE WOOD HAND

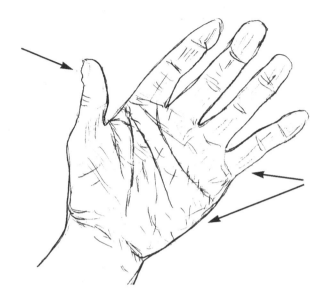

An evenly proportioned size and shape, with many lines on palms and ventral fingers. Excess yang is reddish, dry, with thick grooves and nails. Excess yin is cold, clammy, pale, possibly tingling or numb. Fragile or horizontal grooved nails indicate poor calcium absorption. Nervous or emotional Wood persons often bite their nails.

supple joints we move forward and bend smoothly.

The emotional energy of the Wood element also involves movement. These people hate being stopped, delayed, or frustrated. They love to create, move, dance, and travel. They can be impatient, perfectionistic, and demanding, or inhibited, depending upon the emotional blocks they find or create for themselves. They need to find constructive ways to live their dreams.

If you are a Wood type, try to avoid excessively oily and rich food and drink. The resulting liver pain and nausea inhibits the free flow of *chi* circulation and possibly your tolerance of others. Your karmic issue is power. Movement gives you the capacity to create, but with wise use of your personal strengths you can gain insight and move mountains. As you

develop compassion for others, all doors will open for you and you will move smoothly through life.

THE WATER PERSON

Persons with a Water-type hand often have edema (water retention) in the hands and elsewhere in the body because of weakness and fatigue. Often there is dark skin circling the tops of their fingernails. Their energy and vulnerability are located in the kidney and adrenal area of the lower back. Fatigue for them can be crushing. It can feel like a heavy weight pulling them downward at the waistline. They may feel demoralized or hopeless when exhausted. They may descend to self-pity or find it hard to move at all.

THE WATER HAND

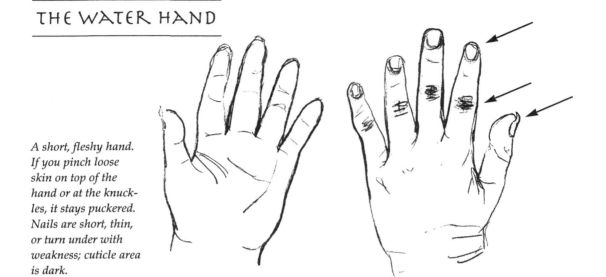

A short, fleshy hand. If you pinch loose skin on top of the hand or at the knuckles, it stays puckered. Nails are short, thin, or turn under with weakness; cuticle area is dark.

When *chi* is in excess in the Water element, Water persons may feel overly courageous and daring, or, alternatively, claustrophobic and paranoid. Their karmic issue then becomes the need to develop steady, smooth energy. That gives them a sense of stability that helps them to overcome fear. Often, Water types tend to work hard enough to blow a fuse, then remain exhausted for a long time. Adrenal exhaustion can lead to mental fuzziness, poor memory, sexual problems, low immune strength, and global overweight. (See chapter 15.)

When problems in the Water element are long-term, we should address both the *yin* (urinary function) and *yang* (energy function) of the kidney and adrenal glands. We will cover one such herbal remedy, called **Sexoton,** in chapter 31.

COMBINATIONS

Our energy always involves more than one element. For that reason we are often made up of more than one type. It's fun to conjecture what certain combinations might produce. For example, a combination of Wood and Metal might read, "I'd rather do it perfectly myself!" Metal and Fire might produce the statement, "Things get emotional in my ivory tower!" Fire and Wood: "If I don't get my way, I'll scream!" or "I have to work out every last detail to the letter or I get upset."

Earth and Wood might say, "If we don't make peace, I'll get very angry!" Whereas Earth and Water might ask, "We're all one big happy family, aren't we?"

You'll feel like a gypsy, looking at hands. People will be amazed at your accuracy in discovering personal matters. How-ever, specific illnesses are hard to diagnose by observing hands because the body is more complicated than the types imply. Tongue and pulse diagnosis are used to confirm what we intuit in this way.

It is important also to determine the cause of an imbalance, not just the tendency toward it. In addition, hand diagnosis is inexact because so many of us live under constant stress from pollution, fatigue, or medications that our adrenal glands and immune strength may be threatened whether we have a Water constitutional type or not. Many of us live big-city lives where we tend to eat richly at late hours. Our digestion suffers whether we have an Earth hand or not.

Therefore, the best use of the Five Element constitutional types is to determine your relative health: How is your *chi* doing in terms of your type? In other words, for the Earth person, the following questions should be considered: How is your digestion? Is your vitality impaired by indigestion or pain? Do you crave sweets excessively? Are there indications of blood-sugar imbalances? Is your problem chronic or acute?

Then you have to decide which Earth problems to take care of first. For example, what is more troublesome—bloating from indigestion, or an ungrounded feeling from being "off center"? This kind of observation method may help you get in touch with feelings you did not know you had. Perhaps you did not link chronic indigestion with relationship problems, or

fear with fatigue. Many times, herbal combination remedies treat mind and body problems at once. We shall study many such herbal pills in Parts Four and Five.

The Humors

Another way of observing your constitutional type is with the *humors—wind, bile,* and *phlegm*. This triumvirate is generally accepted by all Asian medical traditions. European medical schools taught four *humors* until the turn of the century: blood, two kinds of bile, and phlegm. A person was said to be "phlegmatic" if there was an abundance of phlegm, or "bilious" if there were problems with the liver.

The *humors,* which pervade all aspects of body, mind, and spirit, can be perceived not only by examining constitutional type but also through other methods of diagnosis such as pulse reading, urine analysis, and questioning. *Wind* is described as quick, cold, light, and dry. It makes communication and change possible. *Bile* is warm and oily. It makes digestion, thought, and memory possible. *Phlegm* is heavy, bland, and sticky. It makes moisture and rest possible.

The character of each *humor* determines the problems inherent to each constitutional type. A healthy *wind* person will have fast energy and a lot of ideas. But *wind* stimulation can go too far. For example, the *wind* type can be remarkably thin and nervous, because its main feature is *wind* energy. A sickly *wind*-type person experiences more nervous sensitivity or nerve exhaustion. In that sense, a modern equivalent for *wind* energy may be the nervous system.

A healthy *bile*-type person has a strong and muscular body with good digestion and a sharp memory. But a tendency to *heat* symptoms from stuck liver *chi* (and stuck bile) can develop. This leads to all sorts of inflammation problems, from rashes to insomnia to rage.

The *phlegm*-type person tends to have slow digestion, with excess congestion. This could lead to asthma, overweight, or cloudy thinking.

THE TRADITIONAL ASIAN VIEW OF *HUMORS*

The ancients used the *humors* to predict everything from physical health to social behavior and life span (also see chapter 37).

Phlegm types are described as having more body fat, thick skin, and oily hair; they sleep soundly and have long memories. Tibetan doctors go so far as to say *phlegm* types are more patient and live longer. They are also supposed to be more greedy and rich.

Bile types can be "bilious," that is, jaundiced, angry, or frustrated. The *bile* person is described as having angular features, reddish hair, a strong physique, good digestion, a gregarious, aggressive personality, and good memory. Tibetan doctors have said that *bile* persons normally "live lives of normal or medium length with moderate wealth."

Wind persons are described as nervous, dark-skinned, curly-haired, thin, and tired. They tend to have more circulation problems and pains all over the body. They shiver and yawn a lot. They have flatulence from poor digestion. Their limbs are stiff from nerve-related problems and poor circulation. According to Tibetan doctors, problems of *wind* or "air" make people "vomit and be short-tempered." Also according to them, *wind* types love music, spend money extravagantly on luxuries, and live shorter lives than the other types, presumably having a good time while doing so.

We have to take this kind of information with a grain of salt—or soy sauce, if you prefer. It's not meant to be prescriptive, only descriptive, and its origins are in a particular time and place. In real life, nothing is static. The types change as easily as our *humors*. That, in fact, is one great benefit in observing them: We can affect the balance of our *humors* with diet and herbs because they are so changeable.

With that in mind, please observe your *humors* by filling out the following questionnaire. Although it's my invention, it illustrates traditional Asian concepts.

Note whether you marked more items for one or two types. That indicates the importance of those *humors* when observing your health. Which ones are at work for you now? Humoral imbalances occur periodically from changes in season, stress, or diet. But for chronic problems related to *humors*, healing foods, herbs, and lifestyle changes are very convenient.

Constitutional Type Questionnaire: Three Humors

MY FIGURE LOOKS LIKE THIS
(mark one):

1.   2.   3.

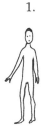 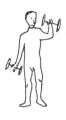

Wind   Bile   Phlegm

1. __ thin or quite variable
2. __ angular, strong
3. __ ample

HAIR

1. __ very fine
2. __ thinning
3. __ thick

SKIN

1. __ transparent
2. __ reddish
3. __ oily

ENERGY

1. __ fast, nervous
2. __ hard-driving
3. __ steady

DIGESTION

1. __ difficult or variable
2. __ effortless
3. __ slow

MOODS

1. __ quite variable (mood swings)
2. __ I don't notice
3. __ stable (moderated)

EMOTIONS

1. __ often depressed
2. __ often angry or frustrated
3. __ often sleepy

SLEEP PATTERNS

1. __ light
2. __ not very much
3. __ deep

DREAMS

1. __ I fly or climb
2. __ sexy or nightmares
3. __ I don't dream

FRIENDSHIPS

1. __ many, brief
2. __ intense
3. __ deep, long

WEATHER PREFERENCE

1. __ I love the heat
2. __ I avoid heat
3. __ I avoid rain or humidity

TOTALS: 1. ___ WIND
2. ___ BILE
3. ___ PHLEGM

REMEDIES FOR THE *HUMOR* BODY TYPES

In chapter 13 we will observe a healing routine that can bring each of the three *humors* into balance. For *wind* problems, the appropriate remedy would be *warming, grounding, nourishing* foods. Herbs would have qualities that balance the overly dry, light quality of *wind.* They would therefore be heavy, *warming,* and oily, and have the appropriate pungent and sweet tastes and sedating effects.

For *bile* problems, the appropriate diet and herbs aim to reduce excess acid and inflammation. The remedies would be bitter, sour, and *cooling.*

For *phlegm* problems, antimucus foods and *warming,* drying herbs are recommended, as well as sweating, which reduce phlegm. We shall study these types of treatments throughout the rest of the book in order to cleanse and balance the *humors.*

THINGS TO CONSIDER WHEN OBSERVING *HUMORS*

Referring exclusively to constitutional types as defined by tradition can be misleading. We each have all the *humors* and energetic tendencies in varying degrees, which makes it hard to recognize exactly what types we are at a given time.

Also, we need an update. The types were determined in antiquity, when it was expected that people would stay more or less the same through their entire lives. Is the person who gets a curly permanent

suddenly no longer a *phlegm* type, but a *wind* type? We can rather easily change our appearance. This might lead a curious health professional to ask, "What would you look like if you had not colored your hair, had plastic surgery, and remodeled your body at the gym?"

We must also recognize what is more important: apparent constitutional type or the actual cause of the problem. Even though you use type analysis, you will still have to judge which problems are more painful or important for you to treat at a given time, then take appropriate remedies.

CONSTITUTIONAL TYPES AND SEASONAL IMBALANCES

I think the best use of constitutional types is in preventing future problems. This can be done by using an important aspect of the Correspondences and Five Element theory: illness according to the seasons. Each of the elements has its associated season. That element is most vulnerable during that time of year and under its related weather conditions. Spring brings wind; summer is hot; Indian summer (late summer) is humid and mild; autumn is cool and dry; while winter is cold. Particular symptoms associated with the Five Elements will surface at that time.

The following chart provides a brief summary. It shows the Five Elements along with their associated seasons and *internal heat* and *internal cold* imbalances, with a possible remedy for each. Like all the charts in this book, it is not written in stone; you'll be able to expand it as you read later chapters.

The Aim of Diagnosis

Shorthand methods of observation may seem like "quackno-tech," but they can and should be confirmed with the best sources of information available. Asian diagnosis may be inexact, but it can make you more sensitive. With a little practice, you'll be able to intuit who among your friends seems slow and heavy from excess *phlegm*; hot and irritable from stuck *bile*; or nervous and scattered from exhaustion and excess *wind*. You will have become sensitive to the movements of *chi*.

CONSTITUTIONAL TYPES AND SEASONAL REMEDIES

ELEMENT	SEASON	PROBLEM	REMEDY
WOOD	spring	Hot: headache, rash Cold: indigestion	aloe, dandelion ginger
FIRE	summer	Hot: heatstroke Cold: weak heart	chrysanthemum flower tea hawthorn
EARTH	Indian summer	Hot: ulcer Cold: nausea	aloe, cumin ginger
METAL	autumn	Hot: cough, thirst Cold: shortness of breath	**Lo Han Kuo Beverage** thyme, clove
WATER	winter	Hot: sparse urine Cold: frequent clear urine	saw palmetto, parsley clove

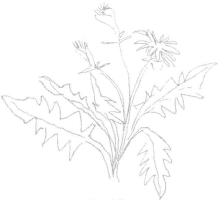

Dandelion

11
Your Tongue and You

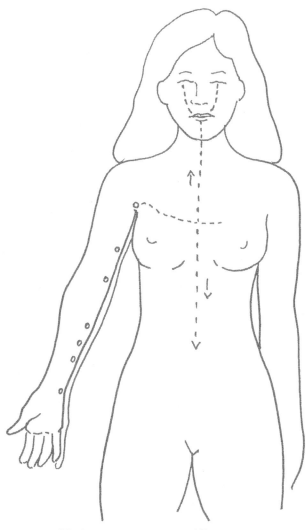

The heart acupuncture meridian

Your tongue is a window to your metabolism. It's the only internal organ you can see directly. Its color, shape, and mobility indicate vital energy and blood production, which affects your ability to digest food, breathe, eliminate toxins, and fight illness. Your metabolism points the way to your future health.

How to Read Your Tongue

Observing your tongue in a mirror can greatly influence your choice of herbs. In the following experiment, I'll ask you to eat several foods in order to illustrate the changes they produce on the tongue. We will observe it for three days, morning and evening.

The best time to observe your tongue is upon rising, before you have eaten, but you can get an even better idea of how your *chi* is doing by observing your tongue again during the day. Try to observe the tongue in adequate, but not direct, sunlight. Relax the tongue to avoid extra tension that changes its shape. Just let it hang out flat, noting its color, shape, and texture. It will help to draw and describe your tongue.

When observing the color, notice the body of the tongue itself, ignoring any coating. Its color may range from very pale —nearly white—to bright red or reddish purple. The body of the tongue shows longer-standing conditions, whereas the coating varies with daily digestion. The coating can range from watery and clear to thick and yellowish or even darker.

The shape of the tongue can be rounded or oblong, regular or irregular. Its texture also varies quite a bit, from rough and bumpy to smooth. Note every detail, including the location of grooves, marks, dots, shiny areas, or cracks. Everyone's tongue is unique. Our health constantly goes in and out of balance to varying degrees. The person who is ill remains out of balance longer and to a greater degree than the healthy person.

A healthy tongue looks not remarkably different from healthy flesh: It is neither waterlogged nor burned in appearance. The tongue should be moist and pink, with no unusual markings except perhaps a thin white coating resulting from a healthy meal being digested. In other words, the tongue shows no signs of *internal heat* or *internal cold*. But the tongue of a sick person is easy to spot, varying greatly from what we expect as the norm.

The coating of the tongue shows temporary acid or alkaline conditions from digestion. Whitish or clear phlegm can indicate excessively alkaline conditions (*internal cold*), and thick yellow or brown phlegm shows excess acid (*internal heat*). To better discern a healthy tongue, let's study the deviants from the norm.

INTERNAL HEAT CONDITIONS: A red, dry tongue.

If the entire tongue is red, indicating a state of *internal heat* from excess acid, dehydration, inflammation, or infection, this *heat* will likely appear as symptoms in other areas. Some of us are already overheated or dehydrated from stimulants, smoking, blood or fluid loss, and illness. Additional use of *heating* stimulants, foods and herbs, exacerbates the imbalance.

Drinking large amounts of water will not correct this condition because the metabolism is too fast, which leads to dehydration. Instead, use *cooling*, moisturizing herbs and foods. Some of these may slow metabolism or increase retention of water or blood in the organs themselves. This kind of remedy applies to both adults and

Observation of the Tongue

DAY ONE

Morning observation   Late afternoon
Draw and describe   Draw and describe

Relax the tongue. Is it long or narrow? Wide or puffy? Does it have grooves at the sides where your teeth have been? Is the tongue itself pale or white? pink? reddish? purplish?

Does the color or shape change somehow in the afternoon? Make a note of your level of energy or fatigue as you observe the tongue in the afternoon.

DAY TWO

Morning observation   Evening
Draw and describe   Draw and describe

Is the tongue the same color as the previous day? For the morning observation, note what you had for the previous dinner and before bed. Is there a coating on the tongue? Is it white, gray, yellow, black? Is the coating thick or thin? Do you have lots of saliva or a dry mouth?

In the evening, eat hot, salty, or spicy food or popcorn, then note the tongue. How did it change? Often its coating will change after you eat. Coatings correspond to the acid-alkaline balance in the digestive tract, which can change quickly.

DAY THREE

Morning observation   Before bed
Draw and describe   Draw and describe

Note the color and coating of the tongue. Are there any other marks such as spots, grooves, bumps, cracks? Where are they located? Before bed, eat a bowl of steamed fresh greens, such as dandelion, spinach, or kale, without other seasoning. Drink the cooking juices. Is it soothing and relaxing? Does it change your tongue the next morning?

---

children. If your child has a red tongue and is fussy or insomniac, giving him pepper or garlic could make him more "overheated."

The coating of the tongue can range from thick white to yellow. It can represent a temporary condition caused by spicy or acid-producing food, or a chronic condition if you notice it for more than a day. A thick white or gray coating indicates excess *phlegm*, but a yellow coating indicates excess acid. Most often in *internal heat* conditions with a reddish tongue, we see a yellow coating. The total absence of coating—a bald, shiny tongue—also indicates serious internal dehydration. A black-coated tongue indicates dehydration or disease conditions.

The following chart will help you to understand *internal heat conditions* as observed on the tongue. The color refers to the body of the tongue itself, and indicates the chronic condition of blood and energy production. Moving left to right, from a normal pink tongue to greater dehydration, the tongue gets more and more red.

TONGUES INDICATING *INTERNAL HEAT*

TONGUE COLOR AND COATING

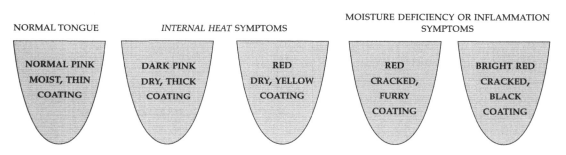

NORMAL TONGUE	*INTERNAL HEAT* SYMPTOMS		MOISTURE DEFICIENCY OR INFLAMMATION SYMPTOMS	
NORMAL PINK MOIST, THIN COATING	DARK PINK DRY, THICK COATING	RED DRY, YELLOW COATING	RED CRACKED, FURRY COATING	BRIGHT RED CRACKED, BLACK COATING

A DRY RED TONGUE: THINK *COOLING*, MOISTENING HERBS

If you have a dry, red tongue, *heating* herbs, such as ginger, Chinese ginseng, or echinacea, would cause further inflammation. Chinese banlangen (in Latin, *isatis;* in English, wild indigo), honeysuckle flower, or other *cooling* antibiotics should be used as needed instead of echinacea. This is because moisturizing, *cooling* herbs and foods are required to balance your metabolism.

The choice of moistening, blood-building, or anti-inflammatory antibiotic herbs varies according to the illness. But in each case you must monitor the changes in your tongue to determine the correct herbs, according to their type and temperature. Ignoring Asian tongue diagnosis leads to trouble. By ignoring imbalances in metabolism, we interfere with the body's ability to heal itself. By analyzing the tongue, as well as other signs and symptoms, while taking an herbal remedy, we can monitor our progress and correct our individual dosage.

INTERNAL COLD **CONDITIONS:** A large, pale tongue.

The tongue that shows *internal cold* is pale and often larger than normal. It might have indentations around the edges left by the teeth. It is often a big, pale gray tongue that indicates weakness, the result of chronic fatigue, overwork, illness, blood loss, or an excessively alkaline condition leading to weak internal organs.

Below is a chart that shows *internal cold* symptoms as expressed on the tongue. The color of the tongue itself—pink, very pale, or white—shows chronic weakness of the digestive tract and also, indirectly, of *chi* and blood production. The tongue's paleness may also result from a long-term *cooling* diet or other causes of *internal cold.* The grooves left by teeth around the tongue indicate weak *chi.* Internal organs are not working well to maintain vitality.

A generation ago, Western doctors linked a pale, waterlogged tongue to chronic kidney or heart weakness or low vitality of the aged, with deficient blood quality and poor circulation.

A thin white or watery coating can result from cold, raw, or alkaline-producing foods, but causes can be as varied as humid weather conditions and parasites. Excess saliva could lead to nausea after eating rich food. A thick coating, white or yellow, can also indicate excess phlegm in the digestive tract, often leading to pain or indigestion.

Stagnation can occur when our energy is either too fast or too slow to flow smoothly; then our organs do not work well. Ayurvedic doctors say spots on the tongue indicate toxins. This makes sense when we realize that irregular metabolism leads to waste buildup. The spots show poor circulation of *chi.* Aside from indigestion, the spots might indicate some other interruption of *chi* and blood circulation, such as tumors or stones. With proper use of medicinal herbs, even those kinds of energy *stagnation* can be improved.

A PALE TONGUE: THINK *WARMING* HERBS

If you have a pale tongue, digestion can be slow and difficult. Vital energy (*chi*) may be low, leading to shallow breath, fatigue, poor concentration, and depression. A swollen, pale tongue indicates slow metabolism. *Warming* stimulant herbs could

TONGUES INDICATING *INTERNAL COLD* AND *STAGNATION*

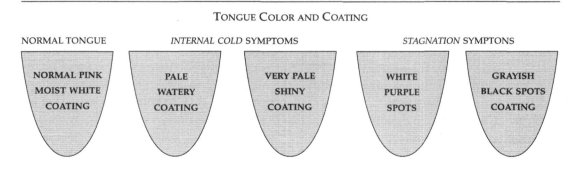

TONGUE COLOR AND COATING

NORMAL TONGUE	INTERNAL COLD SYMPTOMS		STAGNATION SYMPTONS	
NORMAL PINK MOIST WHITE COATING	PALE WATERY COATING	VERY PALE SHINY COATING	WHITE PURPLE SPOTS	GRAYISH BLACK SPOTS COATING

Here the tongue is divided into three parts—the root, center, and tip—each third corresponding to several internal organs. Markings on the surface indicate internal imbalances.

Internal heat—a red, dry, or cracked tongue.

Heat dampness—a thick or yellow coating.

Internal cold—a pale or white tongue, with lots of saliva.

Cold dampness—a white or gray coating.

Stagnation—red, purple, or black spots; also a green or brown coating.

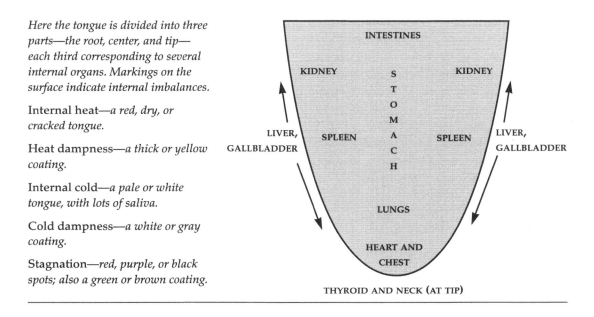

INTESTINES

KIDNEY   S   KIDNEY

LIVER,   T
GALLBLADDER SPLEEN O SPLEEN LIVER,
      M   GALLBLADDER
      A
      C
      H

LUNGS

HEART AND CHEST

THYROID AND NECK (AT TIP)

improve not only digestion but vitality. (See chapters 31 and 34 and the Spice Remedies chart on pages 66 and 67 for *warming* herbs.)

How to Use Tongue Analysis

Both improvements and problems will show up on the tongue. Did you notice that your tongue changed color after you ate popcorn? It's very drying; many people's tongues will become dry and red after eating it. In order to check the progress you are making with any health regimen, periodically examine your tongue.

If you do not know the temperature of a food or herb, eat it for a day and watch your tongue change. People sometimes ask me how many herbal pills to take, or for

how long. I tell them they can find the answer by looking at their tongues.

Parts of the Tongue

Various parts of the tongue correspond to parts of the body. The tongue in the chart above is divided into three main parts: tip, middle, and back. Within these regions are areas corresponding to internal organs.

THE ROOT
Kidneys, adrenal glands, intestines

The part of the tongue closest to the throat, which I'm calling the root, corresponds to the lower body, including the kidney/ adrenal organ functions at the sides and intestines at the center. A thick coating at the center of that area is a likely sign of food being processed in the colon. It indicates a problem for the colon when the coating is very thick and dark-colored or completely absent. The rest of the tongue may be healthy pink, but if the root always has a thick coating, it corresponds to congestion, *dampness,* or other *stagnant* energy, leading to chronic diarrhea or constipation.

THE CENTER

Stomach, spleen/pancreas, lungs

This area is important to notice for digestive problems. The center and sides of the tongue correspond to the organs responsible for digestion: stomach, spleen, and pancreas in the middle, and liver and gallbladder at the sides (see chapter 14). The stomach area of the tongue corresponds to the line from the back of the tongue through the center. In excess acid conditions, such as ulcers, this line can appear dark red, dry, or cracked. Stomach ulcers appear as a burned area in this line along the center of the tongue.

The spleen and pancreas are considered to have a combined digestive function. If digestion is weak, the result is excess fat and cellulite, also a "fat" or waterlogged tongue.

The area between the center and the tip of the tongue corresponds to the lungs. It will appear dry and cracked for smokers or for people who suffer from dry cough and emphysema. Dryness and cracking of

the tongue here show dehydration and possible tissue damage.

THE SIDES

Liver, gallbladder

The areas corresponding to the liver and gallbladder are the edges at both sides of the tongue. Sometimes this area can be red, gray, dotted, or cracked, showing liver damage from *internal heat.* Deficiency of liver shows up as a symptom of weak *chi*— i.e., scalloped edges around the edge of the tongue. If toxins in the liver and blood are significant, inside the body of the tongue will appear dark-colored. Chinese doctors refer to that condition as "fire toxins affecting the blood."

Chi stagnation looks purplish. It can affect the sides or the entire tongue. This is because the liver produces enzymes that make calcium absorption possible. With adequate calcium, the heart can work smoothly. But if circulation of *chi* is poor, healthy blood will not reach the tongue. Thus, blue or purplish signs on the mouth and tongue indicate blood *stagnation.*

THE TIP

The heart and thyroid

The tip of the tongue corresponds to the heart area. Sometimes congestive heart problems or heart weakness can show up here as a crack at the tip, but confirmation by a health specialist is necessary. If other symptoms, such as chest pain or numbness in the arms, are present, there is a possibility of circulation problems in the heart area.

We cannot easily tell by looking at the tongue whether problems are chronic or temporary, although chronic fatigue is usually associated with a large, pale tongue. The entire tongue is pale because chronic adrenal fatigue is associated with chronic heart weakness and low *chi.* In other words, chronic fatigue is not limited to only one area of the body. Chronic fatigue may be associated with slow metabolism, illness, or weakness.

On the other hand, chronic global inflammation from infection or dehydration is seen as a dry and cracked red tongue. The entire tongue may be affected, or just the areas that correspond to inflamed internal organs. I once observed the tongue of a man who was later diagnosed with thyroid cancer. He was overweight with an excess *phlegm* condition affecting the entire body. His large tongue was coated with gray mucus, but at the very tip was a protruding red bulb, indicating severe inflammation at the thyroid.

ANYONE FOR TONGUES?

There are a number of fine Chinese tongue diagnosis texts available in English translation, including one from Beijing, by Professor Song Tian Bin, that has more than two hundred color photos of diseased tongues. Arg! Meant for the Chinese health practitioner, it contains technical medical termi-

nology. Most interesting is its comparison of tongue types used in Chinese medical diagnosis with corresponding diseases according to Western diagnosis. Thirty-seven different examples of pale tongues are provided, with corresponding illnesses such as anemia, malnutrition, chronic kidney weakness, cardiac deficiency, pulmonary heart disease, asthma, leukemia, and arteriosclerosis. Of the ninety-six examples of the "pale red tongue," many different kinds of coatings are illustrated, including "thin, white, and shiny," "fatty," "soya cheese," or "yellow, sticky, fatty," and so on. The corresponding "damp heat" illnesses range from chronic gastritis to ulcers, chronic inflammation of the gallbladder, hepatitis, herpes, serious infections, nephritis, and hypertension. The forty-six "red tongues" are even more serious. From the "red shrunken gleaming tongue" to the "red tongue with black coating," we have everything from cerebrovascular disorders, cirrhosis and liver cancer, infections, rheumatoid arthritis, to allergic reactions to medications. Then, just when we think the tongue can't look any worse, the book goes on to scarlet and bluish mauve tongues.

For our purposes, all we have to recognize is the difference between a red, dry, or yellow-coated tongue and a pale, wet tongue. The first kind corresponds to *internal heat* conditions, the second to *internal cold.* By observing your tongue, you can avoid making the condition worse. You can judge how well an herbal regimen is working, and how long to pursue a given treatment.

INTERNAL HEAT AND *COLD* ON THE TONGUE

ORGAN (Element)	AREA OF TONGUE	*INTERNAL HEAT*	*INTERNAL COLD*
TONGUE		red, dry, cracked; thick dark coating	pale, scalloped; excessive saliva
HEART (Fire)	tip	palpitation fast heartbeat excitement	slow heartbeat low energy depression stuttering
LUNGS (Metal)	near tip	dry cough thirst laryngitis anxiety	phlegmy cough shortness of breath low energy depression
STOMACH (Earth)	center	ulcer burning excessive hunger mania	excessive mucus slow digestion hypoglycemia overweight
SPLEEN (Earth)	center	craves sweet obsessive thoughts	no appetite diarrhea whining
LIVER (Wood)	sides	insomnia anger red eyes headache allergies high sex desire menstrual pain	nervousness indecision poor muscle tone greenish skin low enthusiasm anemia
KIDNEY (Water)	root	dark urine sparse urine insomnia high sex desire	clear urine frequent urine insomnia weak sex desire and strength amenorrhea depression poor concentration exhaustion low immunity
INTESTINE (Metal)	root	burning diarrhea frequent urge pain, spasm	watery diarrhea with exhaustion pain better with massage

CORRESPONDING INTERNAL SYMPTOMS

Internal heat and *cold* conditions (the acid/alkaline balance) may vary in different areas of the body. The chart shown opposite summarizes this, showing which internal organ is affected, and the corresponding area of the tongue. For a more personal comparison, check your responses to the Diagnostic Questionnaire (chapter 8, pages 76–79). Do those conditions apply to your tongue?

What can we do if *internal heat* and *internal cold* affect the same organ system or energetic group, such as several digestive organs, at once? For example, a person may experience excessive hunger along with slow digestion.

The answer is to use a combination of herbs that treat *stagnation* of the organ systems involved. These are some of Asian medicine's favorite household remedies. **Xiao Yao Wan** (page 36) treats irregular digestion, breathing, and energy all at once. Another remedy, **Curing Pills** (page 341), treats nausea, diarrhea, morning sickness, carsickness, and the common cold by improving *chi* circulation. This is because when the flow of *chi* is smooth, everything improves. Thus, fewer *hot* and *cold* imbalances can occur.

Throughout the rest of this book, we will refer back to Asian tongue diagnosis. The traditional herbal remedies we'll cover are quite varied, depending upon the imbalances, but you'll witness improvements as they apply to your own tongue. In that way, you'll be able to use this form of diagnosis while studying many illnesses.

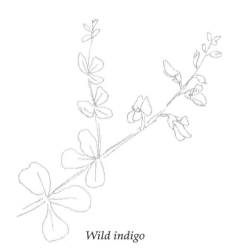

Wild indigo

眞氣眞氣眞氣眞氣眞氣眞氣眞氣眞氣眞氣眞氣眞氣眞氣眞氣眞氣

[zhenqi]

Vitality; genuine energy: the combination of the inborn original vital energy and the acquired energy derived from food and the air, serving as the dynamic force of all vital functions

12
Putting It All Together

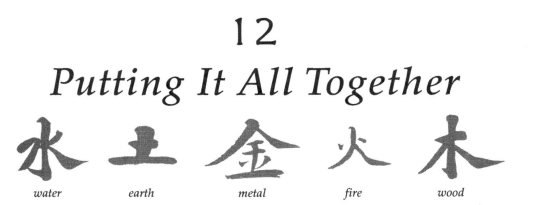

water   earth   metal   fire   wood

After reading the last four chapters on traditional Asian diagnosis, noticing everything from the cracks in your tongue to the color of your sputum, you may be wondering how an Asian practitioner *ever* reaches a diagnosis. The answer is that we deal in minutiae, building a mosaic of signs and symptoms. The trick is to put the observations together and find out where *chi* is trapped. Let's do that now for you.

If you have been a bench-sitter with self-diagnosis thus far, now is the time to fill out the questionnaires in earlier chapters and observe your tongue. Note that if you are experiencing a cold or flu when filling out the questionnaires, that will influence your responses. Since your immune system is fighting infection, many of your answers will seem more *hot*. Take this into consideration and do the questionnaires again at another time, so you can get an idea of how your *chi* functions normally.

In this chapter we'll use the information gathered from previous ones to get a working idea of what's happening with your *chi.* Then, in Parts Three, Four, and Five, we'll apply your diagnostic information to a number of specific health problems you may have.

Most Asian doctors don't believe that you can understand enough about your symptoms to reach a diagnosis, and Western doctors don't care enough about your individual differences, as long as laboratory tests prove a medicine safe. In short, the experts don't trust us to know ourselves. They are both wrong. An herb can be perfectly safe but inappropriate for your problem. If you use an herb based solely on lab test results or traditional usage, or if you choose an herb based upon what you've read about it in herb books, that herb will certainly be ineffective unless your particular symptoms require it. Most people self-medicate every day, knowing nothing about their symptoms. In the previous chapters, you have learned how to observe your symptoms with some care. With practical experience, you'll use herbs with confidence, watching for improvements on your tongue or with your energy, facial color, or other signs from the Correspondences.

How to Begin

In analyzing the array of information you have gathered in your observations, we'll proceed in the order most useful for you. We'll observe your constitutional type first, then create four large categories—*hot, cold, phlegm,* and *stagnation*—to see where your symptoms fit. It is important to realize that they are *not* a picture of your health *forever.* Emotions and physical states vary because *chi* changes constantly.

Please assemble your observations of hands and tongue, and your questionnaire responses. You should have before you the Diagnostic Questionnaire (pages 76–79); The Correspondences Applied to You (pages 92–93); the constitutional type observations, including the questionnaire called Constitutional Type Questionnaire: Three Humors (page 115); the pictures of hands inspired by the Five Element constitutional types (pages 108–112); Observation of the Tongue (page 120); and finally the pages on *internal heat* and *cold* on the tongue (pages 121–122, 126). You won't always need to gather all this information, but I am going to show you how it fits together.

First look at your hands and decide which Five Element–type hand looks like yours. Yours may actually be a combination of two or more hands, but see which of them you notice first; that one will be the most important. Make a note of this. We're keeping score. Then notice if your hand looks a bit red, pale, or dark and purplish. Red signifies *heat;* paleness or color deficiency shows *cold;* and purple shows *stagnation.* If, for example, you have an Earth hand that is reddish, write, "Earth, *internal heat.*" If the hand is not particularly colored, just write "Earth" and go on to the questionnaires.

The Diagnostic Questionnaire describes *internal heat* and *internal cold* among the Five Elements. Notice the summary of your checks at the end of the questionnaire. Does it correspond to what you noticed on the hand? In other words, if you have an Earth hand, did you check more responses for Earth? If so, are there more checks for *Heat, Cold,* or *Stagnation*? Which elements seem to be challenged by more imbalances? Do you tend to have more symptoms of *internal heat* or of *internal cold*?

At the end of the Diagnostic Questionnaire, I asked the question, "During what season have you filled out this questionnaire?" That is because seasonal changes also affect our *chi.* In spring, our Wood element will have more symptoms; in summer, Fire; in Indian summer, Earth; in autumn, Metal; and in winter, Water. Take this into consideration as you look over your responses. You may be an Earth type with an Earth hand, but you may also have some Water-related problems because it is winter.

Then glance back at the list of the Five Element Correspondences on page 89. Review your responses to the questionnaire The Correspondences Applied to You (pages 92–93). After reviewing the two questionnaires, do you still agree with the decision you made about your hand type? Remember, body type analysis is inexact; all we need to establish at this time is which

of the Five Elements most applies to you at this time. Do you have mostly Wood symptoms, or those of Metal or Water? Are they mainly *heat, cold,* or *stagnation* symptoms? You may wish to make a list of each significant element, for example: "Wood, *heat*" or "Fire, *stagnation,*" while ignoring the elements that have few responses.

With the next questionnaire, Constitutional Type Questionnaire: Three Humors (page 115), we are introduced to *wind, bile,* and *phlegm.* Many of the responses apply to the previous questionnaires. For example, the *bile* type tends to have reddish skin, hard-driving energy, and angry or intense emotions originating from *internal heat.* Some of the responses of *wind* apply to *internal cold*—for example, depressed mood and difficult digestion. This *humor* is said to be "cold and dry in nature." Make a note of which *humors* are at work for you at present.

Now review your tongue observations. Notice the parts of your tongue for signs of *heat, cold,* or *phlegm.* See if the problem parts of your tongue match the symptoms of the Correspondences. You may decide, for example, that you have *heat* and *phlegm* troubling digestion because you see a red area with yellow phlegm in the middle of the tongue. Do you also have the *internal heat* symptoms listed in the chart *Internal Heat* and *Cold* on the Tongue? Those are ulcer, burning, excessive hunger, mania, craves sweets, and obsessive thoughts.

By observing the tongue and comparing it with the symptoms in the questionnaires, we can put together a composite of internal symptoms and outward appearance on the hands, body, and tongue.

All you need to know at this point is in what part(s) of your body the problems are located, and the nature of those problems. From this knowledge you will be able to form a working hypothesis. Remember that the simplest way to notice imbalances is by observing the tongue. The questionnaires are added here to refine your observations.

For the present, form a working opinion about your vitality. This will be refined as you study further.

I have signs of *internal heat* or *stagnation* affecting
____ Wood (liver, gallbladder)
____ Fire (heart, pericardium, small intestine)
____ Earth (stomach, spleen)
____ Metal (lung, large intestine)
____ Water (kidney, bladder)

I have signs of *internal cold* or *stagnation* affecting
____ Wood (liver, gallbladder)

____ Fire (heart, pericardium, small intestine)
____ Earth (stomach, spleen)
____ Metal (lung, large intestine)
____ Water (kidney, bladder)

____ My tongue is reddish and dry or has a yellow or brown coating (*heat*).
____ My tongue is pale and puffy, with a watery coating (*cold*).
____ My tongue is purplish or has dark spots on it (*stagnation*).
____ My tongue shows lots of phlegm (*phlegm*).

Most of us already know we have indigestion or headaches, but do not understand how they came about. Noting the symptoms of *internal heat, cold, phlegm,* and *stagnation* gives us a better idea.

Asian diagnosis uncovers imbalances that maintain physical and emotional discomfort. It can give you a clear idea of proper, individual diet and lifestyle, because it is based on your observed vitality, not on the energy you *think* you should have.

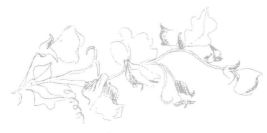

Sweet pea

PART THREE

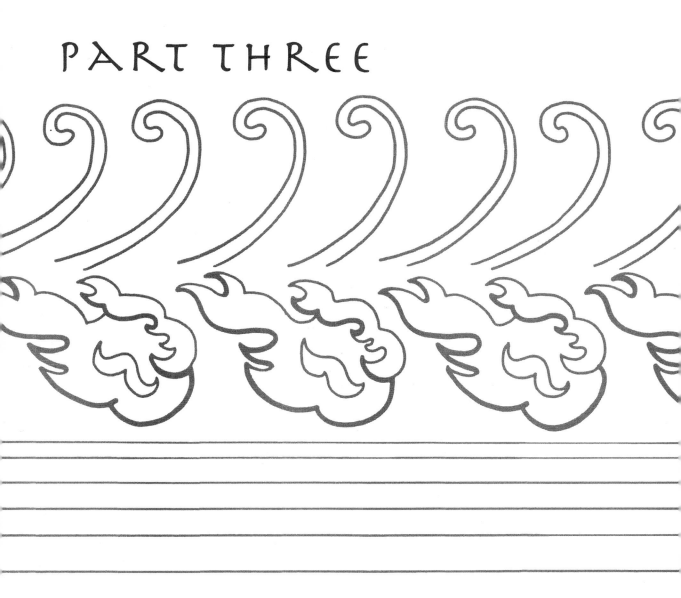

Bringing You into Balance

SONG OF THE VERMEIL PHOENIX

See you not Heng Mountain towering over Hunan hills,
From its summit the vermeil phoenix murmuring leans
Over to gaze, forever seeking his comrades?
His wings are folded, his mouth is closed, but his mind is working
With pity for all the birds that are caught in nets,
From which even the tiny oriole hardly can escape.
He would dispense to them ants and fruit of bamboo,
Provoking hawk and vulture to scream their threats.

—Tu Fu (A.D. 713–770)

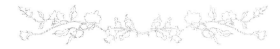

ཀླུ་ན་རྟུག ཀླུ་ན་རྟུག ཀླུ་ན་རྟུག ཀླུ་ན་རྟུག ཀླུ་ན་རྟུག ཀླུ་ན་རྟུག ཀླུ་ན་རྟུག ཀླུ་ན་རྟུག ཀླུ་ན་རྟུག

[tanaduk] Attractive to behold. The Internal Tanaduk is the place where you yourself are the Teacher of Medicine. (from a Tibetan medical text)

13
Achieving Balance: A Three-Part Cleansing Program

There is an innate harmony of body, mind, and spirit that makes us an integral part of nature. Holding true to that philosophy is, in itself, healing. Herbs enhance beauty, health, and inner peace. With them you can create the freedom necessary to become kind. The importance of cleansing impurities goes far beyond personal health practices. When you are free from physical and emotional pain, you can become more receptive to others. When you become responsive to their needs, your own capacity for well-being increases. Who can doubt it? Merely thinking a loving thought, saying a kind word to someone, opens your heart. The response is immediate. But think a mean thought, say an angry word, and muscles tense, digestion suffers, energy becomes stagnant and grinds into a spasm. Sadness costs you vitality and creates stupor. Fear scatters your energy and defenses so that you become sick. Illness is made from negative emotions frozen by time and bad habits.

Because it presumes the correlation of body, mind, and spirit, natural healing always affects more than one person. That's why the following healing practices include more than a simple diet plan. Meant to clarify on all levels, the threefold program in Achieving Balance is offered as a celebration of total health.

This chapter gives you direct experience in creating balanced energy, emotions, and actions. It offers tools for times of stress and for prevention of illness and aging. Using these three multifaceted cleansing programs, following them in the order presented, you'll first clear phlegm so that digestion, vitality, and mental clarity improve. Then you'll cool inflammation to soothe aches, rashes, bad tempers, and frustrations. Finally, you'll settle nervous irritability in order to relax, breathe deeply, and see more clearly around you. Then you will be able to turn your attention, like the vermeil phoenix with wings folded and mouth closed, to all those caught in the nets of suffering. To feel

compassion is the highest form of health and balance.

Our Healing Aims and Methods

This three-part program can heal the whole person: Herbs, purifying diets, and special baths will treat imbalances. Increasing circulation will improve *stagnant chi* and tone internal organs while easing pain. I'll take you through guided visualizations and activities that engage your healing powers.

This routine involves learning what to cleanse, as well as how and when. It may be best to read the entire chapter first to gather herbs you may need and to understand what you will be asked to do. It is important that you proceed consecutively with each step in order to cleanse in the most effective manner. Try not to create shortcuts, but respect the order I've described. There's an optimal order to follow when cleansing. We follow this order with sections I, II, and III. First we reduce phlegm, then inflammation, and finally nervous irritability; thus we ensure that cleansing can progress from the most intractable toxins to the most subtle. Many of my readers and students have benefited greatly by this program.

CLEANSING: HOW MUCH AND FOR HOW LONG?

Cleansing should always be flexible and individual, never weakening. This three-part program does not require a set amount of time for cleansing for everyone, but gives you a table of Goals and Guidelines in each section. This lets you know when it is time to stop and go on to the next section or back to the previous one to clear up any problems. That way you can eliminate any unpleasant side effects from cleansing.

Not everyone has the same leisure or desire for cleansing. I have found from experience that people usually fall into one of two categories, or somewhere in between. They are "ho-hum" cleansers or "gung ho" cleansers. The "ho-hums" might observe each part of the chapter for one day, for a total of three days. The "gung hos" might observe each part for up to one week, for a total of three weeks. That method would be suitable for a weekend or for a scheduled period of time, say, for example, during the season(s) that corresponds to your constitutional type. (For example, Fire corresponds to summer, Earth to early autumn, Metal to late autumn, Water to winter, and Wood to spring.)

However, the best way to organize this schedule is by paying attention to your improvements, using the guidelines I offer at the beginning of each section. As you develop skill in Asian tongue diagnosis, you will want to repeat the cleansing program, paying particular attention to your specific needs.

You may wish to note your progress and impressions in a diary. Be sure you give yourself enough time to process your emotions. This may mean adjusting the cleansing period to accommodate particular needs. Here is where you'll put your personal diagnostic information from the questionnaires into practice.

Later, after you've experienced its benefits, you may enjoy adding sections of this chapter to your daily routine. You will also recognize how sections of the diet will be more appropriate at certain seasons of the year.

GROUND RULES

If you are weak, you might feel worse from cleansing too long. To guard against this, I've included purifying foods, grains, and vegetables. This is *not* a white-knuckle, nothing-but-water fast. There is little to be gained from extreme diets. For most people they result in depression, illness, or a sweet binge afterward. You'll benefit more from simplifying your meals, eating as much as you want of one or two cleansing foods each day, without suffering the weakening effects of privation. That way it becomes a strengthening diet.

Another way to maintain health during cleansing is to continue taking your usual vitamin and mineral supplements. Trace minerals, especially zinc and chromium, help maintain healthy blood-sugar balance and reduce cravings for sweets (useful for Earth types). Manganese helps us absorb calcium (useful for Wood types). Taking lecithin is important to ensure proper digestion of fats and healthy brain function. Coffee and black-tea drinkers need twice as much lecithin as most other people do, up to 1,000 mg daily.

Harmful food combining, or eating one meal too quickly after another, accumulates toxins that can lead to disease. I have avoided problem combinations by stressing one grain and one or more cleansing vegetables for each of the three-part cleansing routines.

It may be convenient to take the suggested foods and teas to work. Try not to eat leftovers, since they encourage the growth of yeast. If the atmosphere at work is too tense, try to isolate yourself when eating, and do quiet deep breathing before and after. Remember, "eating" negative emotions gives us indigestion.

MY PERSONAL PROFILE

Individuals vary according to stress, age, and other temporary conditions. The following chart offers a shorthand method to assess your present energy balance so you can decide which part(s) of the cleansing routine to stress at this time, I, II, or III.

	I Antiphlegm	II Anti-inflammation	III Antinervousness
CONSTITUTIONAL TYPE	*Phlegm* type Earth, Metal, Water	*Bile* type Wood (*heat*) Metal (*heat*)	*Wind* type Fire, Water, Earth Wood, Metal
SYMPTOMS	overweight slow digestion sinus congestion phlegmy asthma parasites depression poor concentration poor memory	chronic headaches inflammatory pain allergies (skin) diabetes high blood pressure anger, frustration insomnia	exhaustion frequent urination low sexual energy depression spacey feeling
TONGUE	Body: pale, wet, scalloped Coating: thick mucus	reddish, dry yellow, green, brown	pale or red dots, shaking
URINE	thick, flaky	dark, oily, odorous	clear, frequent

HOW TO PROCEED

Each night of the three-part program, unless you have diarrhea, take a laxative as described in detail later.

Start each day of the cleansing diets with the suggested hot tea. If you are constipated, add aloe juice or gel, drinking enough to start cleansing. I often drink a whole pot of hot green tea first thing in the morning, to refresh the senses and clear wastes. A cup or two may be sufficient. If early-morning tea makes you feel queasy, add a slice of raw ginger to the cup. Continue with the special diet I recommend after the morning voiding.

Try to do ten minutes of bending and stretching and deep breathing during the day, to relax tension. This will be a good time to visit the gym, as well as health practitioners such as massage therapists, acupuncturists, and chiropractors. Your cleansing diets will make their work easier and even more beneficial.

You may have to do the visualizations at night, during or after the recommended bath. Make sure you do the programmed activity along with each diet routine. Foods and herbs enhance body and mind, but the emotions and spirit are also engaged by visualizations and activities.

I. The Antiphlegm Cleansing Program
GOALS AND GUIDELINES

𝒫 Reduce *phlegm,* improve breathing and digestion.

𝒫 Notice the mucus-coated tongue.
𝒫 Take antiphlegm herbs at mealtimes, during humid weather, and in spring and fall.

When to change section I:
𝒫 When white or gray mucus is reduced, go on to section II.
𝒫 If you have yellow or dark mucus, also drink one quarter cup of aloe juice daily.
𝒫 Stop when mucus is reduced, or after seven days.

The Asian medical definition of *phlegm* encompasses problems far greater than those created by mucus. Mucus is a discharge from anywhere in the body, but mainly from nose, mouth, or genitals; it can be watery or thick and sticky. *Phlegm (dampness),* however, refers to a large category of mental and physical problems associated with faulty digestion and slow metabolism, including mucus but also fat, cholesterol, and tumors. Excess phlegm clogs the works.

HOW *PHLEGM* AFFECTS THE BODY, MIND, AND SPIRIT

Section I is designed to rid the body of excess phlegm. Of the people who need this part of cleansing, most are *phlegm* constitutional types or often have a coating on the tongue. Sometimes the entire body is slim, but the abdomen becomes distended and painful. Do you digest slowly, or experience fatigue and bloating after meals? Do you have a sweet tooth, put on excess weight, or have parasites? Do you have a rattling, wet cough? Because phlegm makes breathing difficult, section I can reduce asthma or bronchitis and improve breathing made difficult by a head cold, pneumonia, or TB.

Humid weather retards the functioning of the liver, a major detoxification organ, so that cells become waterlogged with impurities. I have seen pollution cause allergies, insomnia, and depression more frequently among my clients in recent years.

Phlegm, at times, is hard to see, although we suffer from its severe aches. The antiphlegm cleansing program reduces arthritic pain aggravated by damp weather or by eating "sticky" foods such as pasta, sweets, and cheese. It is especially useful for rheumatoid arthritis. The pains most relieved from this stage of cleansing are heavy and dull, with joints that feel congested and movements stiff.

Excess *phlegm* from poor digestion makes the mind dull, the body heavy and lazy. This cleansing fast is beneficial for people who feel heavy or experience congestion, dulled senses, or pounding sinus headaches.

According to traditional Asian doctors, the negative emotional states associated with *phlegm* (as a *humor*) are depression, greed, possessiveness, or obsession. There is an obvious connection between *phlegm,* reduced breathing capacity, and mental sluggishness. Digestive *phlegm* leads to indigestion, low energy, and possibly blood-sugar imbalances. These all affect depression because weakened vitality, breathing, and digestion all affect mood and brain function.

Perhaps rumination is the futile attempt to "digest" present circumstances, or the inability to lift ourselves out of the past to take a breath of fresh air.

The tendency for obsessive ideas can be developed over a lifetime of work that demands intellectual or artistic perfection. But anyone can develop bloating, cloudy thinking, and stomachache by consuming rich foods and alcohol, and from a lifestyle of stress and little exercise.

As we cleanse, old ideas and energy patterns break apart. I've heard of cases where people furiously clean house or reevaluate stale relationships as they clear phlegm.

Preparation for the diet

WHAT YOU WILL NEED

- An herbal laxative (trifala, cascara sagrada, aloe, or other)
- Bancha twig, oolong, or green tea
- Schuessler's tissue salts: **Acne** and natrum sulphate or equivalents
- Raw barley, raw ginger, black pepper, fresh parsley, dulse seaweed
- Raw vegetables: radishes, carrots, beets, squash, cucumber, lemon juice
- (Optional: garlic, onion, lemongrass, Chinese fu ling, millet, Chinese yams, lotus nuts, dried orange peel, thyme, basil, cinnamon)

Before beginning

The evening before the fast, put a handful of uncooked barley into a quart of spring-water. Leave it overnight in a warm place

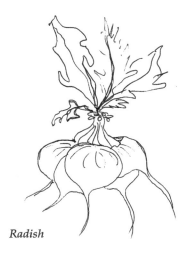

Radish

so that it will ferment. Later you will drink the fermented juice as a cleanser. (Optional: For pungent flavor, add two slices each of raw ginger and dried orange peel.) After one day, you can stop the fermentation by storing the juice in the refrigerator at night and adding fresh water as you drink it during the day. Drink a glass twice a day, one half hour before meals or at bedtime.

The fermented juice will provide healthy intestinal bacteria. Some people find it to be laxative. I recommend you take a laxative each night during the three-part program, but the dosage must be according to your comfort.

How to use laxatives

In the Ground Rules section, I recommended that you take a laxative nightly, unless you have diarrhea. This is because with a light, bland diet, the colon is less apt to eliminate toxins. Laxatives work in various ways, some almost immediately, others

in several hours or overnight. For example, aloe vera, an anti-inflammatory, relaxes tense muscles and moisturizes, while stimulant laxatives such as cascara sagrada create peristalsis the next morning.

To speed cleansing, you can take one capsule of cascara sagrada the evening before beginning. Start with only one capsule, since its effects can be strong. Or take a milder remedy, such as one or two capsules of **Trifala.** This is an American version of a well-balanced Indian cleansing remedy made from three dried fruits. **Triphala churna** powder is the original, less expensive version from India. One **Trifala** capsule equals approximately one-half teaspoon of **Triphala churna** powder. (Add the powder to one-quarter cup of cool water and swallow.) Either version of triphala is wonderfully healing, with long-term benefits such as improved vision and voice. Cascara sagrada tones weak muscles to improve bloating.

Trifala and cascara sagrada capsules are available in many health-food stores. **Triphala churna** powder is available in East Indian groceries. If you cannot find the recommended herbs locally, please refer to the Herbal Access appendix. (Also see page 226 for **Trifala Guggul.**)

Day one

On the first day, drink a cup or two of hot bancha twig, green, or oolong tea. If you are constipated, add homeopathic natrum sulphate or aloe vera juice to the tea. Other cleansing remedies can be conveniently added at this time. I recommend a homeopathic preparation for speeding metabolism, Dr. Schuessler's tissue salt remedy called **Acne.** These tiny pills, available from health-food stores, contain various forms of potassium and silicea. You can add ten of them to the quart of barley water and sip the mixture between meals, or add four pills to melt in your morning tea. That way, each teacup is a dose of Schuessler's **Acne** remedy. Even if you don't have acne, the potassium and silicea will help dissolve impurities and phlegm. If you can't find this brand of cell salts, you can duplicate it by taking four pills each of kali mur., kali sulph., calc. sulph., and silicea at 6× strength.

After morning tea, begin the cleansing diet, drinking fermented barley juice in the afternoon, between meals, or before bed.

Make a pot of cooked barley soup, enough to last all day. Add carrots, pepper, ginger, and parsley, but no mushrooms, because they increase the growth of yeast. (Optionally, add dried lemongrass, garlic, onion, or miso for flavor.) Once a day (afternoon or evening), make a raw salad of antiphlegm vegetables, including radishes, carrots, beets, celery, squash, cucumbers, and no sprouts. Eat enough to keep you satisfied, not stuffed. The cleansing effect comes from greatly simplifying the diet, not from starving yourself. Avoid eating leftovers or too many raw foods if you are weak.

VARIATIONS

Those wishing to increase the slimming effects of the barley soup can simmer it with a handful of dried juniper berries or a handful each of several Chinese medicinal herbs: fu ling, fox nuts, lotus nuts, and Chinese yam. See page 184 for details on Four Ingredient Barley Soup. When cooked until soft, don't throw the Chinese additions away. They can be eaten, although the soup tastes very bland. Fu ling's action is diuretic. It works best for people with cellulite or edema (water retention) in the face or entire body. They are likely to have a thickly coated or greasy-looking tongue, indicating phlegm in the digestive tract.

SUBSTITUTIONS

If you tire of barley, try steaming millet. It's easy to make: Add a cup of raw millet to a thermos, add boiling water to cover, and replace the top. In twenty minutes you have steamed millet. Season with salt substitute, black pepper, or antiphlegm herbs such as raw radish, ginger, juniper berries, or thyme.

Another substitute for cooked barley is boiled lotus nuts, which come from the lotus plant stem. Sold dried in Chinese groceries, or by mail order, they have to be cooked until soft, which could take a couple of hours. In South China they are served with raw honey as a dessert.

Although the cleansing fast features a grain and vegetables, for those who wish to use fruit, the best kind to get rid of phlegm is a dried fruit. Of them, the one with most beta-carotene, to build immune strength, is dried apricots. You might try a snack of dried apricots and green tea, but separate it from other grain or vegetable meals by at least several hours, for easier digestion. Better yet, one day eat only apricots or barley soup. The simpler the better.

Warming, drying herbs and spices such as basil and cinnamon are helpful in reducing phlegm because they increase sweating. Drink them as tea, or use them in cooking (see pages 66–67 for others).

Cooked seaweed is a nice complement to boiled grains. People who continue the diet for more than a day can add dulse, a source of potassium, or hijiki, the best source of calcium, which is more easily assimilated than that in milk.

SUPPLEMENTS

Continue taking your usual vitamins and minerals. Herbs useful for ridding the body of phlegm and its by-products, such as tumors and arthritis, are myrrh and its Indian cousin, guggul, dry, aromatic tree-gum herbs used in India as incense. You must buy a pure form that can be taken internally. I like boiling a few pieces of edible guggul in water, along with a Chinese slimming tea, but capsules are available.

You can take a lot of these pungent tree-gum herbs to help clear breathing and rejuvenate the body and mind, as long as you do not suffer from dry mouth or other signs of dehydration and fever. Start with two capsules a day of myrrh. If you tolerate it well, you can increase the dosage to six.

If you desire something sweet, add dried orange peel, vanilla, fennel seeds, or cardamom while cooking grains. Here is a sample menu for one day. All quantities are as much as you wish.

One half hour before breakfast: Hot oolong tea; add 4 pills each of homeopathic natrum sulphate and Schuessler's tissue salt **Acne** per pot of tea

Breakfast: Warm barley soup with ginger and parsley
1 capsule myrrh

Midmorning: Steamed carrots and squash
1 cup fermented barley and ginger water

Lunch: A big raw salad, melba toast
Hot green or oolong tea and 1 capsule myrrh

Midafternoon: A few pieces of dried dulse seaweed

Evening: Millet cooked with orange peel, cinnamon, and clove
Cucumber and cilantro salad, add lemon juice
Warm mint tea with 1 capsule myrrh

Before bed: 1 cup fermented barley and ginger water, add a dash turmeric
1 capsule cascara sagrada (optional laxative)

Here is a possible cleansing routine for one week. (Between meals each day, take barley water and myrrh capsules.)

Monday: Oolong tea, barley soup, and raw salad
Tuesday: Bancha tea, steamed millet, carrots, squash, dulse
Wednesday: Mint tea, dried apricots, cooked lotus nuts with raw honey
Thursday: Bancha tea, Four Ingredient Barley Soup, salad

Friday: Green tea, cooked barley, nori seaweed, radish
Saturday: Oolong tea, vegetable soup,
salad
Sunday: Oolong tea, vegetable soup,
cooked millet, salad

Progress checklist

Here are some indicators to let you know
whether your cleansing diet is proceeding
in the right direction. Cleansing sometimes
entails temporary discomfort as your
energy struggles to maintain imbalance.
You may experience a few days of extra
phlegm, indigestion, or cramps. If that
happens, add more hot ginger-and-mint
tea. The following questions illustrate the
aims we are hoping to achieve.

- Does your tongue show less mucus?
- Is sinus congestion reduced?
- Is bloating and indigestion better?
- Do senses feel more clear?
- Is breathing easier?
- Do joints have less dull ache and
  stiffness?

If these positive changes have started,
go on to section II when you feel comfortable, or after no later than one week.

If you feel too dry, thirsty, constipated, or irritable, go on to section II after
one day.

A SWEAT BATH

After a day of drinking barley soup and
tea, take a special cleansing bath. You'll feel
light and breezy after soaking in ocean
minerals. To prepare, put a few handfuls of
baking soda, Dead Sea or kosher salt, and
dried seaweed into an old sock, and place
it in your bathwater. Rub the souls of your
feet with Dead Sea salt. You might enjoy
listening to taped ocean waves or doing the
visualization I'll describe in a moment.

Instead, you might add one-quarter
cup of dried ginger powder to the bath and
drink a cup of hot cinnamon tea. The resulting sweating action will break up phlegm
and congested circulation as you feel warm
and tingly all over. After you are dry, wrap
up in warm sleepwear for the evening.

Another good way to increase sweating is with a daily workout in the gym, one
half hour before eating. Make sure to take a
dose of the Schuessler **Acne** remedy before
the workout to increase metabolism. The
homeopathic silicea it contains will cancel
unpleasant body odors. Then eat your
meals no later than one half hour after a
workout, while your metabolism is fast.

ACTIVITY AND VISUALIZATION

Each part of this chapter aims to heal past
and present imbalances. This phlegm-
reducing campaign involves more than a
purifying diet of *warming* and *drying* foods
and a sweat bath. *Phlegm* also involves
mental sluggishness and its cousins, depression and apathy. For that reason, the
following activity and visualization are
added to reduce the sticky drain on your
life force that comes from too much *phlegm*.

Activity

Since section I rids the body of solid wastes and congestion, now is a good time to give away clothes you haven't used in years. Leave them on the street for the homeless, or give them to a church. Consider what is valuable in your life and what is not. In that way, everyone benefits from your cleansing.

Visualization

The following visualization can be done anytime during section I. For some people it will help dissolve grief, dependence, or other "sticky" feelings. If those emotions are an issue for you, you'll benefit from doing the visualization often. As you practice it more frequently, you won't need to spend a long time on it. Sometimes it will be refreshing simply to remember the visualization for a moment.

If possible, prepare a quiet, sunny space in your home or office for this visualization. Light a stick of spicy incense, or inhale the fragrance of an opened capsule of myrrh or a lavender oil. These pungent aromas balance *phlegm*, which corresponds to the sweet taste. If you feel particularly stuffed up, sniff a little of the contents of a gotu kola capsule like snuff. Put four drops of **Bach Flower Remedies** homeopathic chicory into a cup of water and sip it during the visualization to ease the flow of energy through your center.

At a time and place where you can be alone and relaxed, sit quietly in a chair. Imagine a line that stretches down the cen-ter of your body connecting the top of your head to your feet. Feel this line gently lengthen the space between each vertebra. Place your hands at your navel and breathe gently there. Do not move your chest as you breathe. Then gently exhale quickly and lightly about ten or twenty times, taking in only small catch-breaths. Yoga practitioners call this a "fire breath." Then inhale and exhale slowly into the abdomen. If that was comfortable, do it again. Try not to stiffen your shoulders or neck and jaw. Alternate the slow and rapid breathing several times.

As you inhale quietly and deeply into the lower abdomen, imagine a bright flame under your navel. This "digestive fire" burns away impurities and negative thoughts during the visualization. As you breathe rapidly, visualize the flame becoming larger to engulf your entire body. Invite a deity or other healing power into this flame. You may wish to imagine a flame made of pure love.

As you breathe quietly and slowly, the flame remains steady and bright at your center. Then imagine that through the left nostril you can inhale pure light. Exhale through the right nostril, ridding yourself of illness and negative thoughts. You may wish to say quietly to yourself, "Inhale clear light, exhale anger. . . . Inhale light, exhale envy. . . . Inhale diamonds, exhale sadness. . . . Inhale blue sky, exhale loneliness. . . . Inhale sunshine, exhale grief. . . ." Continue until you feel calm and clear.

Now slowly raise the flame at your abdomen to the top of your head, then pass it back through your body to your feet. Slowly move it through all the areas of your body until the flame melts you to liquid gold. As each part is melted, memories and emotions may arise. Let the flame dissolve these until nothing is left of your body but a brilliant outline. Your "light body" is pure and sacred. It is always with you. Let it float up through an opening at the top of your head to merge with your ideal of perfection, love, or a deity.

End the visualization by imagining the silver radiance of the full moon floating above your head. Its glow will ground you, relax you, and extinguish the fire as it passes from your head to your feet. Continue to imagine that you are outside on a clear night of blue sky and stars, that the moon's silver light is cooling and balancing as it passes through you until you are empty of everyone and everything. You are pure light, air, and movement of electrons. Let all negative influences pass through your feet into the earth.

With this visualization you have used your mind to create the healing benefits of *heating* and *cooling* energies. The healing energy most useful for clearing *phlegm* is like a flame. Fire purifies and makes light that which is dense, heavy, sticky, and polluted. It lifts body, mind, and spirit to greater clarity.

ARE YOU READY FOR SECTION II?

Continue with the antiphlegm program as your energy and time allow, until your tongue loses its sticky, thick coating. The "ho-hums" who do the fire visualization,

the cooked barley and bancha tea fast, and the sweat bath for only a day may feel lighter and happier. The "gung hos" who do that for a week will lose significant phlegm from lungs, digestive tract, and joints. They will start to feel clear. They may even start singing.

Before you go on to the next part, answer these questions:

- Did your energy improve?
- What memories or emotions surfaced during this part of cleansing?
- Where in your body do you feel those emotions were held?
- What part of the program felt the best?

If improvements in breathing, energy, and joint flexibility were significant, *phlegm* may be an important issue for you.

II. The Anti-Inflammation Cleansing Program

Inflammation assumes many forms in the body, mind, and spirit. In chapter 8 we discussed its origins and consequences (see pages 76–77). In brief, its source can be either external (from wounds) or internal (from energetic imbalance, infection, moisture deficiency, and troubled emotions).

When the cause is external, inflammation can be treated locally to reduce discomfort and speed healing. With internal symptoms, such as fever, pain, or irritability, herbs can reduce *internal heat*, dehydration, and infections (sometimes called fire poisons). The Anti-Inflammation Cleansing Program aims primarily to reduce problems related to *internal heat.*

GOALS AND GUIDELINES

℘ Reduce inflammatory pain, muscle spasm, rash, and irritability.

℘ Notice red tongue, reddish complexion, itchy rash, dry eyes.

℘ Take anti-inflammatory herbs, as needed, in springtime.

When to change section II:

℘ When you feel more cool and relaxed, digestion and elimination are comfortable, and rash disappears, begin section III.

℘ If you become pale or begin to feel weak or chilled, begin section III after one day.

℘ Stop when *heat* is reduced, or after no longer than seven days.

HOW *INTERNAL HEAT* AFFECTS BODY, MIND, AND SPIRIT

Internal heat happens when you get locked into high gear, when you process too fast. It results in red, itching rashes, painful swelling, pounding headaches, and brittle dryness of skin and hair, but also in hot emotions such as hatred and jealousy. Frequently, *heat* originates from physical or mental frustration. For instance, when the normal flow of bile is prevented by rich foods or troubled emotions, digestion becomes stuck. This leads to poor circulation and stabbing or burning pain, because acids and poisons are unable to leave the body by the normal routes. Otherwise, when feelings or actions are stuck as a result of disease, *stagnant chi*, or life's circumstances, hot emotions signal an energetic and psychic impasse.

This part of the present chapter is designed to rid the body of excess acid, stuck *bile*, and inflammation. With these blocks removed, *chi* can flow smoothly. Dam a river, and the result is a reservoir that can turn fetid or light an entire city. Dam the flow of *chi*, and you get pain, swelling, or compressed rage. What you do with the *heat* is the issue.

WHO NEEDS THIS PROGRAM?

The *cooling* diet and herbal recommendations found in section II are most suitable for persons whose problems require prevention, not immediate treatment. They are especially useful for people with eczema, herpes, cloudy vision or dry eyes, allergies, and arthritic aches made worse by hot spices and the so-called nightshades —acidic foods such as white potatoes, tomatoes, green peppers, eggplant, onions, and garlic.

This type of anti-inflammatory diet helps symptoms for which Western doctors recommend cortisone and drugs for high blood pressure, headache, allergies, and hepatitis, as well as laxatives and hemorrhoidal ointments. It can eventually reduce the need for many over-the-counter pain and itch remedies, as well as medications for chronic fevers, night sweats, and menopausal hot flashes. In Asia, anti-inflammatory herbs have been used to treat malaria and encephalitis, as well as to reverse liver and lung damage from addictions.

Persons who benefit the most from the following *cooling* diet will show signs of *internal heat* such as a red tongue and rapid pulse. Other symptoms, such as chronic thirst, excessive hunger, and dark or burning discharges and urine, are associated with dehydration and inflammation, sometimes with infection.

Accumulated toxins at the joints can provoke inflammatory arthritis. Many people suffer after exercise because poor removal of uric acid results in spasms and soreness. The types of pains most associated with inflammation are burning, itchy rashes, stabbing pain at the joints, sharp jabs in the abdomen, shooting "electric currents" running down the legs, and throbbing migraines. If the problem is acute, pain may be serious enough to require immediate attention.

The *cooling* diet in section II serves as a fine adjunct to precede or accompany chiropractic treatments, because adjustments hold better with less muscle tightness and spasm. Hot emotions associated with stuck *bile*, such as nervousness, anger, and frustration—experienced as tight shoulders and neck, and pains in the chest and ribs, improve with a *cooling* diet. Thyroid and heart irregularities augmented by high emotions and hot spices will lessen. This is especially helpful for people with liver damage from chemical poisons, drugs, and alcohol.

Each of us at one time or another has become too hot. Acid inflammation and toxic liver conditions combined with life's glitches can provoke outbursts of rage or jealousy. The result is insomnia and other *internal heat* symptoms. For these, Asian doctors provide herbal liver cleansers. In the West we have called them "spring tonics."

Springtime is the time when the Wood element is said to be most active. Inflammatory conditions originate then, from what some Asian doctors call "rising fire of the liver." I advise my clients to avoid quitting jobs and marriages in springtime, also to eat the following *cooling* diet. By the time they finish with a week of bitter cleansing herbs, cooked oatmeal, and green vegetables, a lot of their hot issues will have blown over.

Preparation for the diet

WHAT YOU WILL NEED

- Fermented barley water
- Green tea
- **Trifala** powder or aloe vera gel
- Acidophilus capsules
- Oatmeal, white basmati rice, peeled, soaked almonds
- Asparagus, broccoli, artichoke, yellow squash, cucumber
- Olive or canola oil
- Cumin, coriander, fennel, dill, mint
- Capsules of dandelion, sarsaparilla, yellow dock, burdock root, nettle, alfalfa, and myrrh
- Optional teas: Chinese chrysanthemum flower, prunella vulgaris,

Essence of Tienchi Flower Instant Beverage

🍃 **Wuchaseng** liquid extract (see page 393)

The healing energy most useful for reducing inflammation is *cooling*. This seems obvious, but *cooling* herbs are not simply anti-inflammatory. They are often not sedative: Their action is indirect. They do not necessarily slow metabolism or shrink swollen membranes, but reduce inflammation by killing germs or eliminating acid. Therefore they might be antiseptic herbs, antibiotics, laxatives, or diuretic herbs. This chapter covers primarily the latter two, which encourage acids and toxins to leave the body by way of the urine and stools.

Before beginning

Each night before bed, take a laxative such as **Trifala** or one capsule of wheat-germ oil.

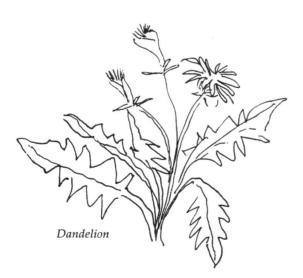

Dandelion

People with chronic inflammation develop dryness that can be improved with wheat-germ oil or a natural source of beta-carotene. If stools are dry, take one or two capsules of either of these oils. Stimulant laxatives such as senna or cascara sagrada may be too strong for people who tend to have spasms.

OPTIONAL: AN ENEMA

If the idea appeals to you, and if possible, one morning of the fast, on an empty stomach, do a warm **Trifala** tea enema. You will need the following:

3 cups lukewarm springwater or purified water

1 level teaspoon Trifala powder or ¼ cup aloe vera gel

Make the tea using **Trifala** powder as though you were going to drink it. You can whip the powder into boiling water, then strain the tea and let it cool to room temperature. Or, instead, add one quarter cup of aloe gel to three cups of warm purified water or springwater. Do not use tap water, because it may contain chemicals or lead. Remember, whatever goes into the colon passes through large blood vessels there, directly into the blood.

I prefer this method to colonics, since you control the flow of water. Be gentle. Use a smaller amount of water, only what is comfortable, and retain it forty-five minutes for good results. Lie down and give yourself a gentle stomach massage while taking deep breaths.

After the enema has worked, end the

cleansing session by taking a capsule of acidophilus, either orally or as a suppository, to replenish intestinal flora.

Day one

Start each day of the anti-inflammatory cleansing program by drinking plenty of hot mint tea and aloe. Aloe vera (gel or juice) works as an excellent antacid, taken in green tea or apple juice all day for constipation, skin blemishes, menstrual cramps, stomach ulcers, and bad breath.

"Ho-hum" cleansers will fast for one day on cooked oatmeal or white basmati rice made with *cooling* spices and mint or green tea, while "gung ho" cleansers can fast for up to a week. Oatmeal is full of minerals. Horses live on it. But a week of cooked oatmeal can slow metabolism and increase *phlegm* for some people. It lowers blood sugar and is an excellent food for persons with diabetes, rheumatoid arthritis, or hot flashes. If you feel weak from too much oatmeal, change to white basmati rice and steamed vegetables. Basmati rice is both nourishing and *cooling.*

Avoid all hot, spicy, oily, or fried foods, especially garlic, onions, and peppers. *Cooling* spices, such as cumin, coriander, fennel, mint, tarragon, and dill, are delicious antacid additions to grains and salads, or drunk as teas. For a healthful and slimming salad dressing, I add a handful of fresh tarragon to a bottle of balsamic vinegar and use no oil.

Other good foods to eat during the *cooling* diet are cooked or raw asparagus, a diuretic food, and blanched almonds, a source of protein. Sweeten meals with fennel seeds, cinnamon, or culinary rose oil (available in Indian shops).

Broccoli is a source of chromium, and an anticancer food. When foods in the cabbage family are hard to digest, simmer them with caraway seeds and bay leaves. When done, add a little cold canola oil.

"Gung ho" cleansers can add pumpkin seeds, steamed green vegetables, artichoke, and yellow squash. The latter tend to be laxative. Avoid carrots, beets, radishes, peppers, garlic, and onions. Anything green is okay. If you wish to use a fruit instead of vegetables one day, apple is the best because it clears inflammation and *phlegm.* Instead of butter, use unheated canola or olive oil and dried herbs.

Cooling *teas*

These can be ordered from Chinese groceries and herb shops. (See Herbal Access and chapter 5 concerning medicinal teas.) Ju Hwa is a delightful, sweet-tasting tea made from Chinese chrysanthemum flowers recommended for headaches and to clear cloudy vision. You can drink it between meals during the fast. Chrysanthemum flowers make a wonderful summer tea that helps prevent heatstroke. One big pinch of flowers in a glass pitcher expands when brewed to make a decorative tea. Avoid the instant form, which is very sugary.

Another flower tea, more bitter than chrysanthemum, is prunella vulgaris—in Chinese, *xia ku cao.* It cures red, dry "computer eyes" and also helps remove lumps in the neck from poor circulation. It comes as dried flowers, and in an instant sugar-cube form. Steep the flower tea the same way you would leaf teas.

Essence of Tienchi Flowers is an instant sugar substitute in the form of crystals. It cools high-blood-pressure headaches, hot tempers, and insomnia. Recommended for those who grind their teeth while sleeping, it's available in many Chinese grocery stores. You can add it anywhere you use sugar.

Chinese chrysanthemum flowers, prunella, and **Essence of Tienchi Flowers** are relaxing because they're anti-inflammatory, not sedative. They do not contain caffeine.

Cooling *herbs: bitter cleansers*

Herbs taken during the anti-inflammatory fast are bitter cleansers that eliminate excess acid through laxative and diuretic effects. They should be taken during the day, using a dose that feels comfortable, not one that provokes prolonged, harsh cleansing.

The following are all important spring tonics. Take any one or several of these as needed after meals while you follow the diet in section II. Your body will guide you. Observe your tongue. Add one new herb at a time, starting with a small dose such as two capsules after meals. Then, when ready, you can increase the dose to three or four after meals. They are all sources of vitamins and minerals that will not drain the body. Think of them as concentrated salad full of sunshine.

Drink adequate water to replace flu-ids. Reduce the dose if you get watery diarrhea or very pale urine. Much stiffness and pain can be eliminated with adequate cleansing. If you have persistent aches and red, itchy bumps, you will want to continue taking these herbs for some time, perhaps a month. You'll feel lighter, fresher, and younger as your discomforts disappear.

Dandelion, a laxative and diuretic cleanser, taken over a period of time, rids the body of fibroids, stones, and lymphatic congestion. Many of my clients have taken a dozen capsules per day (in three doses of four pills) to reduce breast and uterine lumps or eliminate excess body fat. It is especially suited for persons who crave sugar, because it reduces water retention in a healthy way.

Sarsaparilla, a diuretic, cleanses the urinary, reproductive, and nervous systems of toxins and excess acid. Sarsaparilla has been used to treat venereal diseases, herpes, skin rashes, arthritis, gout, epilepsy, and indigestion. It reduces thick, oily-looking, lumpy, or odorous urine by dispelling infection and inflammation while purifying the blood. During the fast, take up to six capsules a day or until the urine becomes clear, pale yellow. Make sure to add this one if you have chronic yeast or kidney infections.

Another stimulant diuretic is the juniper berry. The fruit of the juniper tree rids the body of acid as it strengthens digestion. You can chew a handful, or cook them with grains each day.

Yellow dock, a blood and lymph cleanser, is important at this time. It clears skin rashes and is an excellent source of iron. Burdock, a well-known blood cleanser, will be useful for those with red, itchy skin rashes. If you have inflammatory arthritis, add 8 to 10 alfalfa capsules per day. Alfalfa is a wonderful source of high nutrition. (Also see chapter 19.)

But cleansing isn't everything. Another bitter tonic reduces tension and chronic skin rashes by soothing the nervous system. Gotu kola is the best all-around remedy to revamp a brain burned out from overwork. It is a *cooling* herbal stimulant that provides steady energy throughout the day, and it will not keep you awake if you take it before bed. Take six or eight capsules a day as needed between meals.

A coffee substitute

No coffee or decaf is allowed during the cleansing programs because it drains us of vitamins, minerals, and homeopathic remedies. But you can make a delicious coffee substitute by boiling roasted chicory. I make it strong, like espresso, by boiling one teaspoon of chicory per cup of spring-water. Then add **Essence of Tienchi Flowers** or fennel seeds to sweeten. For added zip, add a dash of cardamom powder, a sweet-tasting stimulant.

CLEANSING AND CIRCULATION

Another important consideration in anti-inflammatory cleansing diets is blood and energy circulation. We want to avoid cleansing so quickly that poor circulation (*stagnant chi*) results. Therefore add herbs and spices that increase blood circulation to liver-cleansing recipes. For example, add a small pinch of turmeric to the chicory coffee substitute or to cooked grains. Turmeric, a hot spice, is a gentle antibiotic that strongly stimulates circulation. It's found in herbal combinations that dissolve cysts and tumors.

Myrrh is another *warming* antistagnation herb I often combine with aloe or dandelion. It heals wounds and is rejuvenating. The ratio I use is 1 capsule of myrrh for each half cup of aloe or 6 capsules of dandelion.

There are a number of Chinese herbal combinations specifically used for poor circulation leading to joint pain. One is **Guan Jie Yan Wan,** which translates as "close-down-joint inflammation pills." It treats heavy, dull pains that shift from one area of the body to another. It's great for arthritis, rheumatism, cold sensations in the limbs, aching joints, periodic flare-ups of sciatica, and early rheumatoid arthritis. Sold in herb shops in Chinatown, it contains 20 percent erythrina bark (in Latin, *Cortex erythrinae var.*), which stimulates circulation in lower back and knees, promotes urination to remove excess acid, and reduces edema (water retention). **Guan Jie Yan Wan** also contains small amounts of cinnamon, ginger, and ephedra to stimulate circulation, as well as barley to help with *phlegm* conditions.

This combination can be taken during the *cooling* fast or at any time to help prevent and treat aches in legs and knees associated with poor circulation. Here's a sample menu for one day:

(Drink 1 cup of barley water between meals per day, if not too laxative.)

Breakfast: Hot mint or green tea, 1 teaspoon **Trifala** per pot
Cooked oatmeal sweetened with fennel seeds
Capsules of *cooling* herbs: dandelion, nettle, burdock, and alfalfa

Midmorning: A handful of almonds
A bunch of raw asparagus or celery

Lunch: Steamed rice and vegetables
Mint and cucumber salad with canola oil and tarragon vinegar, *cooling,* cleansing herbs

Midafternoon: Chicory coffee substitute with **Essence of Tienchi Flowers,** gotu kola, or cleansing herbs

Evening: A big green salad or steamed spinach and almond rice
Hot green tea

Before bed: Gotu kola, **Wuchaseng** liquid extract (see page 393) (no laxatives or cleansers)

Here is a typical menu for one week:

(Optional barley water and cleansing herbs between meals.)

Monday: Mint tea, almonds, oatmeal, and spinach salad

Tuesday: (Trifala) green tea, almonds, cardamom rice, broccoli

Wednesday: Mint tea, asparagus, broccoli, squash, rice cakes

Thursday: Chicory coffee, raisin oatmeal, artichokes, creamed squash with fennel

Friday: Green tea, vegetable soup, green salad, rice pudding

Saturday: Mint green tea, tofu vegetable soup, rice cakes

Sunday: Mint tea, baked squash, almond rice (with rose oil), cucumber

Progress checklist

- Do you feel cooler, calmer, lighter?
- Is your tongue less red and dry?
- Are you sleeping better? Feeling less irritable?
- Is your rash gone or much improved?
- Do you experience less constipation, bad breath, body odor?

If these positive changes have started to occur, go to section III when you feel comfortable, or after no later than one week.

If, after cleansing for one or two days, you felt chilled or developed diarrhea, shortness of breath or nausea, or caught a cold, drink a cup of fresh ginger tea. If necessary, go back to section I for a day or so to clear cold symptoms. Then return to section II for one day before going on to section III.

If you always have chills, diarrhea, or shortness of breath with a very pale tongue, drink a warming tea three times a day during section II (for example, ginger or clove).

A *COOLING* BATH

After eating *cooling* foods all day, enjoy a refreshing bath of Epsom salts and pure essential sandalwood oil. Add one-half cup Epsom salts (magnesium sulfate) to the hot bathwater and soak for twenty minutes. At the same time, put a drop of pure sandalwood oil behind and in front of your ears, on the jawline. Epsom salts soothe sprains, sore muscles, and poor circulation. Sandalwood oil can be added to sunflower or canola oil to massage swollen, inflamed joints.

ANTI-INFLAMMATION CLEANSING: ACTIVITY AND VISUALIZATION

The time during this *cooling* fast is perfect to develop some clarity on unresolved issues, angers, and jealousies—a time for emptying the trash. I have found it quite effective to write letters or poems to people living or dead with whom I had painful, unfinished business. You may want to write a few yourself, forgiving those who have hurt you or apologizing to those whom you feel you have disappointed or betrayed in some way. Send the letters to those who are alive, and burn those intended for the dead. If you are unable to forgive them now, you might at least state your intention to forgive them someday. This can free you to move on.

A *COOLING* VISUALIZATION

This visualization can facilitate your relationships with important others. Our opinions are most often veiled by strong emotions. When we lift the veil by creating calm, we can see more clearly.

All Asian healing traditions teach breathing practices to relax the mind. This facilitates deep cleansing by balancing metabolism while increasing oxygen intake. It helps rebuild beauty and calm that brings clarity. You will find it makes a fine addition to your *cooling* bath.

Prepare your meditation space by lighting a quieting incense such as sandalwood or rose. To a cup of springwater add four drops each of the **Bach Flower Remedies** holly and beech. Sip this throughout the visualization to facilitate healing anger.

Make sure no clothing constricts your breathing. Breathe slowly and deeply into your abdomen. Imagine you are in a crystal blue river that stretches far in both directions above and below you. The cool water rushes over your shoulders and down the back and legs, refreshing every muscle. Some distance beyond your feet is a waterfall. The air is cool and light. The only sound is running water.

Visualize your friends and family seated behind the waterfall. Include old enemies, alive or dead. Slowly watch them fade as the water washes them away, until all emotions associated with them are bathed, leaving only clean water.

During this visualization, inhale and

exhale gently. With each exhalation, think of a part of your body. Starting from the head and moving down to the feet, feel each part in great detail as you exhale, thinking, "Hair . . . relax. Scalp . . . relax," all the way down past your feet.

The water will liquefy memories in all areas of your body. Put them all underneath the waterfall. Let anger dissolve. Your only connection with past events is a faded memory. They exist only in your mind, and you've just washed them clean. Continue this visualization until your mind and body feel cool and empty.

ARE YOU READY FOR SECTION III?

Continue with the anti-inflammatory diet and *cooling* practices until your dry, red, and yellow-coated tongue becomes a more normal pink, until you lose your hot burning pains and emotions. With the anti-inflammatory program, after only one day of the visualization, the *cooling* fast, and the refreshing bath, "ho-hum" cleansers will feel a bit mild and mellow. After a week of *cooling* and cleansing, the "gung ho" cleansers will have lost nervousness, inflammatory pain, and excess weight. They might consider a career change (modeling swimsuits?).

Before you go on to the next part:

- Did your energy improve?
- What memories or emotions surfaced for you during section II?
- Where in your body do you feel that those memories or emotions were lodged?
- What worked the best for you in section II?

If aches, stiffness, rashes, and irritability improved for you, if your menstrual period became easy for the first time, or hot flashes lessened, inflammation may be a health issue for you.

III. The Antinervousness Cleansing Program

We are held together by a network of nerves, bound on one side by all we've seen, heard, tasted, and touched, and on the other side by all we desire to accomplish and all that we do. We're a million-dollar light show, invisible to the naked eye, tingling and vibrating the song of life force. But sometimes, like an incandescent bulb, we burn out.

This program is designed to end pain, fatigue, and melancholy. Nervous exhaustion is the stupor that feels better with quiet, darkness, warmth, and sleep. To these we'll add grounding and nourishing herbs.

GOALS AND GUIDELINES

- Reduce mental and physical exhaustion and lower-back pain; improve concentration, mood, and sleep patterns.
- Notice red, purple, or pale tongue, black dots, scalloped edges.

🖉 Take herbs for nervous exhaustion between meals and at bedtime, late autumn and winter, or as needed.

When to change section III:

🖉 When tongue turns pink and clear of blemishes, when fatigue and mood improve.

🖉 If you become logy and phlegmy, or if you still have a coated tongue, go back to section I for a day.

🖉 If you become too slow and calm, eliminate sesame oil and nutmeg from section III.

🖉 Stop section III when you feel fully refreshed.

Nervous exhaustion can be signaled by the pain of the arthritis and neuralgia of winter, pain made worse by cold weather or cold, raw food. Or it can be the excruciating fatigue aggravated by jet lag, coffee, cocaine, too much sex, or even too much chatter. It's that drained feeling we get from excessive work, worry, advanced age, or too many parties. It leaves us feeling be-

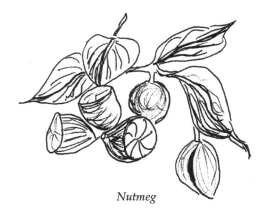

Nutmeg

fuddled, vacant. The associated emotions locked in aching backs and chests are depression, fear, and anxiety.

The chronically nervous person's tongue is reddish purple from *stagnant chi.* It is more serious if gray areas appear in the body of the tongue or dark spots are on the surface. These show a buildup of toxins. The tongue will quiver from nervous tension. The pulse will be weak and irregular because the heart is troubled.

Preparation for the diet

WHAT YOU WILL NEED

🖉 **Trifala** powder or capsules, valerian capsules, sesame oil

🖉 Green tea, basil, clove, nutmeg powder

🖉 Tofu, millet

🖉 Your choice of these cooked vegetables and fruits: asparagus, spinach, beets, peas, okra, leeks, sweet potato; dried apricots, bing cherries, banana

🖉 Myrrh; one adrenal tonic from among: ashwagandha, **Sexoton, Liu Wei Di Huang Wan,** or **Thousand Year Spring Nourishing Syrup**

🖉 (*Optional:* **Wuchaseng** liquid extract, gentian extract)

The healing energy most suited to rebuilding strength after nervous exhaustion is nourishing, *warming,* and sedating. For some people that can mean a delicious meal, a hot bath, and a good night's sleep, but sometimes we can become too overwrought to rest. When we've worked and played too hard, we become locked in high gear. All the warning lights start flashing. Our thoughts scatter and memory fades. We feel weak, depressed, and achy.

To heal ourselves we need easily absorbed proteins; moistening digestive herbs that are heavy and oily in quality; and nerve sedatives and rejuvenating tonics. This ensures protection for our nerves and quality rest.

Before beginning

The night before the fast and thereafter, take **Trifala** or wheat-germ-oil capsules as a laxative. If you can't sleep, rub raw sesame oil on the soles of your feet and wear old socks. If you still can't sleep, take a capsule of valerian, an herbal nerve sedative available from health-food stores.

Day one

Begin the day of the fast with your favorite hot laxative tea as needed, followed after morning evacuation by a strong cup of tea made from basil leaf and clove powder—up to one quarter teaspoon of each. This increases, lifts, and purifies *chi* by scattering it toward the surface. That is why it should be taken only after morning voiding, when we have fewer toxins to send to the surface.

For the fast, choose one or two of the following cooked vegetables: asparagus, spinach, beets, carrots, peas, okra, cooked onion, sweet potato.

The protein source for this program of nourishing and cleansing is soy. *The New York Times* (August 2, 1995) reported that soy protein reduces harmful cholesterol and may be valuable in preventing cancer. Tofu can be served plain or simmered with vegetables. When served plain, cut it into squares and eat it at room temperature along with a dash of soy sauce and lemon juice. It can also be enjoyed warm and sweetened with maple syrup and a pinch of nutmeg. The *warming*, nourishing, and grounding quality of this recipe makes it sedating.

People who experience too much *phlegm* can substitute steamed millet, sweetened with a pinch of nutmeg and vanilla.

Add a few drops of unheated oil to vegetables and grains. Oils that benefit the nervous system are safflower, walnut, canola, and corn. No raw cold food or caffeine-containing stimulants are allowed during section III.

Stewed fruits should be eaten alone, and grains, vegetables, and tofu should be avoided so they don't interfere with digestion. Fruits can include apricots, sweet cherries, and bananas. Choose them according to your needs: apricots are laxative, sweet cherries are a good source of iron, and bananas are balancing but slightly sedative.

Since most fruits sedate digestion, a good time to enjoy them is long after a meal, or before bed. I do not recommend fruit fasts because modern urban men and women do not tend to have stable blood sugar. Fruit is broken down into a simple sugar that turns very quickly into alcohol. Debility combined with too much sweet fruit can cause spacey feelings, even hallucinations for some.

REJUVENATOR TONICS AND ENERGY

Because exhaustion is aging, it's important now to consider prevention and rejuvenation. We've already cleansed the body of phlegm that clogs digestion and breathing. We've cleared the body and mind of excess acid inflammation that causes pain and agitation. Now we need to solidify strength and bolster prevention of illness with herbs that activate the body's powers of repair and rejuvenation.

The tonics most useful for exhaustion treat blood and energy deficiency simultaneously, along with *stagnant chi,* because all these suffer after a long period of stress. Such tonics are well rounded, containing many ingredients that maintain balance, although some individual diagnosis is required. I will suggest several from which you can choose after looking at your tongue.

Take the one that seems the best for you, starting with the lower recommended dose I describe, twice a day between meals. Then continue to observe your tongue as your energy improves.

Reddish-purple tongues, or tongues with dots

Mauve is not an attractive color in tongues. It shows *stagnation,* and requires herbs that are stimulating and rejuvenating. Myrrh is an excellent herb used for activating circulation, healing wounds, and rejuvenating tissues. For the person with nervous exhaustion, it can be used for arthritic pain made worse by cold, damp weather, but must be accompanied by other, more nourishing herbs to support strength.

If you have a mauve-colored tongue, take 1 or 2 myrrh capsules daily during section III, if you do not have inflammation signs such as fever, dry, red tongue, and thirst.

Pale tongue

The pale tongue requires *warming* rejuvenation herbs. Myrrh is very helpful. You can take as many as 6 capsules a day, depending on your comfort. You will also need quite a bit of help with your energy. There are excellent Indian and Chinese patent remedies for this. In general, they are considered stimulant tonics because they support weak adrenal glands, lungs, and spleen to treat a variety of complaints ranging from fatigue and poor mental clarity to sexual impotence.

For example, an Indian rejuvenator, ashwagandha, available in Indian food markets, health-food stores, or by mail order, helps rebuild blood, nerves, muscles, and sexual strength. It is a tonic suitable for men and women similar to Chinese ginseng (ren shen), though less *warming.* It's great for muscle weakness and exhaustion. We'll study it more closely in chapter 34, when we consider sexual tonics.

In Chinatown there are many wonderful tonics. **Sexoton,** unlike what the name implies, is not just a sexual tonic, but a nourishing, rejuvenating herbal combination that treats fatigue, insomnia, shortness of breath, and asthma. It reduces cold hands and feet and profuse, clear urine. It is well suited for persons with pale tongues, because it alleviates weakness of lungs and adrenal glands.

The recommended dosage for tonics is often high, 10 to 20 pills twice a day. But your own dosage, based on experience, is always the best. Start with half the recommended dose and go from there, until your tongue regains its pink color and your discomforts are reduced.

Red, dry tongue

If you have diabetes, chronic fevers, or hot flashes, you don't need a *warming* tonic, no matter how tired you are. You require nourishing, moistening herbs that support your lungs, liver, and kidneys while easing tension.

One such blood tonic is called **Liu Wei Di Huang Wan.** It treats insomnia, a hot sensation in the soles of the feet or the palms, mild night sweats, dizziness, tinnitus, sore throat, high blood pressure, diabetes, lower-back stiffness, and restlessness.

The dose can be 6 to 16 pills, three times a day. Start low and increase the dose as needed.

I have taken **Sexoton** or **Liu Wei Di Huang Wan** at various times for fatigue. They are each very safe tonics that rebuild adrenal, kidney, and liver strength and blood. They have a similar formula. The difference is that the first is *warming* and the second is more *cooling* and moisturizing. We will study many tonics such as these in later chapters on blood-building and fatigue remedies.

REJUVENATION TONICS AND PAIN RELIEF

There are many Chinese herbal combinations that tonify and invigorate the blood and circulation, but for nervous exhaustion or problems of aging, we need something much stronger. Chapter 19 of this book is devoted to arthritis remedies, but here are a few suggestions for now. You can take one of the following combinations, according to directions on the package, between meals as needed. All are useful for the weakness underlying arthritis and rheumatism.

A good tonic for older persons is **Wan Nian Chun Zi Pu Ziang,** translated as "Thousand Year Spring Nourishing Syrup." It contains 80 percent royal jelly, plus energy tonics such as ginseng and the blood-builders tang kuei and he shou wu.

If you wish to make a soup at home to tonify energy and blood circulation, simmer the following herbs in a quart of springwater for one half hour. Drinking a cup of the soup several times a day will help joint and muscle aches. It is also recommended in early rheumatoid arthritis.

1 pinch ma huang (ephedra)
2 handfuls barley
1 small piece of tang kuei
1 handful of peonia root
2 pieces of atractylodes
1 cinnamon stick
A few pieces of licorice root

These *warming* and stimulating herbs build blood and increase circulation. Used in conjunction with a raw sesame oil massage, they can help overcome anxiety or fear due to weakness. Persons with high blood pressure should avoid ma huang.

Optional

For special problems, there are two optional herbs, one for diarrhea, the other for insomnia.

If you have chronic diarrhea, shortness of breath, and depression, Chinese doctors say it may be a result of "weak spleen." (This is more likely if you are a weak Metal or Earth type, or have colitis.) One easy-to-use remedy for this type of watery diarrhea is gentian extract. Put 10 drops of this extremely bitter herbal extract into a goblet of sparkling water after meals. It's an ingredient in many European digestive liquors that helps prevent low blood sugar spaceyness.

If anxiety or stress leads to insomnia, take one teaspoon of Siberian ginseng extract (**Wuchaseng**) before bed. It does not have the usual sledgehammer effect of Western sedative drugs, but quiets the mind by rebuilding damaged nerves (see page 393).

Progress checklist

🌿 Do you feel more rested and grounded?

🌿 Is your tongue a more normal color and texture?

🌿 Do you experience less lower-back discomfort, less fatigue?

If these positive changes have started to occur, continue with section III until you have gained its full benefits.

If, after a day of section III, you have developed too much phlegm or feel too sedated or depressed, repeat section I for one day, then return to section III. If you always have too much phlegm, substitute barley or millet for tofu in section III.

If you have caught a cold, stop section III, return to section I, and take herbal cold remedies (see chapter 30).

End section III when you feel nourished, rested, centered, and calmed.

ANTINERVOUSNESS ACTIVITY AND VISUALIZATION

People who suffer from nervous exhaustion need to feel grounded in order to renew their connection with their bodies and with the earth. Often they work and play so hard they lose their sense of limits. Then exhaustion can lead to anxiety, making them nearly hysterical. To begin this program, it helps to take a night off, pamper yourself a bit, listen to quiet music, care for a loved pet or plants, or call a loved one. After rest, healing can begin on a profound level. Even though you are taking all the right vitamins and herbs, if you do not comfort your spirit, you will remain sick.

If you are miserable and suffering, it will help you to help someone less fortunate. Generosity opens our hearts for ourselves as well as for others. The guided activity for section III is to place some canned or packaged food on the street each day. Your spirit will feel uplifted to help the hungry. No one deserves to be ignored. And you will be feeding a part of yourself that has been ignored a long time, restoring your spiritual connection with every other person and animal.

Then you may find that doors within you and around you will begin to open. Positive experiences can come your way when you're more generous with yourself and others.

A GROUNDING BATH AND VISUALIZATION

This will bring you back to the garden from which you came. It can be done in a sweetly perfumed bath or during a raw sesame oil massage.

Make the room dark, or light some candles. Make sure it is quiet. We want to eliminate stimulation. Use a very sweet incense or flower perfume, because it quiets the nerves. For example, hops, magnolia, and jasmine are all heavy, oily, and sweet in quality. Certain kinds of musk are very grounding. Dab the sweet essential oil in the middle of your chest or on the insides of your wrists.

To a warm bath, add a little raw sesame oil or massage some into your shoulders, elbows, knees, and feet. Play a tape of forest or swamp sounds. For extreme anxiety, put one drop of sesame oil into each nostril with a dropper. This is very quieting because the nerves in your nose go right to the brain.

A GROUNDING VISUALIZATION

To a cup of warm springwater add four drops of **Bach Flower Remedies** elm, used to soothe an overwhelming sense of responsibility. Sip this during your bath or before the visualization.

Imagine you are sitting on the forest floor, near a pond. On your body, visualize the following aromatic flowers as you breathe their fragrance. It is the energy and spirit of the flowers that heal us. The sun, earth, air, and water give the flowers their life, so you can respect the spirit of each flower with your mind.

At your seat, imagine blue iris and lilac, also jasmine, a large vine sending roots into the ground. Their lush, sweet fragrance warms summer nights. Imagine the roots spreading, grounding you to the earth.

Visualize at your navel a golden bowl of red hibiscus and yellow chamomile. Relax that area as you enjoy the aroma.

Imagine at your heart spicy lavender flowers and lily of the valley. Both of these stimulate and soothe. In your lungs, the bright orange daisy echinacea grows wild, filling the breeze with pungent freshness. Honeysuckle flowers are there as a cooling balm, and holly expands your chest and increases your breath.

At your throat imagine the mints—peppermint and spearmint—to cool and cleanse.

At your third eye, in the middle of your forehead, see and feel a white rose slowly opening.

At the crown of your head imagine a lotus, a huge, pale pink flower with a diameter of five feet. It floats on quiet ponds, sending its root downward through the water. This one sends its root through you into the pond beneath your feet. It grounds you to the earth.

This root joins you with all those who have lived on earth and loved nature. It's as though we're all holding hands together right now, all who have loved the flowers and trees. Every bird, every cat or dog or tiny insect, everything in nature is part of you. Your breath is smooth and long. You are the sweet earth, generous to all of your loved creatures, your flowers, and yourself.

After the bath, rub the bottoms of your feet with raw sesame oil, put on warm socks, and rest.

Before you end section III:

- Did your energy improve?
- Do you feel more rested and calm?
- What emotions or memories surfaced for you during section III?
- Where in your body do you feel they were lodged?
- What worked best for you?
- Do you feel stronger and more optimistic?
- Are you facing certain people or situations from a different perspective?

If you feel much improved from the nourishing and grounding herbs and activities in section III, nervous tension is an issue for you.

Do you need to continue with Achieving Balance? What part(s) of Achieving Balance felt the best for you at this time?

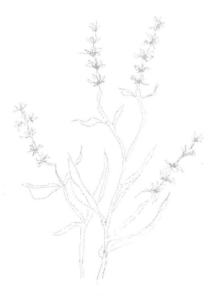

Lavender

ACHIEVING BALANCE—A SHORTHAND REFERENCE

	SECTION I (antiphlegm)	**SECTION II** (anti-inflammation)	**SECTION III** (antinervousness)
LAXATIVES	**Trifala** cascara sagrada	**Trifala** aloe	**Trifala**
TEAS	oolong, bancha twig	green tea, chrysan-themum, prunella, chicory, **Essence of Tienchi Flowers**	green tea, aloe, **Trifala,** basil/clove
GRAINS	barley with parsley	oatmeal, basmati rice with soaked almonds	millet with nutmeg
VEGETABLES	dulse, hijiki, kelp	cabbage, asparagus, broccoli, yellow squash	tofu, spinach, beet, peas, okra, sweet potato
FRUITS	dried apricot	apple	dried apricot, cherry, banana
OILS	flaxseed, olive	canola, olive	sesame, canola
HERBS (after meals)	pepper, ginger, juniper berry, dulse, fu ling	cumin, coriander, fennel, dill, mint, aloe, dande-lion, sarsaparilla, parsley, yellow dock	nutmeg, myrrh, gentian, ashwagandha, **Sexoton, Liu Wei Di Huang Wan**
HERBS (between meals)	myrrh	gotu kola	**Wuchaseng**
BATHS	sweat bath: sea salts, ginger	*cooling* bath: Epsom salts	relaxing bath: sesame oil
INCENSE	spicy, patchouli	sandalwood	lavender, lily of the valley
ACTIVITIES	give away clothes	write letters	give away food
VISUALIZATIONS	bright flame	cool blue river	relaxing flowers

Supplements for all sections: daily vitamins; minerals; trace minerals and lecithin; fermented barley water as needed between meals with optional tissue salts (kali mur., kali sulph., calc. sulph., silicea, natrum sulph.).

PART FOUR

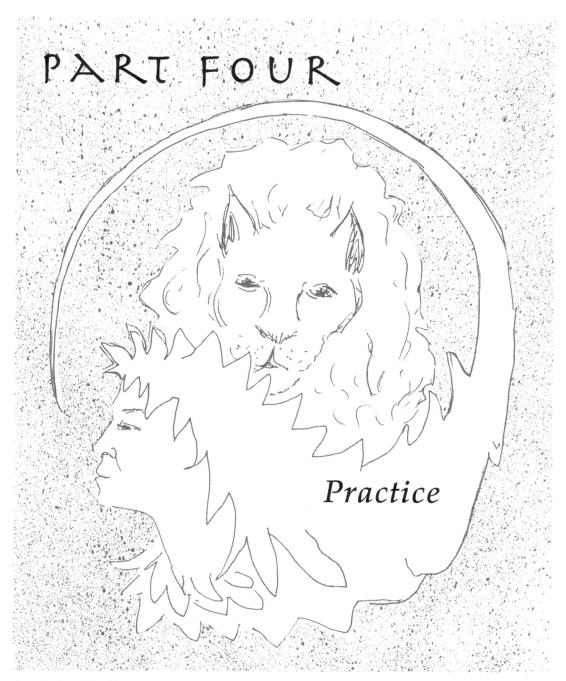

Practice

A symbol used in alchemy is the serpent or dragon swallowing its own tail, the blending of base metals and quicksilver to make gold. The healer must refine all senses, tastes, and passions in order to make himself or herself into gold.

Thus far, this book has given you a general background in Asian energetic medicine. You have learned how the taste, temperature, and type of an herb affect your energy. You've studied healing teas and foods, gaining insight on how they bring you into balance. Most people choose their foods or natural cures without paying attention to diagnosis, but this book has given you experience in observing yourself as an Asian healer does.

Now is the time to apply those observations to your specific needs. To become adept at choosing herbs takes knowledge gained from a great deal of experience. This part of the book offers you practice in applied diagnosis. Even though you won't have all the maladies covered in Parts Four and Five, you will be able to study their herbal remedies while sharpening your diagnostic skills. Guided by the following descriptions of my health clients, you can learn to become your own health practitioner, at least to whatever extent you are able to observe yourself. That takes practice. I, too, try to refine my skills each day.

Practice makes perfect, so it is said. My practice involves helping you find your own perfection. I look at you, listen to you, feel what you feel, and suggest herbs. Your experience requires using the herbs correctly while paying attention to their energetic effects. If you don't learn to observe yourself and others carefully, you can never know how herbs help you.

Over the years I've met countless people who have opened their minds and hearts to the healing ways of Nature. Whether in hospitals, jungle huts, or mansions, they have become friends. I've watched in awe as they've revealed themselves in a hundred ways, and I have learned something from every one of them.

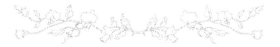

EATING
DISORDERS

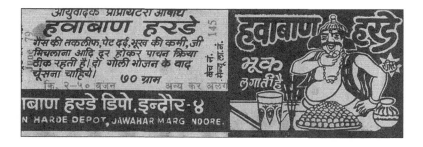

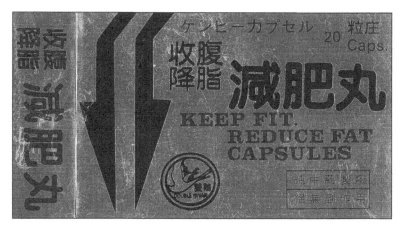

殼氣 殼氣 殼氣 殼氣 殼氣 殼氣 殼氣 水殼之氣 水殼之氣 水殼之氣 水殼之氣

[qǔqì]

Food energy

[shuǐgǔ zhī qì]

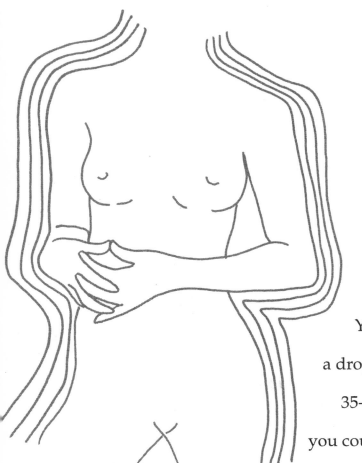

14
An Asian Approach to Weight Loss

"Is It Fat Yet?"

You may be twenty-five without

a drop of cellulite. You may measure

35-24-34 and be a gym fanatic, but

you could still have a weight problem.

You may have given up smoking cigarettes

and drink only one cup of coffee a day, or take ginseng and

lots of vitamins, but there's more to becoming fat than you know.

In short, you may not be aware that age, physical weakness, stress, and poor diet can set you up for weight gain later. I call it "potential fat." It's not only a result of the calories you eat, but also of how well your body uses them.

Energy is the basis of good health. When adequate, it fuels metabolism so that food is transformed into energy and blood instead of waste. But when *chi* is deficient, digestion and elimination are poor, and we retain water and accumulate phlegm, fat, and cysts.

STAMP OUT POTENTIAL FAT!

Sixty million Americans are overweight. Recently, Western medicine has developed new drugs to reduce appetite. These only maintain hazardous addictions. What good can come from eating one junk food instead of five or ten? None of them build vitality or beauty. They only maintain weakness, so that the drugs themselves become addictions.

The Asian energetic way to reduce and prevent fat and cellulite is to improve *chi.* We can't see weak *chi* directly, but only its effects: An increase in clothing size corresponds to a decrease in energy. Movement becomes an effort because we feel puffy, slow, and heavy, with a large waistline or global water weight. These three chapters offer a detailed approach to eliminating present and future fat.

The organization of the weight-loss chapters ensures the correct order to follow in dealing with potential and long-term

weight problems: First strengthen the body, then reduce weight. I will provide guideposts to measure your progress.

If you are slim but live a high-stress, fast-paced, coffee, cigarettes, ham sandwiches, and chocolate sort of life, you need to follow the advice in both chapters 15 and 16, dealing respectively with global water retention and poor digestion leading to excess fat.

If, on the other hand, you have a severe or long-standing weight problem accompanied by weakness, you will also need to follow the diets and herbal regimes described in both chapters but should spend a longer time developing strength by using the suggestions in chapter 15.

If you have managed to reduce daily stress and eat a perfect diet (like a gym instructor in Hawaii), but you still get some aggravating water retention around your period time, then follow the advice in chapter 15 if you feel exhausted, or chapter 16 if you crave too many sweets.

How the Asian Approach to Diet Is Different

Some experts advise weight-loss diets that are low in fats; some stress raw foods; others recommend diets high or low in carbohydrates; still others say everything should be done in moderation. All these good-for-everybody diets ignore you as an individual. Although certain foods are accepted as healthful or beneficial for weight loss, your digestion and energy are not like everybody else's. With an Asian approach to weight loss, your optimum diet is determined by traditional diagnosis.

A diet that assumes everyone is the same is part of the Western medical mindset. Ultimately it is product-oriented, not process-oriented. Western nutritionists study digestive acids and enzymes so that they can either supplement or reduce them. Put another way, scientists observe reactions that are easy to quantify. This helps doctors set dosages for medications, and helps drug companies sell pills. With that approach, the outcome—an enzyme, a protein, or whatever—becomes more important than the digestive process. This ultimately suits Big Business: A diet plan that simply stressed eating less, with no product to purchase, would probably never become popular. Who would advertise it?

An Asian medical approach is process-oriented. The difference is that effective weight loss is best achieved not with extreme diets or medicines, but by enhancing energy itself. As we have learned, digestive *chi* varies from person to person. It even varies from time to time in the same person. That is why there is no universal weight-loss diet that works for everyone. The best diet for you strengthens your weak *chi*. In this way, Eastern medicine links digestion with other life processes, such as breathing, circulation, and immune strength, in a holistic perspective.

Another way in which a holistic approach to weight loss is process-oriented is that the activity itself can become an opportunity for self-learning. Our eating habits are part of a bigger picture of our en-

ergy. This becomes clearer when we consider our constitutional type.

EXCESS WEIGHT AND CONSTITUTIONAL TYPES

In chapter 10 you determined your constitutional type among the Five Elements: Fire, Earth, Metal, Water, and Wood. Although your constitutional type indicates tendencies for health problems associated with a particular element or combination of elements, many people suffer from overweight no matter what their element, because of stress, poor diet, and emotional factors.

Chinese medicine views overweight specifically as a sign of weak *chi* of the Water and Earth elements. Therefore, diet is not the only factor to consider when losing weight. It depends upon your constitutional type. I am not saying that we can give up eating a healthy diet. No one loses pounds by eating cookies, but some people need to build strength *before* they can lose weight. Chapters 15 and 16 detail two different approaches geared to the most common causes of overweight, weak *chi* in the Earth and Water elements.

EXCESS WEIGHT AND THE WATER ELEMENT

If you have a weakness in the Water element, you may be one of those people who put on extra pounds when eating nothing at all. You tend to have water retention. You may feel waterlogged and tired before your period or when overworked. Your digestion is poor, and you are prone to allergies, hormone imbalances, or mood swings. You don't need fewer calories as much as you need rebuilding and rest. Herbs can help you do both, so that your digestion and elimination have enough energy to work properly again (see chapter 15).

EXCESS WEIGHT AND THE EARTH ELEMENT

People with weakness in the Earth element often put on extra inches at the waist and hips. If your Earth element is weak, you tend to crave sweets or heavy foods. This makes you suffer from excess phlegm that congests sinuses or results in headaches, abdominal bloating, or stomachaches. Weak Earth leads to cellulite. Blood-sugar problems can make you feel tired or spacey. Even if you are not overweight but tend to feel unhappy, unsettled, and ungrounded, or if you feel weakness or emptiness in your center, your Earth element needs help (see chapter 16).

CHRONIC OBESITY

Long-term stress and imbalance can result in global weakness, hormone imbalances, and chronic obesity. This is more serious than potential fat. It can even be life threatening, because all of the Five Elements become affected. You have to strengthen first Water, then Earth. You can alternate the diet plans in chapters 15 and 16 for a long time—six months or more—so that you strengthen your baseline energy while you lose weight. You will be able to use some of the dieting herbs found in those chapters from now on to ensure weight loss. I have also included several wonderful immune-strengthening herbs in order to build health while reducing.

Even if you have remained overweight for a very long time, it pays to reduce fat and protect yourself from further gain. It is especially true because we all have the potential for weak *chi* and future illness. Many health professionals believe that diet is an important factor in the prevention of heart disease, stroke, and cancer.

THE FIVE TASTES AND EXCESS WEIGHT

An Asian approach to successful weight loss assumes healthy cooking, not starvation diets or appetite-reduction pills. The main thing is to strengthen the body, not weaken it. With carefully chosen foods and herbs, we can stimulate *chi* in order to facilitate strength, good digestion, and elimination. That way fat is treated as a toxin.

In chapter 6 we examined the Five Elements along with their corresponding tastes. Some tastes stimulate the *chi* of internal organs associated with those elements, and other tastes drain or cleanse them. In the following chapters we'll use the flavors most associated with weight loss.

Bitter, sour, and a dash of hot

Bitter, sour, and hot flavors all work together to affect digestion. Hot spices melt toxins, while bitter and sour flavors move them along the path of elimination. These flavors work well together because they stimulate and move stagnant digestive *chi*. Bitter, sour, and hot tastes are cleansing.

However, sweet, oily, and rich foods slow digestive *chi* and the nervous system. They are sedatives. You will always feel more energized after eating a salad made with leafy greens, lemon juice, and radish (bitter, sour, and hot) than after eating creamy, fat, and sweet dishes. Such sedating foods cause us to put on weight because cleansing is impeded.

LONG-TERM EFFECTS

An Asian approach to weight loss is wiser than crash dieting in the long run, because using cleansing and tonifying herbs daily helps the body work better. You will see that certain slimming herbs, when used every day, prevent fat, fatigue, and depression as well as asthma for some people. If you have experienced yo-yo dieting, losing weight only to gain and lose again, you will greatly benefit by continuing your specific weight-loss program after attaining an ideal weight. It will help you stay trim, fit, and young because herbs improve *chi*. Slimming herbs will even help you crave healthier foods because *chi* and food cravings are related: The healthier your *chi*, the healthier your cravings.

Whether you are overweight or only have "potential fat," taking cleansing herbs to reduce *phlegm,* fat, and water retention lowers your risk of serious health problems.

THE GOOD EARTH

When your Earth element is healthy, the stomach, spleen, and pancreas organ systems work smoothly. The resulting good digestion yields energy, blood, and balanced emotions.

But weak Earth *chi* can lead to excess toxins and mucus in the body. According to traditional Chinese doctors, an excess *phlegm* condition (*she*) is the underlying condition in illnesses that can be as varied as parasites, tumors, cysts, or mental disorders. By reducing digestive wastes, we reduce not only an ample waistline, but also the "stagnant digestive *chi*" that leads to cloudy thinking, poor memory, and im-

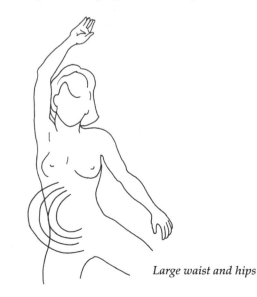

Large waist and hips

paired concentration. It is hard to think clearly while struggling to digest; it is also hard for the heart to beat smoothly and to feel comfortable in our emotional center.

We cannot separate smooth, effective digestion from our production of blood and energy, the basis of immune strength. In other words, poor digestion leads to other problems besides indigestion, bloating, and pain—it slows the whole works.

THE WATER OF LIFE

When our Water element (made up of kidney and adrenal organ functions) can maintain a healthy balance of body fluids, hormones, and brain chemistry, we have good energy, healthy emotions, and immune strength. When the *chi* of our Water element is healthy, we experience fewer extremes in dryness and moisture affecting many parts of the body. With adequate lubrication, our internal organs function

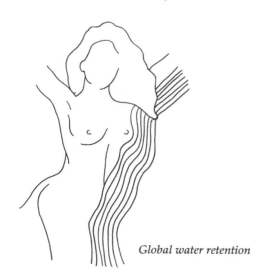

Global water retention

smoothly. With too much water retention, we experience not only excess weight but also the physical and emotional imbalances that accompany hormonal irregularities such as depression and sexual problems. We need enough water to keep us moist, not submerged.

Western doctors and researchers are just now exploring the connections between mind and body. Some scientists, for example, feel that weight problems are part of our genetic heritage or hormone balance, while others maintain that overweight is a result of conditioning. If we accept this explanation only at face value, we deny all the benefits of cleansing, and we maintain the cravings for foods and substances that can drive us to addictions and depression.

Weight gain is only part of a larger energetic picture. To be healthy, strong, and slim, we need healthy *chi,* the energy of metabolism. *Chi* is subtle yet powerful. It permeates our entire being, energizing all that moves. It flows like a river. Where it is dammed, there is friction, heat, and pain. Then it becomes *stagnant* and spoiled. It turns to toxins and fat. There are many means to move *chi* again, including thoughts, herbs, fragrances, and colors. Everything that affects *chi* affects body, mind, and spirit.

TRACKING YOUR PROGRESS

In order to determine your constitutional type for the purpose of weight loss, decide which of these two types most resembles you at the present time.

Global water retention

Global water retention, or chronic puffiness under the eyes or at the ankles, is most often a problem related to weakness affecting the Water element. If this describes you, turn to chapter 15 for diet and herbal advice.

I recommend that you proceed slowly. Before you can possibly lose weight, you must regain your lost strength. It may take several months of building adrenal strength before you lose weight, but by then your new vitality will keep those pounds off. You will also find that the tonic herbs in that chapter lift your spirits.

Large waistline

A large waistline is symptomatic of weakness in Earth. It can indicate long-term low energy from poor eating habits and blood-sugar problems. Chapter 16 presents the approach most suited for your needs because it helps balance sugar cravings and spacey or scattered energy. You will find that taking the slimming herbs covered in that chapter improves dips in your energy level after meals.

Your Diet Journal

You will achieve your ideal weight more easily when you set personal goals. Decide the period of time that you'll spend on your reducing campaign, and set a weekly target amount you can achieve—for example, to lose two pounds a week.

I recommend that you record your progress in a diet journal. Keeping a record of foods you consume, along with times and locations, helps you become aware of hang-ups. For instance, do you always eat cookies while reading the Sunday paper in your favorite chair? If so, it may pay to change not only your diet but also the time and location. On one page of your journal, record your impressions along with the number of pounds you lose each week.

Make sure to pay attention to the five tastes: bitter, sweet, hot, salty, and sour. Note the number and kinds of sweets and oily things you eat each day, because they increase water retention and impede digestion. This will be explained in detail in the next two chapters.

WEIGHT LOSS BY CLEANSING

Cleansing and strengthening is the best way to lose weight. Starving ourselves with extreme methods only damages immunity against illness and depression, while low-fat, high-energy foods, along with cleansing and strengthening herbs, help us look and feel great. Any person with "potential fat" or actual obesity will benefit from the cleansing routine that follows. It includes a basic slimming diet along with herbs and recipes for specific problems. You don't have to feel that this is your diet plan *forever*. I will offer you ways to simplify meals in order to reduce toxins, fat, and cholesterol and help you live longer and better. You may want to use these suggestions to overcome an occasional bout of rich eating.

Discomforts from cleansing

You may experience temporary discomfort from dieting, such as mild diarrhea or frequent urination. Do not be concerned unless it lasts for more than a day or two. If you begin to feel weak, make sure to eat warm, cooked, nourishing foods from among those suggested in the diets.

If you feel discomfort while taking slimming herbs, you might have to change the time of day you take them, or do additional gentle exercise to smooth circulation. It's best to avoid taking diuretic herbs immediately before going to bed.

EMOTIONAL FACTORS AND WEIGHT LOSS

Sometimes emotions are trapped in excess weight. As you cleanse, personal issues may arise for you. While dieting, keep a record of your feelings, memories, and dreams in your journal. You may want to use them in later chapters, because poor digestion and *phlegm* underlie many health problems.

Some people carry extra pounds as a form of protection, to insulate their feelings. They may feel vulnerable losing weight, as if they were shedding an old self. To reverse such feelings, I recommend they mark their progress with a loving contribution. One of my favorites is, for every day I diet, I buy seeds to feed the birds.

Helpful Hints to Lose Weight and Live Longer

- Promise to live longer and better by drinking green tea every day.
- Don't starve yourself—the body naturally responds by slowing metabolism. Instead, eat smaller meals throughout the day, while speeding metabolism and cleansing with herbs.
- Bitter-tasting cleansing herbs reduce the craving for sweets. Eat lots of dandelion and dark leafy greens. For a healthy sweet treat, try bee pollen or royal jelly.
- If you have a phlegm-coated tongue, eat a raw or cooked radish daily. If you have a reddish tongue, chew fennel seeds or licorice sticks. If you have a pale tongue, chew cloves. Or use them as teas.
- Never start the day with cold raw foods or drinks. These weaken digestion and can cause headache and nausea.
- Body fat keeps us warm. In its place, during cold weather wear lots of clothes and have warm, cooked foods and drinks.
- Exercise before you eat. Sweating speeds metabolism. Try to eat no later than one half hour after your gym workout. Drinking cinnamon tea also increases sweating.

15
Lose Pounds by Gaining Strength

Angela sat before me, a mother of five, a former restaurant owner now turned real-estate executive. She had money, love, and acclaim; she owned homes all over. All she wanted was enough energy. She also badly needed to lose about 70 pounds. Years of working hard hours, coupled with big responsibilities, had left her weak but not

176

defeated. When her husband died, she took over the restaurant business single-handed. She flashed a cheerful smile. "I cooked too well," she said, referring to her weight.

I have seen this type of weight problem in a large number of my health clients. I've even created a category for them: "superwoman" or "superman." They have tremendous drive, often working under extreme conditions. By the time they are middle-aged, they have driven themselves with careers, marriages, and life's challenges so that they are too weak to lose weight. Serious illness or difficult childbirth can also produce it. I call this pattern "weak Water element edema."

WEAK WATER ELEMENT EDEMA

Tongue: large, scalloped, pale or red
Figure: global water retention and fat throughout the body
Early warning signs: puffy under the eyes or at the ankles
Energy: low or irregular
Emotions: depression, anxiety, or unrealistic confidence

In this chapter we'll study cures for water retention arising from weakness in the Water element. Early symptoms manifest themselves as puffiness and swelling of the face or ankles. You can see this if your finger leaves an impression when you press the flesh near the ankle. Eventually swelling spreads throughout the entire body. This condition is water retention, also known as *edema.* It happens when stress and exhaustion impedes *chi,* and fat cells become gorged with fluids because the organs of elimination work inefficiently. There may also be weakness, long-term illness, or hormone imbalance.

Often this kind of edema is accompanied by signs of kidney and adrenal gland weakness leading to urinary problems, such as urination that is too frequent or scanty, as well as menstrual irregularities, sexual weakness, and depression. Please check the pertinent statements to see if this type of edema applies to you.

WATER ELEMENT EDEMA CHECKLIST

____ I often crave salty or rich foods and chocolate.

____ When tired, I eat lots of whatever is available.

____ I'm extremely tired in late afternoon or most of the day.

____ I have a swollen tongue.

____ My whole body feels bloated.

____ I can gain weight just thinking about food.

____ Healthful cooking bores me.

____ I'm always up for a challenge but lack energy.

____ I perspire for no apparent reason.

____ I always demand the best from myself.

____ I work or play until I drop.

____ I have always given my all to others.

____ I have an aching, tired lower back.

____ I'm depressed.

____ I often can't fall asleep until early morning.

____ I start the day with strong coffee.

_____ I use cocaine.
_____ My sexual energy is low.

The statements above apply to a personality type that could be described as "Tired Type A." If you checked five or more of these responses, chances are you're overweight or can become overweight because you tend to abuse your adrenal energy.

Stress and Excess Weight

Weak Water element edema is most often related to chronic illness and overwork, precipitating adrenal exhaustion. According to Chinese medical theories, the Water element contains our inherited source of *chi,* or vital energy, and also the foundation of our sexual energy and immune strength. When you think about it, you will probably realize that you crave harmful and fattening foods when tired, depressed, or during premenstrual hormone changes.

One factor often linked to edema is thyroid irregularities. (The thyroid indirectly affects metabolism and heart rhythm.) Thyroid problems have been known to un-

derlie poor concentration and borderline depression. When such far-reaching imbalances occur, it becomes even harder to lose weight, because depressed people easily get trapped in addictive eating habits. But improving *chi* can break the cycle of fatigue, overeating, poor digestion, and depression, leading to addictions.

Health problems related to a weak Water element might include heart trouble, high blood pressure, or immune-threatening disease such as cancer. This is because adrenal energy is indirectly related to circulation (the Fire element) and the production of white blood cells. The bottom line is that reducing weight by strengthening instead of weakening the body can go a long way toward preventing disease.

What to Do About Global Edema
STEP ONE: STRENGTHEN

If you have excess water retention in the face or the entire body, it is wise to start a weight-loss program with herbs that build kidney and adrenal *chi.* Such stimulant

Key to Step One
Tongue tends to be large, possibly with scallops around edges

	USE	SLIMMING TEAS
PALE TONGUE	*warming* stimulants clove	Bojenmi or The Well-Known Tea for all categories
RED TONGUE	*cooling* cleansers	
PHLEGM-COATED TONGUE	*drying* tonics	(add 1 sliced radish)

herbs will give you energy to lose weight. You will soon feel added vigor in late afternoons or when climbing stairs. You will also have more drive to push away pies and rich sauces. By strengthening detoxification, we eliminate many problems of weak *chi*. Stimulant herbs are not in themselves weight-loss herbs, but you can't lose weight without them. They give you the strength to cleanse. It is best to take adrenal stimulant herbs between meals for added vitality, because they do not directly speed digestion.

According to your tongue

PALE TONGUE

Use: *warming* adrenal stimulant herbs
Flavors: hot and sweet
Add clove powder to slimming teas
Herbs: Sexoton

If you have edema along with a pale tongue and low energy, use clove, a *heating* adrenal stimulant. One dash of this popular cooking spice added to a cup of boiling water makes a spicy, delicious tea. Clove warms adrenal and lung *chi* to counter fatigue, shortness of breath, and asthma with watery phlegm and wheezing.

You know clove is the right spice for you if, the minute you drink a sip of this tea, you feel wonderfully energized and can breathe better. If it makes you feel too hot, thirsty, or nervous, it is too *heating* for you. You need to drink fennel seed tea instead, while reviewing chapter 11.

Another possible adrenal stimulant is damiana, available in capsules at health-

food stores. It is less *heating* than cloves. Start taking one capsule a day, then increase the dosage to three to six a day as it feels comfortable.

If you prefer pills, two Chinese patent remedies, available by mail order from addresses in the Herbal Access appendix, can be used instead. They are **Sexoton** and **Ping Chuan Wan.** Either formula builds *chi* for the Water element and is useful for fatigue, shortness of breath, and asthma. Start by taking five pills of either remedy, three times daily between meals. Observe your improved energy and continue taking the remedy as you monitor changes in your tongue.

RED TONGUE

Use: *cooling,* cleansing foods and herbs, laxatives
Flavors: bitter, sour
Add fennel seeds to **slimming teas**
Herbs: 10–12 capsules of dandelion daily

If you have a dry, red tongue or dark urine, do not use *heating* stimulants. Instead, eat a bowl of Four Ingredient Barley Soup (page 184) along with a tea made from cilantro leaves. Cilantro and fennel seeds are both *cooling,* stimulant herbs. Fennel seeds are somewhat laxative, while cilantro increases urination. Either one makes a tasty daytime tea.

Other teas for water retention with a red tongue are dandelion (herb or capsules) and teas made by boiling cornsilk or corncobs. These are usually considered weeds and garbage, but they provide safe and effective stimulation to the liver and kidneys. When taking such stimulant cleansers, take a dosage that is effective to increase urination and movements, but avoid severe diarrhea. For example, take 6 to 12 capsules daily of dandelion or a maximum of 3 cups of cornsilk tea. If you start to cleanse too much to be comfortable, cut back the dose.

IF YOU ARE EXTREMELY WEAK OR SICK

Use: *chi* tonic herbs
Flavors: bitter, sweet, hot, salty, sour
Add: astragalus powder to tea or soup
Herbs: Shen Qi Da Bu Wan

Clove can help regain your strength if your weakness lies in the Water element, especially in the adrenal glands. This is good for temporary fatigue. But some people are chronically exhausted by long-term illness or low immune strength. They may be troubled by allergies or even life-threatening illness. For them a strongly *heating* stimulant or diuretic may be unwise. In that case I recommend astragalus (in Chinese, *huang qi*). Recommended for preventing and treating cancer in China, it is better known as a *chi* tonic but also has diuretic properties.

Many people with water retention are very weak; astragalus is the best herb for them because it strengthens and builds immunity. Add a teaspoon of astragalus powder to a cup of hot water as tea or in soup two or three times a day. Or drink the delicious liquid extract as a pick-you-up that won't let you down.

A combination made of equal parts of codonopsis root and astragalus root, available in pill form, is called **Shen Qi Da Bu Wan.** Eight pills three times daily are recommended for general debility, fatigue, poor digestion, and blood deficiency. Since these herbs strengthen immune response, they are best taken *before* allergy or cold and flu season strikes, in order to prevent exhaustion, depression, illness, and resulting weight gain.

Signs of improvement

You'll know things are improving because you look and feel better, you're able to think and breathe more clearly, and you might even crave fewer sweets. Your urination will also change as your kidneys and adrenal glands begin to heal. People with *internal cold* (pale tongue) urinate too frequently because of weakness. After they take adrenal-strengthening herbs such as cloves for a while, their urine will turn from clear to pale yellow and will regain a normal frequency—for example, not every twenty minutes. People with *internal heat* (red tongue) don't urinate enough. Their urine tends to be dark and odorous. Drinking cilantro or cornsilk tea will increase urination to reduce water retention.

Eventually a pale tongue should become pinker, and a red tongue should be lighter, without spots or coating. If you develop a coating on the tongue after using the stimulant herbs, it shows that your body is starting to cleanse. This is a good sign. If you tend to have headaches or constipation, take four capsules of dandelion with each cup of clove tea to improve the action of the adrenal stimulant.

How long to take herbal stimulants

You should take herbal tonics for as long as you need them, but when losing excess weight due to weakness, you can take them even longer. The better your energy becomes, the more quickly you will lose weight and keep it off. You should begin taking weight-loss herbs only after your energy has improved from stimulant herbs. For most people, that could take as long as two weeks. Then weight-loss herbs (see page 187) can be taken along with your stimulant herbs to provide a full range of cleansing and building.

How much to lose

When you finally start to lose weight, you should aim to lose no more than three pounds a week. If you have weak kidney *chi*, most of the excess weight is due to water retention. Losing fluids too rapidly will result in weakness (or shock) so that you will not be able to maintain the improvement. Thus, taking the above adrenal stimulants ensures strength but also helps keep weight off.

STEP TWO:
SLIMMING DIET AND HERBS

Key to Step Two
Observe these changes before beginning weight-loss herbs:

- Energy improves.
- Pale tongue becomes slightly more pink.
- Red tongue becomes less dark, dry, and red.

The following is a daily diet plan together with explanations of herbal ingredients and suggestions for useful daily supplements. I have also provided a few examples from my experience.

DAILY PLAN

Start off your day with a pot of hot oolong or green tea, or with a slimming tea such as Bojenmi. Following the directions on the bottle, add one dose each of two homeopathic remedies, kali mur. 6× (potassium chloride) and natrum sulphate 6× (sodium sulphate). They reduce fat and decrease water retention while helping to relieve constipation. Drink 3 or 4 cups of unsweetened tea, then have breakfast. Even if you do not wish to eat breakfast, have some fresh or candied ginger and a twist of lemon with the tea.

During the day, take your herbal stimulant tea or capsules (clove, damiana, or dandelion) as needed.

Take weight-loss pills (see page 186) after meals or one half hour before a gym workout.

Eat at least one bowl per day of Four Ingredient Barley Soup (page 184).

Choose one item in each of the following categories, and have as much of it as you like for each meal.

BREAKFAST OR LUNCH WITH GREEN TEA OR A SLIMMING TEA

- Rye toast, a baked or boiled potato with olive oil, tarragon, sage, or rosemary; add lots of parsley, cumin, and (optional) salt substitute
- Rye toast, steamed asparagus or broccoli, a few blanched almonds or sunflower seeds
- Four Ingredient Barley Soup, with fresh parsley (Optional: add 100-percent egg-white protein powder.)
- Rice cakes, a few sheets of raw nori seaweed, raw tofu with soy sauce, vinegar, lemon juice, parsley, scallions, and sesame seeds
- A can of tuna, sardines, or salmon (packed in springwater), rice cakes, and nori or dulse seaweed
- Two boiled eggs, a dab of mustard, rye toast or sprout bread, green salad
- 100-percent egg-white protein powder in vegetable or pineapple juice (half juice, half water)

LUNCH WITH A SLIMMING TEA OR SPRINGWATER

- Cooked vegetables, grains (barley, millet, quinoa, or basmati rice), salad; candied ginger or lemon
- A fish simmered in lemon juice (no butter); salad or cooked greens with vinaigrette
- Enchiladas with vegetables or beans (no meat or cheese), a mild green sauce; rice, salad; mixed vegetable juice

- A soup of vegetables, chicken, or fish (no cream sauce)

MIDAFTERNOON SNACKS (CHOOSE ONE)

- Sunflower or pumpkin seeds
- Fresh popcorn made with a dash of turmeric and olive oil
- Bee pollen or royal jelly
- Sprout bread; rice cakes; nori seaweed
- Fennel seeds, cinnamon, or cloves (chew or steep as tea)
- Plain or vanilla yogurt (add cumin, coriander, or parsley, not fruit)
- A cup of ginseng tea if you have a large, pale tongue
- Cloves or thyme tea if you have shortness of breath with a pale tongue

Take evening primrose oil and other slimming pills, chromium picolinate, and chickweed capsules, even if you don't eat lunch.

DINNER

Try to eat heavy meals earlier in the day, when you have better energy, and foods that require less digestion later. Eat lightly when fatigued. Choose one of the following, along with a slimming tea:

- Fruit or vegetable salad
- Watercress or spinach soup made with half water, half soy milk
- Pasta cooked with fu ling (see pages 184–85), a nonfat sauce, salad
- Tofu cooked with vegetables (no grains)
- Steamed dandelion greens (add gin-

ger, **Lo Han Kuo Instant Beverage,
Ling Zhi Instant** cube or other healthy
sweetener, lemon, salt, and pepper) ⟩

EVENING
(OPTIONAL: CHOOSE ONE)

- Raw or baked apple
- Steamed spinach with a pinch of turmeric
- Yogurt with turmeric, rose oil, and cumin
- Warm almond milk

How to Make Your Cooking Light

WEIGHT-LOSS INGREDIENTS FROM YOUR KITCHEN

Often there are ingredients in your kitchen
cupboard that can be added to recipes in
order to make them slimming. Several slimming ingredients are explained below,
along with sample recipes.

Diuretics

Make sure to use parsley if you use more
than one diuretic herb per meal, because it
replaces potassium lost in urination. Take
diuretics until oily, dark-colored urine becomes more normal, and dark circles or
puffiness under the eyes is reduced. Add to
cooking:

a pinch of cream of tartar
*up to 1 teaspoon dried juniper berries per
day*

1 teaspoon coriander seeds or cilantro leaf
handfuls of fresh parsley
*fresh corncobs or cornsilk (a tea simmered
at least 20 minutes)*

Cream of tartar (used in meringue
dishes) is used medicinally, one dash to a
glass of water, as a strong laxative and
diuretic cleanser. Made from grape seeds,
it is a folk remedy for the prevention of
cancer.

Other diuretic herbs include capsules
of sarsaparilla and herbal combinations
such as **Cellulite Capsules** by Thera,
which combines the diuretic herbs buchu,
couch grass, cornsilk, hydrangea, uva ursi,
and juniper. Follow directions on the label,
or start with one pill after meals, and then
adjust the dosage.

A special Chinese herbal diuretic

Fu ling is a Chinese medical herb (also
known as poria or hoelen) that is very useful for water retention from weakness. See
a puffy, thickly coated tongue. It is recommended for difficult or painful urination.
Sometimes fu ling comes in thin slices, or is
cut into small squares. Boil one square or a
handful of slices at a time.

This dried white fungus, when boiled
at least one half hour, can be used in making teas, soups, or pasta. Eventually, when
cooked, it can be eaten and has a neutral
taste, a bit like chalk. It cleans toxins that
could turn into stones and cellulite held in
place by water retention. Fu ling is sold in
groceries and herb shops in Chinatown.
(See the Herbal Access appendix.)

RECIPES

ALMOND MILK
One serving

Make almond milk by boiling a handful of peeled almonds a few minutes. Blanching the almonds or soaking them overnight removes excess acid. Discard the water, then whip the almonds in a blender along with one cup each springwater and soy milk. Add a dash of turmeric. Store it in the refrigerator only a day.

FOUR INGREDIENT BARLEY SOUP
Two servings

Traditional Chinese doctors recommend this soup in spring, because the season encourages *she* (*phlegm*). But some people need this soup year-round. To lose excess water weight, eat at least one bowl daily. The original Chinese medical recipe is not eaten for pleasure, so I've added some variations, depending upon your tongue.

½ cup Chinese dried barley
½ cup fu ling
½ cup fox nuts
½ cup Chinese white yam (dioscorea)
½ cup fresh parsley
See spices below

For each serving, use about a handful each of Chinese dried barley, fu ling, fox nuts, and white yam. Simmer these in a glass or ceramic-coated pot until all ingredients are soft, approximately one hour or more. Add fresh parsley, a little salt substitute, and black pepper. You can eat all the ingredients, although they're very bland.

Use spices according to individual tongue diagnosis. If you have a white coating, add *drying* and *heating* spices such as orange peel, cloves, or ginger and pepper to taste. Garnish with sliced radish and parsley. If you have a yellow coating (excess acid), use cumin, coriander, tarragon, and fennel.

WATERCRESS OR SPINACH SOUP
Two servings

½ pound fresh watercress
1 cup soy milk
1 dash cumin powder

Steam the greens until they are tender but still green. Use just enough springwater to cover them. Turn off the heat and whip in a blender with soy milk. Season with a dash of cumin powder and (optional) salt substitute and black pepper.

TWO PASTA RECIPES USING SLIMMING HERBS

SVELTE ITALIAN PASTA
Two servings

1 package pasta
1 handful sliced or 1 square dried fu ling
¼ teaspoon cream of tartar

4 cloves minced garlic
¼ cup Italian extra virgin olive oil
½ cup or more fresh chopped parsley
½ to 1 teaspoon peperoncino
½ teaspoon cumin powder

Cook the pasta *al dente,* adding either a piece of fu ling or a big pinch of cream of tartar. While the pasta is cooking, steam the minced garlic in a little water. When the garlic is soft, turn off the heat and add the oil.

Toss the pasta while it's hot with the garlic oil, chopped parsley, and dried hot red pepper called *peperoncino.* (Neither slimming herb will change the taste of the pasta. After cooking, keep the fu ling aside for a second use.) This recipe is spicy, so you can use little or no pepper and add cumin, a *cooling* digestive spice.

SLIMMING SESAME NOODLES
Two servings

1 package pasta
1 tea bag Bojenmi Chinese slimming tea
½ teaspoon cream of tartar
¼ cup hummus beaten with ¼ cup water
¼ teaspoon salt substitute
⅛ teaspoon fresh black pepper
¼ teaspoon turmeric powder
2 tablespoons raw sesame seeds
½ cup chopped fresh parsley

Boil the pasta as you would ordinarily, but add a bag of Chinese slimming tea during the last few minutes. (Bojenmi is so mild in flavor it will not change the taste of the pasta.) I also add a big dash of cream of tartar to the cooking water.

Thin the hummus with water. Whip the mixture until it's light. Add to it black pepper and salt substitute, also a big pinch each of turmeric and cream of tartar. Garnish with sesame seeds and chopped parsley.

SEAWEEDS FOR SLIMMING

An underactive thyroid can encourage water retention, leading to excess weight and cellulite. Low thyroid function has recently been linked with lethargy and depression. If you tend to have slow digestion and elimination, excess catarrh, or sinus trouble, and generally feel down in the dumps during humid weather, seaweeds high in potassium, calcium, and iodine are for you.

For example, laminaria and sargassum are seaweeds that reduce cellulite by stimulating the thyroid gland. They reduce lumps and sticky phlegm in the throat while providing needed minerals. Packages of these edible seaweeds found in Chinese grocery stores are most often identified only in Chinese characters. The seaweed must be carefully washed to get rid of little shells and sand. Steamed, laminaria makes a nice addition to rice or vegetable dishes, but sargassum is a bit like tough string.

Laminaria and sargassum, along with two seashells high in calcium, come in a pill form called **Laminaria 4,** made by Seven Forests and sold by Health Concerns in Oakland, California. The seaweeds are slightly diuretic and reduce cellulite. Ask your health-food store to order it for you.

Kelp, used in salt substitutes, also stimulates the thyroid. If you crave salty foods but find that they cause water retention, try dulse. It is a great source of potassium, which speeds metabolism, increases oxygen levels in the brain, and is an important anti-aging food. Here's how you can use it:

A MODEL
VEGETABLE SOUP

Once a beautiful world-class model consulted me. I'd admired her photos on the sides of buses as they passed, on the covers of fashion magazines, and in clothes ads. Her large, sensuous lips and blond hair were her high-fashion trademark. The pouty smile and graceful eyebrows I'd seen in print gave me no indication of her height. I gazed up at her. She was a giant Venus, a millionairess in her teens.

She wanted to lose ten pounds of baby fat. Her profession demanded slimness beyond the ordinary. Her weight-loss routine would have to be nourishing and energizing, while reducing water retention. She accumulated extra water weight before her period, and it made her feel sluggish and puffy. I suggested a vegetable soup to which she'd add seaweed. Here's a recipe for about 6 servings.

5 pounds raw vegetables
¾ cup raw peanuts

1 cup dried slices or 3 squares fu ling
2 tablespoons juniper berries
1 tablespoon fennel seeds
½ teaspoon cumin seeds
1 tablespoon coriander seeds
1 teaspoon salt substitute
⅛ teaspoon black pepper
Chopped fresh parsley
Hungarian paprika
½ cup dried dulse seaweed

Use lots of vegetables of all colors, including carrots, onions, white potatoes, spinach, yellow squash, green beans, and peas. Avoid turnips and cabbage, because they slow metabolism. Add raw peanuts for protein. Add fu ling, juniper berries, fennel, cumin, and coriander seeds to speed digestion. Season and simmer in springwater until done (approximately one half hour). Then add fresh parsley and Hungarian paprika to taste.

Serve warm or cold along with leaves of dried dulse, which provide a pleasant salty taste and are a rich source of potassium.

For variety and to increase the slimming power, cook this using Four Ingredient Barley Soup as a stock.

WEIGHT-LOSS PILLS THAT REDUCE WATER RETENTION

Most Asian weight-loss formulas are a balanced blend of energy- and blood-building herbs, because we need both in order to be

GLOBAL WATER RETENTION

What makes it worse?

Overwork, caffeine, jet lag, chronic illness, thyroid weakness, hormone imbalance, allergies, and hard-to-digest foods.

What makes it better?

Rest, herbs, and foods that support and rebuild kidneys and adrenal glands.

	HEAT SYMPTOMS	*COLD* SYMPTOMS	*PHLEGM* SYMPTOMS
TONGUE	red, swollen excessive hunger or thirst	pale, swollen	phlegm coating
URINE	dark, oily	frequent urination, clear, bubbly	foamy, flaky
REMEDIES	kidney and adrenal tonics dandelion	clove or astragalus	**Laminaria 4** dulse

Weight-loss herbs and supplements for all categories: evening primrose, chromium picolinate with vitamin B_6. Diuretics for all categories: fu ling, astragalus, juniper berry, cilantro, dulse, **Alisma 16, Cellulite Tablets, Laminaria 4.**

healthy. Such herbal combinations are always safer to take than single herbs because they are formulated to maintain good health. For that reason they are safe enough to be taken not only as long-term remedies, but for prevention. You'll benefit from increased energy and a better mood. As you continue cleansing, cravings for fattening foods will be reduced because they are a sign of imbalance.

The following pills reduce water retention with diuretic action and generally tone the system. Choose one herbal combination, although if you have severe chronic obesity, you will want to combine several herbal remedies at once. For example, **Alisma 16** from this chapter and **Shen Chu 16** from the next chapter are often used together. Evening primrose oil and chromium picolinate are beneficial for everyone, and can be combined with any herbal slimming remedy. Normally you can take them with one of the following remedies. There are directions and dosages in English on the bottle. Your health-food store can order them.

Alisma 16, made by Seven Forests Products, is named for alisma plantago, a diuretic. You can tell when it is best to use it if the tongue is swollen, with tooth impressions at the border and a moist coating. This combination of herbs reduces weight by reducing moisture retention. It is used for edema, digestive disturbance, joint swelling, headaches, diarrhea, urinary tract irritations, pain in the limbs, and prostate swelling. Useful for hypothyroid conditions, it contains alisma, fu ling, polyporus, atractylodes, cinnamon twig, morus bark, ginger, areca seed, magnolia bark, stephania, akebia, pinellia, citrus, astragalus, chaenomeies, and licorice.

Keep Fit Reduce Obesity Pills, from Taiwan, are available in grocery and herb shops in Chinatowns across America. The formula contains blood-builders such as tang kuei and Siberian ginseng to stimulate metabolism for an energy boost that burns fat. It gives a lift to persons who are too tired to digest.

Cellulite Tablets, made by Thera, contain diuretic herbs along with rose hips, iron, and potassium. The formula also has kelp and lecithin to digest fats.

Evening primrose oil, taken in capsule form along with vitamin B$_6$, is said to reduce cholesterol and excess weight in persons who do not process fats effectively. Although it may be most useful for persons with weak digestion, I can think of no reason to avoid taking it. It will also benefit those with weak adrenal strength.

A Word to the Wise

The low-fat, low-sweets diet we've outlined in this chapter, along with herbal pills to reduce water retention and increase adrenal strength, will benefit persons with weakness in the Water element. But to make the most progress in weight-loss programs, remember that you also need to develop some wisdom about *chi:* you must understand that your vital energy affects your weight. Doing gentle daily exercise while eating fewer rich foods may help a great deal; however, overuse of draining stimulants such as caffeine, combined with late hours and overwork, weakens *chi.* With weak *chi* we suffer exhaustion and depression, and we crave unhealthy foods, so that it becomes impossible for us to lose weight. For chronic overweight, we must first strengthen energy.

In the next chapter we'll cover the causes of fat localized at the waist and hips stemming from weakness in the Earth element.

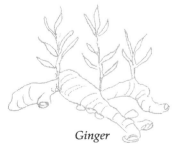

Ginger

氣滯血瘀　氣滯血瘀　氣滯血瘀　氣滯血瘀　氣滯血瘀　氣滯血瘀　氣滯血瘀

[pí wéi shēnghuà zhī yuán] The spleen is the source of nutrients for growth and development, since it has the functions of digestion, assimilation, transportation, and distribution of nutrients.

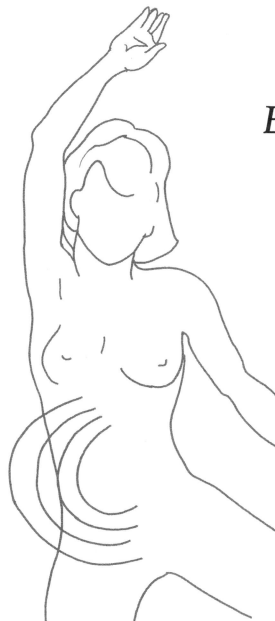

16
Eat Right to Keep Fit

It had been ten years since I'd seen Paris. After a sentimental tour of neighborhoods where I'd lived, I saw tourist town. The Champs-Élysées, Marais, and the Eiffel Tower were all wonderfully the same, I reflected that evening, while admiring rococo cherubs dancing in a kitsch sky. I'd decided to dine at Le Train Bleu, one of that city's high-class *restaurants, before taking the overnight train to Nice.*

Snooty waiters flitted past, carrying trays of rich delights, sweets, wines, everything absent from my usual menu. Sometimes I like to take a vacation from myself; forget health habits and splurge—within reason, of course— on a dinner of many courses. That night it was salmon mousse, baked fish, a salad of delicate white asparagus tips, and wine. Just as I was contemplating dessert, I looked up from the menu at a commotion nearby.

A man directly opposite me, wearing a dark suit and apparently in the middle of a business dinner with another man, turned as red as a beet and fell forward onto the table—a heart attack. The waiters came flapping white linen towels while others carried him away, a victim of cholesterol and chronic stress.

I immediately rethought my dessert decision and soon afterward fled. Perhaps it was the weather, but I felt content chewing raw carrots, cucumbers, or apples and bran flakes for a while after that.

This chapter covers excess weight that originates from too many unhealthy fats and sweets and ends up as a spare tire if you're lucky, or a trip to the hospital if you're not.

WEAK EARTH ELEMENT "SPARE TIRE"

Tongue: puffy, large, possibly coated, spotted

Figure: bloated abdomen, cellulite at waist and hips

Early warning signs: sweet craving, indigestion, stomachache, diarrhea, or constipation

Energy: fatigue after eating, poor concentration when hungry

Emotions: depressed, obsessive, or chronic worrying

Some persons who are otherwise slim have a large waistline that indicates poor functioning of several digestive organs. The waistline is the center of *chi* affecting the liver, gallbladder, stomach, and spleen/pancreas organ systems. If we are fit, it is likely that our digestive *chi* is sufficient and working smoothly. But bloating, indigestion, and abdominal pain are warning signals that something is wrong.

Persons with local excess weight from poor digestion often have a tongue covered with a gray, yellow, or brown coating, which indicates toxins in the digestive tract. They need to use pungent digestive spices as well as detoxifying laxatives and diuretics in order to move stuck *chi* affecting both Wood and Earth elements. Traditional herbal combinations that treat indigestion often contain a variety of such herbs. For example, they may combine herbs that increase bile and stomach acid for indigestion along with others that reduce fat and cholesterol. Such combinations are slimming because they result in less fat and bloating.

In the previous chapter we used teas and herbal tonics to treat exhaustion, an important underlying factor causing unhealthy food cravings and overweight; here we'll strengthen digestive processes and reduce fattening foods. In treating long-term overweight we need both steps, strengthening *chi* and then cleansing to build health from deep problems to more superficial ones.

Do you have weak or stuck digestion? Check the responses below that apply.

WEAK EARTH ELEMENT

_____ I love sweets, desserts, ice cream, and cheese.

_____ I feel bloated or get a stomachache after eating.

_____ I often have flatulence.

_____ My energy is low after meals. I take an afternoon nap.

_____ I have lots of mucus.

_____ I eat on the run, or I eat junk foods.

_____ I enjoy sweets and fruits every day.

_____ I use lots of butter.

_____ I worry about people, problems, or money all the time.

_____ I often have diarrhea or constipation.

_____ Rich or milky foods nauseate me.

_____ I have pain under my ribs.

_____ I often feel anxious, irritable, or depressed.

_____ Pasta and bread are my addictions.

_____ I'd rather buy new clothes than an exercise machine.

_____ I'd rather take a gourmet vacation than go hiking.

_____ My work and hobbies involve sitting and fussing over details.

Did you check five or more responses? Chances are you eat on the run, too lavishly, or too late at night, you crave sweets and fats, and you suffer indigestion from excess phlegm in the digestive tract.

"Potential fat" or excess weight resulting from a troubled Earth element involves blood-sugar imbalances and addictive cravings. All sweet, rich, creamy, or phlegm-producing foods and beer maintain the imbalance by slowing digestion.

Are You an Emotional Eater?

"Retention," or emotional satisfaction from eating, is the dynamic for a weak Earth element more than for a weak Water element; in the latter, hunger is motivated by exhaustion. Weak-Earth-element people often eat to satisfy psychological needs. They literally want to feel good in their center. Food becomes an important way to achieve emotional grounding and satisfaction, a way of dealing with worry, boredom, or loneliness. Because of this, they are prone to food addictions. These people are known as emotional eaters. Are you one?

_____ I eat more when I'm alone.

_____ I eat when I'm upset or nervous.

_____ When depressed, I eat chocolate, cheesecake, or milk.

_____ I always eat too much on holidays or at family gatherings.

_____ Eating keeps me calm.

_____ I hate having an empty stomach.

_____ When dining out, I always pick the most expensive dish.

_____ When hungry, I get angry or upset.

_____ I treat myself to sweets daily.

_____ Before my period, I devour things I usually don't eat.

_____ Milk or ice cream calms me.

What to Do About Weak Earth Element Spare Tire

KEY TO STEP ONE

TONGUE SHAPE FOR WEAK EARTH	puffy, large in the center, spots		
HERBS TO USE	digestive stimulants, and laxatives for all tongues		
TONGUE COLORS	pale	red	phlegm-coated
HERB FLAVORS	hot, sour	bitter, sour	hot, bitter, sour
HERBS OR SUPPLEMENTS	hawthorn	evening primrose oil, aloe	chickweed, chromium picolinate
SLIMMING TEAS (see chapter 5)	Bojenmi	The Well-Known Tea, add aloe	Bojenmi
ACHIEVING BALANCE (see chapter 13)	section I	section II	section I

Did you check three or more? If you reach for food as comfort, you may be an "emotional eater." The error in this is that, in trying to eat troubles away, we get sick. It may be a far better idea to take something to soothe emotional upset directly. For example, a teaspoon of **Wuchaseng** (a Chinese form of Siberian ginseng extract) eases tension and insomnia so that the underlying upset is lessened. Another useful remedy for people addicted to creamy sweets is homeopathic pulsatilla. Taken as directed between meals, it relieves excess sinus congestion and eases sadness and crying. This, unfortunately, is not enough to lose weight. We need to enhance digestion as well. If it goes unaddressed, unwise eating of congesting fats and sweets creates a quagmire of illness.

Health problems related to the weak Earth element might include hiatal hernia, ulcers, blood-sugar imbalances, or heart trouble resulting from poor circulation and excess cholesterol. The bottom line is that eating right improves our energy and chances for health.

How to Proceed

STEP ONE: LOOK AT YOUR TONGUE AND ACT ACCORDINGLY

Your tongue color and texture will visibly improve as you eat foods that facilitate digestion. But not everyone's metabolism is alike. For example, some weight-loss pills containing *heating, drying* stimulants such as ma huang have been known to make certain people feel great and others ill. (It's too *heating*.) Your tongue can show you what kind of digestive stimulant works best for you.

The pale tongue

Use: *warming, drying* foods and stimulant herbs, laxatives
Flavors: pungent, sour
Add: fresh ginger and lemon to slimming teas
Herbs: 1 hawthorn berry capsule three times daily (after meals)

If you have a pale tongue, you need to warm your *chi* with the antiphlegm cleansing diet in chapter 13. Remember to stimulate digestion the first thing in the morning with a cup or two of hot slimming tea, adding a slice of fresh ginger and lemon juice. One capsule of hawthorn berries, taken after meals, helps reduce cholesterol, eases digestion, and strengthens your heart so that you will not feel sleepy after eating.

Vigorous daily exercise and an occasional trip to the sauna or a massage with corn oil will help speed metabolism. This will eventually make the overly pale tongue more pink and less coated.

The red tongue

Use: *cooling,* cleansing foods and herbs, laxatives
Flavors: bitter, sour
Add: aloe vera to slimming teas (enough to be laxative)

Herbs: dandelion, **Shu Gan Wan,** Earth Slimming Soup (see below)

If you have a reddish tongue, you need to cleanse while reducing your sweet cravings with the anti-inflammation diet in chapter 13. Eating daily meals of Earth Slimming Soup, and adding *cooling* herbs such as aloe vera to slimming teas, will reduce toxins, inflammation, and excess weight by cleansing. In time, the overly red or dark-coated tongue will become pink, moist, and clear of spots, cracks, ridges, or bald areas.

The Earth Slimming Diet

Research done in the last few years has shown that people can lose weight merely by sniffing certain fragrances. One of the most effective seems to be green apple. Perhaps it's satisfying and calming. Apples do reduce inflammation and *phlegm.* However, we also need to change our eating habits. Before I give you any diet suggestions, please try the following experiment to observe your digestion:

For five consecutive days, sometime in the morning have one teaspoon of flaxseed, olive, or canola oil. I enjoy olive oil and dried Italian herbs on toast. Keep the oils refrigerated to preserve freshness. In the afternoon, have one or more teaspoons of bee pollen as a sweet energy boost. Then, after five days, observe any differences in your eating habits: Do you enjoy this addition of healthy fat and sweet foods? Do you find that you crave your usual fats and sweets less because of them?

I have found that the best way to change your diet is not to drop all of your favorite bad-for-you foods and add new foods all at once. Instead, let your body become accustomed to new tastes by adding the healthy ones gradually.

STEP TWO: A BASELINE SLIMMING DIET

Our aim is not temporarily to relieve symptoms, but to normalize food cravings and reduce bloating and pain while increasing absorption of nutrients and eliminating wastes. We can begin to accomplish this by establishing a baseline diet that is both cleansing and slimming.

No matter what you are currently eating, if you add these powerful cleansing and slimming ingredients to your meals daily, you will begin to lose weight: two cups of Earth Slimming Soup Stock and a thermos of slimming tea. Otherwise, you can be guided by the daily diet plan in chapter 15. If you still suffer from excess hunger, add one quarter cup of aloe vera gel to green or slimming teas.

EARTH SLIMMING SOUP STOCK
Approx. eight servings

You can cook a large pot of this mild-tasting stock, refrigerate it, and simmer raw soup ingredients in two cups of it daily, or cook grains with the liquid. To mail-order herbs, see the Herbal Access appendix.

1 cup Chinese pinellia
5 sticks magnolia bark
1 piece chen pi (dried citrus peel)
*1 handful dried sliced licorice root or 1
    level teaspoon dried licorice powder*
1 teaspoon sliced raw ginger

Simmer all ingredients in a ceramic-coated pot in one gallon springwater for about an hour, or until the pinellia is soft. The magnolia bark is very bitter, to stimulate the flow of bile. You can sweeten the stock with fennel seeds or other *cooling* sweeteners.

SLIMMING TEAS

Chinese slimming teas help balance blood sugar and are mildly diuretic and laxative, which eliminates toxins. Their bitter taste reduces cravings for sweet and oily foods. They contain little or no caffeine, but are sometimes effective enough to reduce excess weight without further dieting (see chapter 5). Start with one cup daily, then increase it as needed.

The Well-Known Tea contains fu ling, hawthorn, gentian, tangerine peel, and oolong tea. Fu ling, a diuretic, reduces water retention. Hawthorn fruit reduces cholesterol and blood lipids while strengthening the heart. Dried tangerine peel reduces phlegm. Together they combine the energetic properties of bitter, sour, and pungent tastes while being stimulant and *drying.*

Another famous slimming tea is Bojenmi. Its ingredients and action are much the same. Both teas are said to remove atherosclerotic plaque. Such Chinese slimming teas give an energy boost to people who suffer from slow digestion. Bojenmi is light, bitter, and bracing. Its aroma reminds me of Hong Kong on a rainy day.

Take a thermos of Chinese slimming tea to work and encourage the whole office to drink it. Its anticholesterol properties can help reduce the toll of our nation's greatest killer, heart disease. Caution: Overuse of hawthorn can irritate the stomach or cause nervousness.

STEP THREE: HEALTHY SUBSTITUTES

One way to turn fat into muscle is to substitute healthy fats and sweets for unhealthy ones. Avoid butter, cheese, fried foods, pastries, and cream sauces, especially during humid weather, because sweet and oily foods slow digestion.

Healthy fats

The following recipes use pungent, bitter, and sour herbs to speed cleansing. I like to use them as a substitute for butter.

SLIMMING SALAD DRESSINGS

Adding liver-cleansing herbs to oil-and-vinegar salad dressings turns them into healing remedies with a certain zing. To a bottle of canola or olive oil, add 1 teaspoon minced garlic.

You can make a stimulating herbal extract by adding one teaspoon diced orange peel and a handful of fresh tarragon herb to a bottle of balsamic vinegar. The oil and vinegar will be ready to use in two weeks. I like to use such digestive salad dressings on toast or over steamed vegetables whenever possible.

BASIC SEED BUTTER
Eight-ounce serving

Here is another useful butter substitute I dab on vegetables, baked potatoes, toast, or pasta. It's a tangy sauce made with powerful herbal cleansers. This seed butter is different every time I make it, depending on the ingredients at hand, but the basic recipe includes two strongly detoxifying ingredients, pumpkin seeds and garlic.

½ pound raw pumpkin seeds
1 heaping teaspoon minced garlic
½ lemon
¼ teaspoon salt substitute
⅛ teaspoon black pepper
½ cup fresh parsley
1 small red onion
1 teaspoon dried orange peel
2 tablespoons balsamic vinegar
3 tablespoons extra-virgin olive oil
Optional: 1 tiny dash asafoetida powder

Blend the first nine ingredients gradually in a food processor, adding enough water to make a light paste. Then slowly pour in the olive oil for richness. It can be used immediately, but tastes better after being stored in an airtight jar in the refrigerator for about three days.

SLIMMING FLAVORS: PUNGENT, BITTER, AND SOUR

Pungent, bitter, and sour foods and spices make digestion smoother, preventing the full feeling, pain, and lumps that can result from poor circulation and digestive wastes.

Pungent foods include radish, pepper, and hot spices.

Bitter greens

Laxative, stimulant, *cooling,* and cleansing, bitter greens offer a refreshing lift after rich meals. For example, dandelion leaves in a salad, or roasted dandelion root as a coffee substitute, cleanses the liver. Other bitter salad greens, including chicory and endive, are rich in vitamins, yet slimming.

Sour foods

Slimming sour foods include rhubarb, grapefruit, lemon, and naturally fermented pickles. Here is a recipe using lemon juice as a butter substitute.

SLIMMING FISH
Four servings

4 six-ounce skinless fillets of salmon
2 tablespoons fresh lemon juice
2 tablespoons fresh lime juice

3 slices peeled raw ginger
1 chopped scallion
2 tablespoons minced lemon peel
⅛ teaspoon salt substitute
Freshly ground black pepper

Sauce
2 cups fresh cranberries
1 tablespoon fresh orange peel
Juice of ½ orange
⅛ teaspoon clove powder
¼ teaspoon fennel seeds

2 fresh rosemary sprigs, for garnish

Steam fillets of salmon for about 10 minutes in a glass pot with lemon and lime juice, raw ginger, scallion, lemon peel, salt, and pepper.

The sauce: Bring all ingredients to a boil, turn off the heat, and let stand 5 minutes. Garnish the dish with fresh rosemary sprigs. Serve the fish with boiled small red potatoes and lots of fresh parsley.

HEALTHY SWEETS

If you have a serious sweet tooth, you might have acquired it very young. Perhaps it demands foods you've grown accustomed to as a comforting treat. Be gentle with yourself when changing old habits.

Make sure to take the recommended amounts of zinc and chromium picolinate daily to reduce sweet cravings. You can also chew fennel seeds all day if you use sweets to quiet your nerves. You might also start adding these sweet substitutes and watch your tastes change while you lose weight. Chew or brew as tea:

- 🐝 For pale tongue, cloves.
- 🐝 For red tongue, fennel seeds or licorice sticks.

Bee pollen

This food is rich in amino acids, the building blocks of protein. It is more nutritious than steak, milk, or most other protein sources, especially because it is very easy to digest. The bees have already digested it for you. You can enjoy a spoonful of bee pollen or royal jelly anytime without fear of weight gain. Royal jelly is the refined syrup, made from pollen, that is used to feed queen bees. Do not heat either of these, and store opened containers in the refrigerator.

Chinese herbalists combine royal jelly with ginseng to build energy. Chinese ginseng is best used by persons with a pale tongue. This combination is especially useful in the fall and winter, when we need help building immune strength because fatigue and cold weather often make us crave sweets more than usual.

⟨ *Lo Han Kuo with hawthorn* ⟩

This tea and coffee sweetener can double as a sugar substitute in certain recipes. I recommend it especially for weight loss because of the hawthorn. (For more tea sweeteners, see pages 48–50.)

HERBAL PILLS FOR WEAK DIGESTION

Does your work require you to "digest" your words, thoughts, work projects, worries, or other people's problems or money or legal issues? All that sort of "digesting" could weaken your digestion and cause discomfort.

The following digestive remedies are suitable in establishing a baseline digestive comfort. Building from that sort of relief makes it easier to change habits and lose weight. Smooth the digestion first, then take herbs to lose weight. You can use the following pill remedies as directed until stomach pain and upsets subside. Then continue with them from time to time as required, while taking the weight-loss pills on pages 199–201.

CHINESE PATENT REMEDIES

When troubled by abdominal discomfort or obsessive thoughts, it is as though you are trying to digest stuck emotions. Smooth "stuck *chi*" in the abdominal area by taking the following Chinese patent remedies after meals.

Shu Gan Wan increases circulation to ease digestive discomfort. Take 6 to 10 of the small round pills after meals. Doses of Chinese patent remedies tend to be higher than those of health-food store capsules because using the combination of herbs is like eating a dish prepared from several healing foods.

Shu Gan Wan contains cyperus and turmeric, along with herbs for pain (cordalis rhizome) and digestive herbs such as cardamom, bupleurum, and citrus peel.

Another good mealtime remedy is **Xiao Yao Wan,** which, according to traditional Chinese medicine, treats indigestion, poor circulation, hypoglycemia, anxiety, and depression. When taken along with a liver cleanser, **Lung Tan Xie Gan Wan,** the two remedies treat problems of headache, constipation, and anger. Take 6 to 8 pills of each after meals. It is safe to take either or both **Xiao Yao Wan** and **Lung Tan Xie Gan Wan** together as long as needed. The former is *warming,* the latter *cooling.* Watch for improvements in your energy and mood. If you develop diarrhea, you no longer need **Lung Tan Xie Gan Wan.** None of these combinations contains sedative or habit-forming herbs. (Also see chapter 35.)

HERBAL LAXATIVES

Once, in China, I witnessed an interesting acupuncture weight-loss treatment. An obese woman was a frequent patient in the Shanghai hospital where I studied with the chief doctor. Medical costs are minimal in China, so that people come for everyday ailments. The doctor placed four thin needles, one on each side of her navel and above and below it, as well as one at the inside of each ankle. To the four needles at her abdomen he attached wires connected to an electrical device. The gentle motion created by the slight electric current passing through the needles made it look as though the needles were wobbling in a bowl of jelly.

It occurred to me that the treatment increased local muscle tone to stimulate the colon. It was a slimming treatment because it got the fat literally to move. This effect can be duplicated in other ways. Aside from trips to the gym, there is an herbal method: People who are out of shape in the middle can benefit from stimulant laxative herbs to move sluggish digestion.

A stimulant laxative

Do you eat too richly and get little exercise? Do you often eat a heavy meal, then take a nap? A stimulant laxative will speed digestion while it strengthens your muscle tone. My favorite stimulant laxative remedy is cascara sagrada, available in capsules. It tends to have a delayed reaction time ranging from several hours to overnight, and can be taken one capsule at a time after meals or before bed. It works by encouraging peristalsis (natural movement of the intestine) and is very bitter so that it helps normalize liver and gallbladder by increasing bile. I take 2 capsules at bedtime after an evening of rich eating.

A cooling *laxative that quiets hunger*

Drinking aloe vera juice reduces stomach acid and hunger. Its slightly bitter taste and alkaline quality make it *cooling* and refreshing. You can add it to slimming teas. If you use about one quarter cup per day, it becomes laxative. It is also the safest way to reduce hunger. Hunger is not just a matter of time and habit, but of energy, which can be affected by herbs.

Appetite is increased by hot foods and spices such as ginger, pepper, cardamom, anise, caraway, and garlic, because they stimulate acids and enzymes (digestive *chi*). Many times, what we experience as hunger is just excess acid or nervous irritability. We then eat to settle our nerves or quiet a hunger we have *created* with spicy cooking. We can even make ourselves emotional eaters with too much spice.

To reduce gnawing hunger, use *cooling* spices such as cumin, dill, mint, and fennel in cooking or as tea. Look at your tongue. If it is reddish, cut out all pungent foods and spices, and use aloe vera daily. If it has a thick greasy or gray coating, boil a square piece of fu ling for at least twenty minutes and use the liquid to make tea.

MODERN CHINESE HERBAL COMBINATIONS

Herb combinations using Chinese formulas have become widely available. They ease pain and help eliminate that sluggish feeling that accompanies poor digestion. They also reduce unhealthy cholesterol and are safe for long-term use when taken as directed on the package.

CHINESE MAIL-ORDER REMEDIES

Your health-food store or herbalist can obtain these from distributors listed in the Herbal Access appendix. **Shen Chu 16,** a Seven Forests herbal combination, is often combined with **Alisma 16** for obesity. It treats eating disorders and abdominal bloating by speeding digestion and resolving *phlegm* conditions. It is therefore useful for "weakness in the Earth element." This modern combination of Chinese herbs has its origin in three classical patent remedies: **Curing Pills, Zisheng Stomachic Pills,** and **Finseng Stomach Combination.**

Shen Chu 16 contains shen chu, crataegus, fu ling, pogostemon, malt, magnolia bark, saussurea, citrus, pinellia, codonopsis, atractylodes, cardamom, ginger, raphanus, licorice, and platycodon. The antiphlegm herbs such as fu ling and citrus are useful in the treatment of digestive distress. Herbs such as cardamom, ginger, and crataegus (Latin for hawthorn) treat bloating from food accumulation. The herbs warm the digestion.

Lotus Leaf Tablets is a high-powered formula for weight loss, available from Health Concerns. It reduces cholesterol and trigylcerides while supporting the liver. It contains 20 percent lotus leaf, together with hawthorn (which reduces cholesterol), alisma (a diuretic), he shou wu (a blood-builder) for the liver, and cassia seed for obesity, hyperlipidemia, constipation, and tiredness after meals. This remedy can be combined with other digestive remedies from Health Concerns: for example, with **Salvia Shou Wu** for elevated cholesterol; with **Shen Chu 16** for excess phlegm after meals; and with **Diagnostic Tablets** for long-term bloating, constipation, fatigue, and stress-related indigestion.

Astra Diet Fuel, from Health Concerns, comes in pill form and can be used in conjunction with **Astra Diet Tea** in tea bags. It is a popular weight-loss formula for abdominal bloating and is less diuretic than **Alisma 16. Astra Diet Fuel** contains several blood-builders, tang kuei, peony, and atractylodes, as well as ma huang, an energy stimulant. (*Caution:* Ma huang is ephedra, and can raise blood pressure when used to excess.) It also contains laminaria and sargassum to stimulate the thyroid, and other herbs such as citrus peel, magnolia bark, and ginger to facilitate digestion.

Trim-Plex is one of several weight-loss formulas that use lecithin or evening primrose oil to reduce excess weight and nausea by metabolizing fats. **Trim-Plex,** made by Nature's Plus, is widely available and contains lecithin, kelp, vitamin B_6, and cider vinegar.

Evening Primrose Oil Epo, made by Efamol, contains omega-6 fatty acids, cis-linoleic acid, gamma-linoleic acid, and vitamin E. Like lecithin, it processes fats. When taken regularly, evening primrose oil is known to reduce not only fat but such inflammatory problems as headaches and arthritis.

You will notice that none of these weight-loss pills aims to reduce hunger. Their ingredients do not increase nervousness or emotional imbalances. They all improve digestion and vitality by strengthening, not draining, the body.

We enhance *chi,* our vital energy, with food, sunshine, oxygen, rest, and emotional balance. When digestion is smooth, we are able to transform food into life force. *Chi* promotes digestion; digestion promotes *chi.*

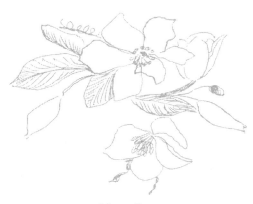

Magnolias

WEAK EARTH SPARE TIRE

What makes it worse?

Fats, butter, fried foods, nuts, tahini, dairy foods, red meats, pork, sweets, pastries, candy, some grains, pasta, sedentary habits, coffee, humidity, afternoon naps, late-night eating, emotional imbalance.

What makes it better?

Salad, bitter-tasting foods, slimming teas and green tea, barley, quinoa, beans, fish, dried fruits, apple, citrus, all vegetables, seeds, rice cakes, seaweeds, tofu, soy milk, wheat bran, healthy oils (canola, olive, flaxseed), bee pollen and royal jelly, plenty of exercise.

HEAT SYMPTOMS	*COLD* SYMPTOMS	*PHLEGM* SYMPTOMS
red tongue, excessive hunger, ulcers, bad breath, hiatal hernia, allergies	pale tongue, cravings for cold or creamy foods, indigestion	phlegm-coated tongue, indigestion, pain, bloating, nausea

All categories strongly crave sweets, especially with fatigue, worry, in cold weather, or from habit.

REMEDIES

RED TONGUE	PALE TONGUE	PHLEGM-COATED TONGUE
fennel seeds	cloves	radish
licorice or cinnamon sticks		

BASELINE DIET

Earth Slimming Soup, slimming teas for all categories

Herbs to speed and ease digestion and elimination

Bitter, sour, and pungent digestive remedies, anticholesterol remedies, laxatives, diuretics

WEIGHT-LOSS HERBS AND SUPPLEMENTS

Evening primrose oil; chromium picolinate; vitamin B_6; lecithin; **Shu Gan Wan** or **Lung Tan Xie Gan Wan** for pain in ribs or abdomen; **Astra Diet, Shen Chu 16,** or **Trim-Plex** for weight loss

PAIN AND INJURY

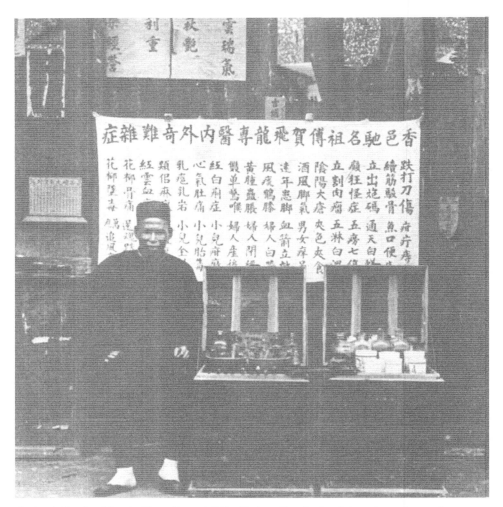

A streetside physician in Hong Kong, 1870, offering stimulants, ointments, and cures for leprosy, dysentery, venereal disease, tuberculosis, and insanity. He also reset bones and removed bullets.

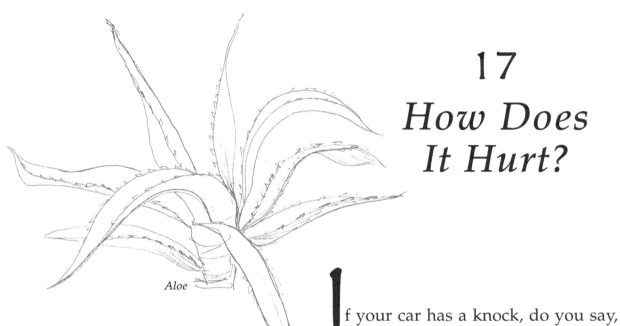

Aloe

17
How Does It Hurt?

If your car has a knock, do you say, "I'll just drive it less," or "Maybe I should drive it slower"? No. You wouldn't "sedate" the trouble; you'd find out what was wrong. Perhaps the fuel is dirty, or the octane too low. We may take splendid care of our cars, but with a headache, a toothache, or other pain, we rarely bother to ask *why* it hurts. Often we just take an aspirin to sedate the problem. But this doesn't really address the *source* of the problem.

Did you ever stop to think that acid foods and meat can cause searing, hot pain? Or that eating cheese can increase dull, heavy aches and stiffness? Or that sweets slow the healing process? Did you ever stop eating hot spices because you found they increased migraines, menstrual cramps, or sciatica? Usually people don't make the connection.

Americans are in pain. According to a June 1, 1993, article in the *Wall Street Journal*, we spend $2.7 billion yearly for painkillers. Many over-the-counter nostrums offer only temporary relief but produce a multitude of side effects. A bad side effect can be a reaction located in the wrong place—when aspirin irritates the stomach, causing ulcers—or one that becomes harmful over a period of time. For example, aspirin's blood-thinning action is useful in some cases, but until now, there have been no studies to determine whether long-term use of blood-thinning drugs can actually weaken immune response or affect fertility. In the view of Asian energetic medicine, long-term use of anti-inflammatory drugs eventually reduces vital energy, affecting metabolism, blood production, and mood.

Does It Burn, Sting, Jab, or Pound?

Asian herbalists take a different approach to treating pain. Their remedies contain analgesic ingredients for the *type* and *location* of the pain. Chinese anatomy and physiology offer a highly developed system for observing the flow of *chi* (and the flow of pain). Herbs are chosen to ease areas most affected by pain. That way a remedy can stop headaches, sinus pain, back pain, or joint aches without dulling concentration. The specific action of herbs is always less damaging than that of anti-inflammatory drugs or brain-numbing medication that affects the entire body. Asian remedies have been safe and effective without side effects for generations.

This chapter will help you recognize types of pain so that you can understand how remedies were chosen in later chapters for arthritis, headaches, and injuries. Understanding the type and location of pain, as well as the choice of painkillers that affect *chi* in proven ways, makes Asian painkillers work so well.

The Internal and External Origins of Pain

To know how to treat pain, you must first understand its origins—both inside and outside the body. Pains resulting from injury come from outside. For example, you may be walking down the street and a runner bashes into you. You may think herbs can't help you. But, as we'll see in the following chapter, herbs can speed healing and reduce pain, bleeding, and bruising from injury.

On the other hand, many pains originate inside the body. For instance, soreness can result from toxins trapped in the body. Dancers and athletes know the stiffness and aches possible after uric acid from eating meat has built up after exercise. This type of muscle discomfort becomes a severe "acid burn" with inadequate oxygen and *chi* circulation. To ease this kind of pain, we must eliminate the acid. Another example is an excessive *phlegm* condition that makes joints ache and head and sinuses feel congested, so that the head pounds and we can't think. To ease this pain, we must eliminate *phlegm*. The trouble with conventional painkillers is that although they temporarily dull discomfort, they allow many underlying toxins to remain.

Pain often comes from stuck *chi* circulation either from trauma or long-term imbalance. Pain is a sign that the smooth circulation of *chi* has been interrupted. This kind of disturbance can be the underlying cause of any malady that is improved by increasing circulation with movement, massage, or a hot bath. What follows is a short exploration of types of pain and their causes.

TYPES OF PAIN

Asian doctors define pain as being either *excess* or *deficient*. This refers not to the severity of the pain, but to its origin. *Excess* refers to pains that come from something extra or unwanted affecting the body, whereas *deficiency* comes from weakness.

Excess *pain*

Excess conditions often originate from outside. For example, cold and flu symptoms are considered *excess*. The pain exists because the body is struggling to eliminate something that should not be there. The symptoms can be hot or cold in nature, but the correct method of treatment is to increase perspiration, to sweat out the pain.

Excess pain can also be due to stuck circulation from internal origins, such as the pain of gallstones. Sharp, stabbing pains are severe and include sciatica, headache, pain from ulcers or hiatal hernia, chest pains, or toothache. In these cases, moving stuck *chi* with herbs that reduce excess inflammation feels soothing and quieting. *Excess* pain feels worse with pressure or massage. It does not want to be touched.

Deficient *pain*

Deficient pain is often accompanied by fatigue or an empty feeling. This pain originates from weakness and feels better with warmth, pressure, and massage, because the person has deficient *chi*. If the discomfort is from temporary stress or a heavy workout, massage can get oxygen to the muscles and joints, relieving pain. But if the condition is chronic, weakness will be profound. The complexion may be pale or sallow, the tongue pale and scalloped, and the pulse slow and deep.

Correct herbal pain remedies increase circulation and warm metabolism to build energy. This not only shortens recovery time after physical exhaustion but also builds resistance to illness.

Deficient pain can be menstrual aches that send you to bed with a hot water bottle, or headaches cured by rest and hot compresses. Sometimes energy becomes so deficient that internal organs slip lower than usual, causing prolapse symptoms. It's that "bottoming out" feeling after childbirth or chronic diarrhea. Certain Asian herbal remedies can lift *chi* and build energy, treating both weakness and pain.

TYPE OF PAIN	EXAMPLE	REQUIRED REMEDY
external *excess*	cold and flu symptoms	increase sweating
internal *excess*	pounding headache	use anti-inflammatory remedies
deficiency, stuck circulation	sciatica after exercise	use tonic herbs that increase circulation
injury, bruising	trauma	use tonic herbs that increase circulation

Excess or *deficient* conditions make circulation worse. In either case, pain is relieved by increasing circulation with *warming* tonics or anti-inflammatory herbs that vitalize the circulation of *chi*. Often flu or allergy remedies, as well as those that address menstrual or digestive pain, contain both *heating* and *cooling* herbs along with herbs that increase circulation. This gets the *chi* flowing—the herbal equivalent of applying hot and cold compresses.

What happens when you use the wrong remedy?

If you use the wrong kind of pain remedy, you might ignore the underlying problem, or even drive the pain deeper to affect internal organs. Here is an example of how taking the wrong remedy makes the pain worse. Nancy has caught a cold but does not know it. She has a headache and stuffed-sinus condition that appeared suddenly (an acute problem). She thinks she is tired or weak (a chronic problem), so she takes garlic or Chinese ginseng, which are *heating* tonics.

The appropriate cold and flu remedy would cause sweating and reduce fever. Instead she has taken foods or herbs that add inflammation without increasing sweating. She has mistaken an acute problem for a chronic one. Her fever and headache become worse. The point is, herbs used for prevention are not always the same as those used for treatment. We will examine this issue further in chapter 30.

THE QUALITY OF PAIN AND REMEDIES

There are different qualities of pain caused by stuck *chi* and toxins. Asian painkillers work by cleansing toxins while increasing circulation, not by dulling the brain and nervous system. The kind of pain is often determined by the type of toxin. For chronic pain, check the tongue.

Phlegm *pain: see a coated tongue*

Dull, heavy pain results from poor circulation and congested *phlegm*—for example, pain that feels better with warmth, movement, or pressure. *Phlegm* can aggravate sinus headaches or allergic headaches after rich food. Such chronic problems can often be cleared by following the antiphlegm cleansing diet outlined in chapter 13.

Remedies for *phlegm*-related pain contain herbs that increase circulation, dry mucus, and clear underlying inflammation and weakness. This approach is especially effective for rheumatoid arthritis, as well as allergic sinus congestions (see chapters 19 and 23).

Phlegm conditions delay the healing of oozing, raw wounds. Slow-healing sores require tonic herbs that move infection out through the surface of the skin. Often such herbs are stimulants, *heating* and *drying* herbs that increase circulation, such as myrrh.

Inflammatory pain: see a red tongue

Hot (inflammatory) pain results from excess acids, nerve stimulation, and other toxins. This type of pain feels better with application of cold or acupuncture. In some cases, hyperactive immune responses lead to skin allergies. Remedies aim to cool inflammation, speed detoxification, move stuck circulation, and, in some cases, build blood and *chi.*

The best prevention for chronic inflammatory pain is a cleansing diet and an herbal regimen like the one described in chapter 13. But herbal remedies for acute inflammatory pain may work as natural

corticosteroid, antispasmodic, antibiotic, anticholesterol, or blood-thinning herbs.

Nerve pain: see a shaking tongue

Neuritis, neuralgia, a shifting pain that travels through the body "like the wind"— all of these describe the sudden electric shock we call nerve pain. It develops into cutting, piercing, or burning pain in drafts, or stiffness and numbness during springtime. Another example is sciatica, a line of inflammation that shoots down your leg. Nerve irritation is aggravated by diet, exhaustion, stimulants, seasonal and food allergies, and tension.

Suitable pain remedies combine herbs that quiet nerve sensitivity, relax tight muscles, build blood, and unlock *chi* and blood circulation. Single herb remedies for nerve pain are often nerve sedatives called *nervines*—for example, valerian or gastrodia. Asian medicine combines gastrodia (tien ma) with other herbs to treat everything from tension headaches to epilepsy. I often take a capsule or two of valerian to settle dizziness and cure a headache after a long flight. An aspirin will not quiet my nerves the way a nervine can.

BE SPECIFIC

Choose a specific remedy for headache or sciatica instead of a general knock-you-out painkiller, because anti-inflammatory drugs can have bad side effects. In the long run they are weakening and make *phlegm* conditions worse because they reduce *chi.*

Whereas antiphlegm remedies can, over a period of time, make nerve pain worse because they irritate, *phlegm* left untreated slows the body's detoxification, inhibiting breathing and digestion or congesting circulation, which encourages stiffness and joint damage.

The best cure for chronic pain addresses not only the pain but also the underlying toxins, irritation, and poor circulation.

Ask ten people what they do for a headache, and nine might say they take aspirin. Perhaps only four of them will have made the right decision.

The next chapter addresses problems associated with injury, pain, bruising, and slow-healing wounds. Most people think of Asian medicine purely as preventive. They might say, "If I were tired or weak, I'd take herbs, but if I had a car accident, I'd use Western medicine." The following chapter may change their minds.

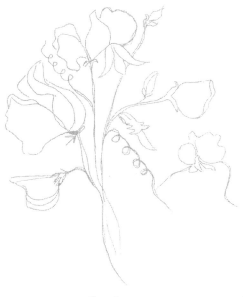

Sweet pea

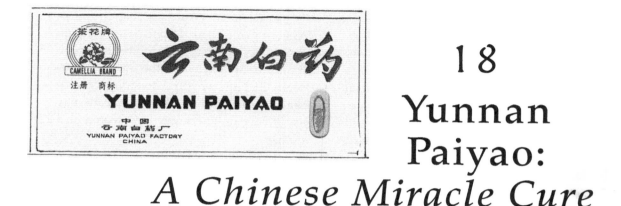

18
Yunnan Paiyao:
A Chinese Miracle Cure

I had just said good-bye to my last client when the phone rang. It was Ashley, but he spoke in such a low voice I could hardly hear him. The music of his Georgia accent was stiff when he asked if I could come to his place right away. He would say no more. The urgency in his voice made me respond. Ashley, a former hippie from Coconut Grove, would never trust a problem to the police when he could reach a friend.

When I got there, he was covered with blood. His long blond hair was wet with it, his white shorts splattered. "I've been mugged," he whispered, gritting his teeth. I was too shocked to cry. I couldn't imagine that he'd been in *a fight. I've never heard him raise his voice. His lanky frame now crouched over, I saw the pathway of a knife wound caught and turned by the chain around his neck. Thank God, it avoided the jugular vein. That afternoon, Ashley had met a moment of fate at the bank. Now blood was soaking his collar.*

*I grabbed a Chinese remedy from my purse, one I always carry with me: **Yunnan Paiyao**. It was a sheet of orange capsules with one small red pill included. I gave Ashley the red pill to swallow. We quickly washed the wound. I then poured the contents of several capsules of the herbal powder directly onto the wound. When we got to the emergency room, we were in luck. A top plastic surgeon was on call. He made a neater scar with many small stitches. Each day, Ashley put more of the same Chinese herbal powder over the stitches and swallowed 12 orange capsules, four at a time between meals. In a week the scar was a thin, light-colored line. The doctor was amazed at the speed with which his repair work had healed. There was none of the usual pain, swelling, and purple bruising. "What miracle has happened?" the doctor asked.*

Even if you are lucky enough to avoid becoming a crime statistic, when you consider the frequency of home and auto accidents, no one is completely safe from traumatic injury. We need a fast, effective way to care for wounds. There have been a number of incredible cases in which victims of attacks or bleeding illnesses have died because doctors could not stop the hemorrhaging or even find the wounds. Patients often die waiting for medical help to arrive, or in the ambulance.

Traditional Chinese medicine offers nothing less than a miracle drug for wounds, pain, and hemorrhage. **Yunnan Paiyao** (Yunnan White Medicine), unlike Western pain drugs, does not turn off pain centers in the brain, but facilitates circulation, bringing oxygen to the injury. It thus forges the body's natural defenses. Considering the $2.7 billion that Americans pay yearly for painkillers, any help would be a miracle.

Extensively used during the Vietnam War years, **Yunnan Paiyao** became a valuable Chinese secret weapon. It quite effectively heals not only gunshot wounds but open cuts and any kind of surgery. It reduces recovery time for surgery by half because it mends injured blood vessels. **Yunnan Paiyao** does not interfere with Western sedative drugs, so it can be used the same day as surgery. By immediately activating blood circulation, it helps resolve bleeding, pain, and swelling. It heals oozing wounds and damaged blood vessels, while expelling pus and counteracting toxins.

The ingredients of **Yunnan Paiyao** powder are still officially secret, although inside sources inform me that the two main herbs are raw and steamed tienchi ginseng. Tienchi ginseng, also called pseudoginseng and sanchi, belongs to the araliaceous family of herbs. According to Li Shih-chen, a famous pharmacologist of the Ming Dynasty (A.D. 1368–1644), its value far exceeded that of gold at that time. It is sold in two powdered forms: raw and steamed. The raw powder is *cooling* and the steamed form is *warming*.

Long-term Use of Raw and Steamed Tienchi Ginseng Powder

Aside from activating circulation to resolve swelling, pain, and blood clots, modern research has found that with long-term use, raw tienchi increases blood flow in the coronary artery, reducing the consumption of oxygen in the myocardium. Raw tienchi lowers arterial pressure and reduces stress on the heart; it can be used to treat angina pectoris from coronary insufficiency. The herb lowers the level of cholesterol in the blood.

The "blood-activating" quality of raw tienchi ginseng makes it an incredible Chinese remedy for conditions ranging from nosebleed to angina. The herb contains saponin A, which strengthens the heart, and flavonoids, which promote circulation. Among my health clients, I have seen raw tienchi successfully reduce bruises from injury as well as heal bleeding gums and colitis.

Steamed tienchi is a *warming,* blood-building, and circulation tonic for anemia, cold extremities, bruises, and irregular menstrual periods with chills and weakness. It is too *heating* for fever, menopause, or inflammation problems.

The combination of raw and steamed tienchi along with other antistagnation herbs makes **Yunnan Paiyao** a balanced and powerful "drug" for pain and injury. The other herbs found in the powder are likely the same as those found in liquid **Yunnan Paiyao.**

LIQUID *YUNNAN PAIYAO*

Yunnan Paiyao Liquor (not a beverage) contains tienchi ginseng, azuga forrestii, dioscorea, chuan shan long, lao guan cao, ku liang jiang, bai niu dan, borneol, and musk. Like the powder, it activates blood circulation, which "disperses blood clots, reduces swelling and eases pain and numbness." Taken internally (3–5 cc per dose) or externally applied with cotton 3 to 5 times a day, it is recommended for "dispersing blood clots [and] easing pain of arthritis, rheumatism and limbering muscles."

DAILY DOSAGES OF TIENCHI

When using tienchi ginseng as a single herb, you have to make sure to use the right one according to your tongue. They are sold clearly labeled as Raw or Steamed.

Use raw tienchi powder if you have a reddish tongue, because it is *cooling.* You can mix ¼ teaspoon in a little cold water twice a day until symptoms improve.

Steamed tienchi ginseng is *warming,* useful as a blood-building tonic for anemic persons with *internal cold* conditions (a pale-colored tongue). You can add steamed tienchi powder to warm tea.

AVAILABILITY AND PACKAGING

All forms of **Yunnan Paiyao** are available in Chinese herb shops and grocery stores, and by mail from the sources listed in the Herbal Access appendix.

Yunnan Paiyao powder comes packaged in a small bottle that contains the loose powder along with a piece of cotton wrapped around a small, round, red pill used for very serious injury. The powder also comes in a more convenient package of sixteen capsules and one red pill.

Yunnan Paiyao Liquor, the liquid form of this remedy, is available in 30 ml bottles with directions in English inside the box.

General Directions for Use

Do not take Yunnan Paiyao during pregnancy. According to the package directions, avoid eating "fava beans, fish, sour or cold foods for twenty-four hours after oral use." Fish seems to interfere with its action. Otherwise you can take it at any time of day or night. Your tongue diagnosis does not matter. This remedy can be taken by anyone, including children. For children, reduce the dosage as directed. (I have also used it for pets injured in car accidents. Pour the powder directly onto the wound and give the red pill or capsule orally.)

DOSAGE

Instructions for use are usually inside the box. Normally, one or two capsules four times a day is the dose for adults, one quarter the adult dose for children two to five years of age, and one half the adult dose for children five to twelve years of age. If you are very weak, take Yunnan Paiyao after meals.

For serious wounds, the red pill can be taken first, with wine, then followed later with capsules. Also take a sip of wine with Yunnan Paiyao if there is no hemorrhage, only bruises and swelling. In case of hemorrhage, take Yunnan Paiyao with lukewarm water, or swallow a red pill.

Some Chinese remedies are taken with wine because that takes the herbs directly to the liver. Circulation is a function of the liver, according to Chinese medical theory. Yunnan Paiyao will still work quite well, however, for persons allergic to alcohol, though they may need to take larger doses in the beginning.

Higher doses and red pills work well during the early stages of injury, while there is still bleeding, oozing, and pain. For that reason I often recommend starting with a higher dose, then reducing it—for example, 1 red pill and 8 capsules daily for two or three days, then only the capsules.

Long-term use (more than three weeks) may leave weak persons feeling a little spacey because so much circulation has been sent to heal the wound. But they quickly recover strength by eating warm cooked food. Try to space the doses throughout the day between meals.

Some Special Instructions and Examples

SURGERY

Immediately before surgery, swallow 1 or 2 red pills; they will neither interfere with anesthesia nor thin the blood. After surgery, for five to eight consecutive days, or until all pain and swelling subside, you can take two capsules three times daily between meals, or the equivalent amount of powder internally.

Even though the directions inside the box say you can take **Yunnan Paiyao** with water or wine, the remedy will also work when swallowed with nothing at all. Here are a couple of examples of how **Yunnan Paiyao** speeded healing after surgery:

A skin graft

I once knew a woman who used **Yunnan Paiyao** after a skin cancer biopsy and skin graft on her nose. She was emotionally paralyzed by the biopsy, fearing loss of beauty more than cancer. Her raving drove her husband crazy for months. All their work stopped, scuttling years of effort. His health suffered, but he remained loyal.

For a week after her biopsy, he cleaned her nose and applied powdered **Yunnan Paiyao** twice daily, which soon stopped the oozing and sealed the small cap of skin at the tip of her nose. Then, to keep the graft softer, he applied pure aloe vera gel for a week, which proved useful for smoothing the color and texture.

She took **Yunnan Paiyao** internally for several weeks. The results were miraculous! There was little swelling; dark bruising disappeared before the bandage was removed; and the skin color became normal. One month after surgery, her doctor was astounded. Normally a biopsy leaves a concave dent in the nose. Instead, hers regained a smoothness closely resembling its original shape and color. The doctor said he had never seen such a rapid recovery.

Facial plastic surgery

Bruising occurs when blood spills into surrounding tissue as a result of injury. Gradually the bruise heals as the "stagnant blood" is reabsorbed. This process is normally very slow, lasting more than one month, with several gradations of color occurring: black bruises become purple, then bright red, and finally yellow or light green. You will see from the following example that such bruises heal very quickly with **Yunnan Paiyao.**

Cynthia was a gorgeous woman who was planning to have plastic surgery. She never liked her nose. Tall, svelte, and dramatic, she could have been a flamenco dancer. Her curly black hair covered her shoulders as she moved with graceful ferocity.

"I hate it!" she said, lifting an eyebrow and pointing to the offending curve. I thought the arch of her nose had a lovely aristocratic shape, but she had scheduled surgery and was now consulting me to help her prepare.

I recommended that she stop drinking and smoking for at least two weeks prior to surgery, and reduce her intake of hot, spicy foods because they impede circulation. If circulation is stuck, blood cannot flow smoothly to the area where it is needed.

On the morning of her surgery, Cynthia swallowed two small red pills of **Yunnan Paiyao.** When she awoke after the operation, she took two capsules, then two

HOW TO PREPARE FOR SURGERY

Before and after surgery, it is important to free circulation while improving the oxygen content of blood. (People who smoke bruise easily because their circulation and oxygen level are harmed from inflammation.)

Therefore, I recommend three doses daily of homeopathic iron (ferrum phosphate) in tea. Increased oxygen in the blood will always speed healing.

Vitamin C in time-release pills (4,000 mg a day) improves immunity by strengthening the adrenal glands and helping detoxify the body.

Zinc is an antistress mineral known to speed healing. Take 100 mg a day. Vitamin E helps circulation and adds extra oxygen. (Take at least 400 mcg a day.)

Vitamin K helps blood coagulation. (Take 60–100 mg daily.)

Avoid foods or supplements such as potassium or aspirin that thin the blood for several days prior to surgery.

Avoid foods that impair circulation—oily and fried foods, butter, tahini, peanut butter, and garlic.

more before bed. For five days after surgery, Cynthia took eight capsules daily of **Yunnan Paiyao.** When her doctor removed her bandages after a week, she was amazed to see that Cynthia had very little swelling and practically no bruises. There was a light yellow tint where there normally would have been a huge purple bruise. Her healing time was reduced to one-third the usual time.

Cynthia was delighted with the results. And there was another benefit of taking **Yunnan Paiyao:** It so dramatically increased her blood circulation during the two weeks after surgery that it reduced the fibroids in her breast!

WOUNDS

You can follow the same directions for internal use when treating external wounds, or pour the liquid directly onto wounds. Recently I recommended **Yunnan Paiyao** to someone who was pulverized in his own building by two thieves with brass knuckles.

He said the attending physician gave him a hundred stitches in his face. The next day he called me for advice, because a friend of his, a movie actor, had used my "miracle Chinese herb" to heal facial plastic surgery. The man was so grateful for my phone recommendations that he bought **Yunnan Paiyao** in Chinatown that same day.

I advised him to take **Yunnan Paiyao** for at least two weeks. The dosage was 1 red pill and 8 capsules (four at a time) throughout the first five days. Then he could continue with capsules. I told him he should eat no salad or fish on any day when he took **Yunnan Paiyao** or the day after.

A week later he reported that his recovery was amazing. "It just looks like I bumped into a door. No one who saw me last week can believe how I look this week. The doctors had to remove the stitches and staples much sooner than expected because I look like I've healed for a month, not a week!"

BROKEN BONES

Yunnan Paiyao speeds the healing of broken bones. When another friend was mugged and had his jaw broken, the attending surgeons were amazed at the speed with which it healed without scars. His jaw was wired together for several weeks while he drank liquid foods. He dissolved the contents of the **Yunnan Paiyao** capsules in water and swallowed them with a straw.

JOINT AND MUSCLE PAIN

Used alone or added to massage oil, **Yunnan Paiyao Liquor** improves rheumatism and sore joints while limbering muscles. Orally, the adult dose is 3–5 cc, three to five times a day, less for children. It tastes bitter.

I prefer taking the capsules internally after a heavy gym workout to speed recovery and eliminate stiffness. **Yunnan Paiyao,** in either powder or liquid form, is an excellent prevention remedy for people with poor circulation and chronic pain. It relaxes and stimulates tired muscles like a massage.

ULCERS AND BLEEDING GUMS

Friends have gotten good results with **Yunnan Paiyao** for everything from bleeding gums (*internal heat*) to weeping, slow-healing sores (from weakness and excess *yin*). This is because tienchi ginseng is *cooling* when raw and *warming* when steamed.

Yunnan Paiyao has been used in China to heal bleeding ulcers and chronic gastritis. Such conditions might also require medical intervention if stools remain black.

In one case, **Yunnan Paiyao** became an everyday remedy for chronic pain. Jack had had a bleeding ulcer. He now had chronic gastritis along with chronic stress. Even though the ulcer had resulted in surgery and he took medication, he feared recurrence. Jack had changed his diet, but not his lifestyle. He was the head of his company, and headed for a divorce. He found that taking two capsules of **Yunnan Paiyao** daily improved his digestion and mood. This helped him work and sleep better. His pain was gone and he felt safe again.

SKIN DISEASES

Aside from its use for wounds, traumatic hemorrhage, and bruises, **Yunnan Paiyao** is indicated for pyogenic infections of the skin such as "red swollen abscess, carbuncles and furuncles [boils]." It brings infection to the surface and dries oozing.

The remedy, as we shall see in chapter 27, is also recommended for certain women's problems related to "blood stag-nation." Here is a brief example from my health practice.

MENSTRUAL PAIN FROM POOR CIRCULATION

Julie sat before me doubled over, having her usual agonizing, flooding menstrual period. Her circulation had been poor for years. Her diet of chocolate, coffee, ciga-rettes, fried foods, and hot spices had done its work to give her a hellish menstrual pe-riod. Angry, she was practically in tears. She said she was losing big clots in the flow. At such times she stayed home in bed. Once she'd read in a magazine that it helped to ease discomfort if we honestly expressed it. After that, during those terri-ble times of the month, she curled up into a fetal position and moaned, thinking it would help. It only gave her a sore throat.

Julie's tongue was slightly purple-blue and overly dark red, indicating *stagnant chi*. Her circulation was bad because her *chi* was "stuck" in her abdomen. *Stagnant chi* leads to *stagnant* blood circulation. She did not ex-perience nausea, but only sharp, stabbing lower-abdomen pain and weakness. Her pulse was hesitant, as though trying to move forward but stopped by a wall.

The day I saw her, I gave Julie one small red pill of **Yunnan Paiyao** to swal-low. In about five minutes she smiled at me and said, "It's incredible. I feel lots better." Her greenish, out-of-sorts coloring im-proved. She relaxed and sat up. Her period became more normal that day, and we could address the issues underlying her *stagnant chi*. Normally, **Yunnan Paiyao** is taken with wine for menstrual pain, but for excess or deficient flow, it should be taken with water. Julie said she couldn't drink anything because she felt sick, so she just swallowed the pill.

EMOTIONAL STUCKNESS

I have another friend who used **Yunnan Paiyao** to cure himself of a real beating. He had married a lawyer, and they never got along. As their marriage got worse, she drank while he beat himself up at the gym. By the time they finally divorced, she'd become a judge and he had a body-building title.

He had started using **Yunnan Paiyao** to reduce muscle pain after the gym, but he noticed it also reduced his psychic pain from the split-up. He told me that it helped him "break apart old patterns and start fresh." He recommends **Yunnan Paiyao** for loss of a loved one, "when you feel bruised and bleeding from emotional pain."

When we study depression in chap-ter 35, we will see how such a Chinese pain remedy works for emotional pain. Obsession is similar to stuck *chi* in that it's a "stuck" emotion. When the flow of vital energy is impaired, we experience conges-tion, toxins, heaviness, pain, and painful emotions.

COMBINING YUNNAN PAIYAO WITH OTHER REMEDIES

Yunnan Paiyao can be taken with other herbal combinations to more effectively take its healing properties to the appropriate area. This will create a stronger treatment, appropriate to the location of the surgery. For example, for facial surgery, combine **Yunnan Paiyao** with herbs that reduce inflammation of the skin and face such as **Kochia 13,** made by Seven Forests, and available by mail order from Health Concerns (see Herbal Access appendix), or a Chinese patent remedy such as **Lien Chiao Pai Tu Pien.**

After surgery, take one dose of either of the above combinations for each dose of **Yunnan Paiyao.** Always take herbs that treat the skin between meals. At mealtimes take digestive herbs if needed, not those that "scatter *chi*" toward the skin.

For combining **Yunnan Paiyao** with herbal remedies for menstrual problems, see chapter 26.

HELPFUL HINTS

🌿 Keep **Yunnan Paiyao** capsules in your purse, wallet, and medicine cabinet.

🌿 Take a capsule of **Yunnan Paiyao** anytime you drink wine, except when eating fish. Long-term use is recommended for chronic gastritis and poor circulation, and is said to help prevent tumors.

🌿 Use **Yunnan Paiyao** powder externally to seal razor cuts or scratches from shaving. Use it both internally and externally for insect bites and stings to reduce itching, pain, and swelling.

🌿 If you cannot find **Yunnan Paiyao** in local Chinese herb shops, you can order it from one of the mail-order addresses in the Herbal Access appendix, or from the manufacturer: Yunnan White Drug-Powder Factory, Xibamilesi, Kunming, Yunnan Province, China. Telephone: 23836. Cable: 3344.

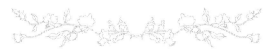

19
Arthritis

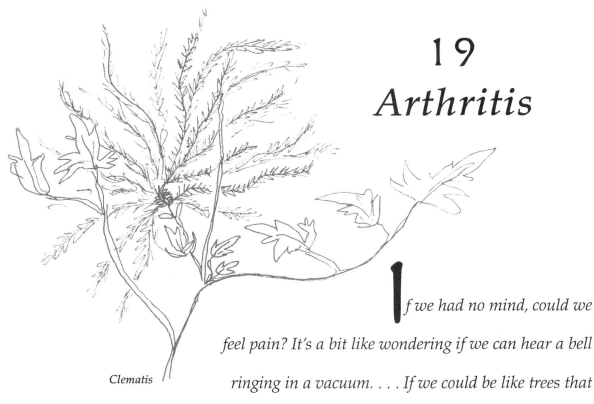

Clematis

If we had no mind, could we feel pain? It's a bit like wondering if we can hear a bell ringing in a vacuum. . . . If we could be like trees that breathe fresh air and bend toward light, perhaps we'd be more free. To inhale, we mustbe empty, ready to be filled. Anger and jealousy are not empty, nor is sadness. They stop the breath. . . .

Lorna lived in a dollhouse. The couch was pale blue with ruffled pink pillowcases. Flowered wallpaper, stuffed dolls, porcelain swans, beer steins, and a cuckoo clock re-created the Black Forest. I expected Lorna to emerge from a *chocolate cake. A singer, she'd asked me to ease the pain of her stiff shoulders, inflamed joints, and sciatica. She was dressed in lace, and her voice was high and melodic. She trilled a hello as she blithely pulled me in the door. Her laugh was an arpeggio. She didn't let up except for a moment when she mentioned her family. Then her voice dropped an octave, her look turned icy, and her body became stiff. I saw the cake beneath the frosting: It was hatred, and it hurt.*

Searing pain, stemming from dietary and emotional toxins, can end up in the joints. This chapter covers an Asian view of arthritis, including its origins: injury, infection, and nutritional deficiency, also specifically rheumatoid and osteoporotic pain. Asian herbal remedies for arthritis are powerful, easy to use, and readily available. Some can even be found in the kitchen or the health-food store. We will consider herbs for both arthritic and non-arthritic pains, so that the formulas in this chapter will be helpful for everyone.

Asian herbal remedies for arthritis remove pain by clearing poisons and increasing circulation, not by dulling the mind. Western medications, which dull pain while ignoring the underlying conditions, only add sugar to poison, making it easier to swallow.

Why Use Herbs to Treat Arthritis?

Does your arthritis painkiller give you ulcers, profound fatigue, dizziness, poor memory, or reduced immune strength?

Long-term use of blood-thinning or anti-inflammatory medicines damages vitality. For example, prolonged use of cortisone results in wasting of bone and connective tissue, and depresses the immune system. What's more, certain Western drugs attempt to parallel the effects of enzymes or brain chemicals, eventually affecting the functioning of cells, which could lead to degenerative side effects. Their full impact might not be felt until much later. It's not clear how your painkillers might someday affect your children or grandchildren.

Asian herbal treatments avoid weakening side effects because ingredients are combined in order to treat specific problem areas without weakening the entire body. They combine herbs that take the painkiller to the pain. Besides, the body accepts herbs like food, so that dietary wastes that aggravate pain can be eliminated. This is uniquely a property of herbal cures.

A Method to Find Your Pain Relief

To use natural arthritis medicines to their best advantage, we will employ personal diagnosis, observing what foods and weather conditions make your joint aches worse. This type of simple inductive method was used by Sherlock Holmes, who said, "Watson, you see, but you do not observe." Holmes's process of elimination was like Asian medical diagnosis—he observed the details first, then reached a decision. By analyzing the type of pain we suffer, along with the accompanying circumstances, we may *observe* more than we *see*.

Finally, we'll uncover an herbal arsenal for knocking out your joint pain that comes from Chinese and Indian traditions, including herbal pills, baths, and balms for external application.

An Asian Definition of Arthritis and Its Symptoms

The traditional Asian view of arthritis encompasses a larger spectrum of discomfort than the Western definition: It is joint pain or deformity arising from an imbalance among the *humors* and *chi,* including not only joint pain but also neuritis, neuralgia, muscle aches, cramps, and joint pain related to food allergies or hormone imbalances.

This definition is so broad because Asian doctors describe the origin of arthritis in terms of toxins, including infection as well as dietary wastes and poor circulation. Indian doctors call such toxins *ama.* They feel that it underlies weakening congestive illness, under which heading they include colds, arthritic pain, paralysis, and cancer.

Arthritis falls into a category of discomforts called "painful obstruction" (*bi,* pronounced "bee") by Chinese doctors, referring to the obstruction of *chi* circulation. Pain and numbness in joints and muscles is the primary symptom, but it is influenced by the *humors* we discussed in chapter 10, *internal wind, heat, cold, dampness,* and unbalanced emotions. A Chinese herbal doctor names specific cases of arthritis, according

to the symptoms involved—for example, *wind-chill-damp* arthritis.

Wind-chill-damp pains migrate in the body—for example, from the shoulder to the wrist, or down the leg. They are aggravated by cold weather and humidity, and also by ice-cold and phlegm-producing foods. As we shall see, these are some of the underlying problems associated with rheumatic and rheumatoid arthritis.

Sometimes the quality of the pain itself can indicate its origins and type—for example, a heavy, dull (*phlegm*), but searing (*hot*) pain that feels worse with acidic or spicy foods (causes of *internal heat*) indicates inflammatory arthritis.

When you know what makes your pain feel worse, you can plan your meals to avoid irritating foods. You can also observe the progress of your illness, because arthritis, like many other weakening illnesses, often progresses from a *cold* stage to an inflammatory one: At the onset, joints feel worse in cold weather, but eventually become inflamed. Therefore, understanding the effects of your diet on your arthritis will help you determine its type and prognosis. We don't merely want to stop the pain, but to reverse the progress of the disease with diet and herbs.

What Kind of Arthritic Pain Do You Have?

Most people make no connection between what they eat and their arthritis, so that they cannot determine its type. Nor have they considered the quality of their pain:

They are not sure whether it feels burning and sharp, cold and stiff, or heavy and dull. They want one pain cure for everyone. But everyone's arthritis is different because we have different habits.

FIND THE ORIGIN OF YOUR PAIN

Foods, weather conditions, and emotions that aggravate joint pain are related to its cause. Finding the right cure requires observing your habits and understanding how they affect your *humors* and *chi*. Please take a moment to analyze what factors underlie your arthritic pain by answering the following question: If you had nothing to eat, what foods would you miss (see table on page 222)? Total your responses. In which column do you have the most circles? Here are the types of joint and muscle pains those foods aggravate:

Wind: nerve pain, soreness, numbness, pain that moves in the body
Hot: inflammatory pain, burning, itching, cramps, worse at night
Cold: fixed, stabbing pain, stiffness, worse in cold weather
Phlegm: dull, heavy ache, stiffness, immobility, malformed joints

Do you have sharp joint pain, inflamed joints, or cramped muscles and crave fat or spicy foods, pickles, and chili barbecue dishes? There is a connection. Don't be surprised if you crave the foods that make your arthritis worse. The body

---

A QUICK TONGUE CHECK

Some people do not notice their food cravings as much as their allergies. Do you consciously avoid certain foods? If so, your body may be revealing an existing problem with *wind, internal heat, internal cold,* or *phlegm.* The best way to check is to observe your tongue.

A tongue that shows *wind* will shake from nervous tension. A reddish, dry tongue points to *internal heat,* while a pale, scalloped tongue indicates *internal cold.* A thickly coated, greasy, or yellow-coated tongue shows *phlegm* along with *internal heat,* but a thin white coating and excess saliva shows *internal cold.*

---

tries to maintain its homeostasis, even in disease.

Arthritis: East Meets West

Putting the energetic fundamentals of arthritic pain together with Western nomenclature helps explain how herbal arthritis remedies work. Most people say they have rheumatoid arthritis, not *wind-chill-damp* pain. But they miss something important: Knowing that caffeine, cold weather, or cheese irritates your arthritis can help prevent future pain. Applying Eastern energetics to our understanding of Western diseases can open up new avenues of prevention and treatment.

ARTHRITIC PAIN AND DIET: AN OBSERVATION

Imagine you are trapped on a desert island without food. Circle the foods you would miss most.

WIND/COLD	PHLEGM	HOT	PHLEGM/HOT
coffee	sweet fruits	barbecued foods	bagel and cream cheese
tea	doughuts	tomatoes	beer
salad	ice cream	oranges	toast and butter
apples	pasta	honey	pasta
white potato	raisins	fried chicken	cheeses
ice drinks	muffins	carrots	beef
alcoholic drinks	soft drinks	beets	pork, lamb
white rice	cookies	vinegar	peanut butter
	bread	garlic, pepper	french fries
	oily foods	potato chips	pizza

RHEUMATIC ARTHRITIS AND RHEUMATOID ARTHRITIS

Rheumatic arthritis

Rheumatic arthritis is an allergic reaction passed through the blood to the joints after a streptococcal infection. Traditional Chinese doctors call it *pi cheng,* "numbness disease." It has a gradual *cold* stage and later an acute *hot* stage with migrating redness of the skin, swollen hot knees, ankles, elbows, and pain at the waist, with limited movement. It affects the large joints at the knees, ankles, elbows, and waist. But the tongue has a thin white or whitish oily coating, indicating *internal cold* and *dampness.* Cold weather and foods are not comfortable.

The problem is that the two stages,

wind-chill-dampness and *feverish and numb,* overlap. For that reason, in the Treatment section of this chapter, I have included several herbal combinations that treat both stages simultaneously.

Rheumatoid arthritis

Chinese doctors call this form of joint pain *li chieh feng,* "rheumatism in joints." It is characterized by chronic systemic symmetrical pains affecting small joints: the fingers, wrists, elbows, or knees of both sides. Even though rheumatic pain is allergic and tends to be sudden and acute, and rheumatoid pain is chronic, what they have in common is that both are aggravated by *wind, cold,* and *dampness.*

WIND-CHILL-DAMP PAIN

- Do your joints hurt worse in cold damp weather?
- Do joints feel better with warmth and movement?
- Do you have a pale tongue with a white coating?
- Do you have slow digestion, indigestion, or fatigue after eating?
- Do you feel bloated in the middle?
- Do you have joint pain that moves around, or that comes and goes?
- Do joints feel heavy, limbs dragging?

If you answered "yes" to these questions, you have the beginnings of *wind-chill-damp* joint pain. Whether it actually turns into rheumatoid arthritis depends on your habits as much as other factors such as your hormones or genes. The most severe joint aches, stemming from an accumulation of dietary toxins and emotional bad habits, are known as inflammatory arthritis.

Inflammatory arthritis

- Do you have red, hot, swollen joints?
- Are your knuckles getting wrinkled and larger, your palms drier?
- Are your joints extremely sensitive to the touch?
- Do your joints feel worse with heat and movement?
- Do you have a reddish tongue with a yellow coating?
- Are you often angry, anxious, nervous, feverish, or thirsty?
- Is your energy fast or insomniac?

Did you answer "yes" to these symptoms? If you have a preference for spicy foods, and experience chronic fever or thirst, you likely have inflammatory joint pain. If you are confused about the type of arthritis you have, here is a little test: Inflammatory joint pain feels better with the application of ice.

JOINT PAIN AND DIGESTION

My general advice for preventing arthritic discomfort is to avoid foods that irritate and use home herbal remedies designed to strengthen digestion and circulation. The specific arthritic remedies we'll cover in the Treatment section aim to eliminate toxins, strengthen weakness, and stimulate circulation in order to ease pain. You have a great advantage if you prevent acid and phlegm buildup in the first place. Remember, because our energetic needs differ, foods that may act as a poison for you may be another person's medicine.

POISONS TO AVOID

For *wind-chill-damp* pain, rheumatism, early rheumatic or rheumatoid arthritis, or any joint pain made worse by harsh stimulants, cold drafts, humidity, cold foods, weakness, fatigue, or depression, avoid creamy, rich, sweet, fat, or sour foods such as dairy products, cheese, sauerkraut, grapefruit, sprouts, white potatoes, pork, red meats, caffeine, alcohol, or pastry.

For *hot-numbness* pain, inflammatory joint aches and arthritis, or any joint pain

A PREVENTION AND TREATMENT PLAN

CRAVING THE SOURCE OF PAIN

Give yourself two weeks to diagnose your joint pain. During that time, observe your tongue and discomforts, recording your progress in a journal. Note what makes the pain better or worse. For example, do you notice joint pain more at night or after spicy foods (inflammatory) or after cold, raw foods and during cold, damp weather?

DIET

As much as possible, during those two weeks cut out red meat, dairy products, alcohol, sweets, hot spices, peppers, onions, garlic, tomatoes, white potatoes, eggplant, green peppers. Those are foods known to increase joint pain.

CLEANSE

Take at least 2 teaspoons of **Triphala churna** powder per day. (Fill eight empty capsules, bought from a health-food store.) **Trifala** is a cleanser and rejuvenator available in Indian grocery stores or from mail-order sources listed in the appendix (see chapter 13). If you prefer, you can substitute ¼ cup daily of aloe vera gel along with one pinch of turmeric powder added to tea or apple juice as a laxative.

NOTICE

While cleansing toxins with this special diet, you'll notice that your body will fight to maintain its imbalances: *You will strongly crave the sources of your pain.* This gives you an excellent opportunity to observe your imbalances.

ANALYZE YOUR CRAVINGS

If you crave hot spices and sour, fat, or fried foods and alcohol, you are more likely to suffer inflammatory-type pains. (Normally, your joints will feel hot. Pain may feel worse at night or with irritation.)

If you crave pastry, ice cream, sweet fruit, and bread, excess *phlegm* is a key factor in your joint pain.

Noticing these cravings will guide you so that you can begin adding non-irritating foods and balancing herbs from among the home remedies and herbal combinations that I've provided.

---

made worse by hot spices, anger, or excess stimulation, avoid honey, fried foods and excess nuts, sesame oil, pepper, garlic, onions, hot spices, pork, red meats, dairy products, alcohol, and nightshades: tomato, green pepper, eggplant.

FOOD ANTIDOTES

For *wind-chill-damp* pain, use *warming, drying* herbs and spices and the antiphlegm cleansing diet in chapter 13.

For inflammatory pain, use the bitter,

cooling, and cleansing herbs and diet from section II of chapter 13.

Treatment

In this section we'll cover home remedies and standard herbal combinations for treating joint pain, based on energetic medicine.

HOW FOOD REMEDIES WORK

Certain foods can ease joint pain because they stimulate digestion, elimination, and circulation to rid the body of toxins. Many pain remedies cleanse the liver: for example, a drink made from a slice of raw ginger along with a teaspoon of apple cider vinegar or fresh lemon juice, added to warm water. The combination of hot and sour flavors provides a balanced cleanser. (See chapter 6.) It's a good remedy after a rich meal or first thing in the morning. Here are some other home remedies especially suited for *wind-chill-damp* and inflammatory joint pain.

Warming *herbs for* wind-chill-damp

Herbs used for early rheumatic or rheumatoid arthritis with *wind-chill-damp* symptoms are teas that are bitter, hot stimulants that dissolve *phlegm* while increasing circulation. In terms of energetic medicine, they burn up *phlegm.* Try one or two of these remedies as you prefer. Increase the dosage as needed in cold weather, and monitor

your tongue changes. Eventually a pale, puffy tongue will turn normal pink.

Diaphoretic herbs to sweat out pain
SPICES

Ginger is expectorant and digestive. It also makes you perspire. The dry powder is more *heating* than raw ginger. Add a big pinch of dry ginger or several peeled slices of the raw root to a cup of green tea. Evenings, add five heaping tablespoons of dried ginger to a bath to sweat out cold. Wrap yourself well and don't go outside.

Cinnamon and turmeric make a spicy tea to warm stiff shoulders. Add ⅛ teaspoon of each powdered spice to a cup of boiling water and drink it between meals.

Juniper berries are diuretic, diaphoretic, stimulant, digestive, and disinfectant. Chew a dozen, or brew them as tea once a day for edema, sciatica, arthritis, rheumatism, and swollen joints.

MYRRH FOR BETTER CIRCULATION

Myrrh heals wounds, detoxifies poisons, and stimulates circulation. Take 3 to 4 capsules a day between meals.

SOUP INGREDIENTS

The Chinese blood-builder tang kuei can be added to soups or stews to increase blood production and circulation for persons with a pale tongue in *internal cold* problems. It eases joint aches for those with *cold/damp*-related discomfort.

The Indian digestive herb asafoetida is extremely *heating*. A strongly detoxifying herb, its main uses are for treating indigestion and killing parasites, but it also warms and energizes the joints. Use only a pinch in soups or when cooking beans.

A SOUP FOR JOINT PAIN

Cook until done 1 cup pearl barley with ½ teaspoon cinnamon, 1 pinch saffron, and 1 piece tang kuei. Add a pinch of the following herbs as needed.

For water retention: 10 juniper berries
For weakness and chills: fenugreek or ginger

Warming *cleansing herbs*

These are health-food store items, not foods. Because of their strong cleansing effects, they form an important part of any herbal regimen designed to reduce joint pain.

Prickly ash bark is a very *heating*, bitter antiseptic cleanser available in health-food store capsules or as a very bitter liquid extract. It is sometimes combined with laxative herbs to rid the gastrointestinal tract of worms and yeast. It can be used for weak digestion, abdominal pain from cold raw food, and chronic chills leading to lumbago, arthritis, and rheumatism, especially affecting the lower body. Add 5 to 10 drops to a small glass of water between meals. (It also combines well with aloe vera gel and water.)

Alfalfa pills or capsules are a must for those who suffer from joint pain or deformity augmented by nutritional deficiency. Calcium is needed to prevent arthritis, but the body is most often too full of toxins to absorb it. Alfalfa pills or capsules provide an excellent source of organic calcium, magnesium, phosphorus, potassium, chlorophyll, and nearly all known vitamins. They are very detoxifying when taken in medicinal doses rather than as foods. I chew about a dozen pills a day with water. Alfalfa can be combined with ginger tea for those troubled by acid regurgitation or nausea.

The Indian healing tradition offers guggul, a high-performance cleanser/rejuvenator used to cure joint pain and eliminate body fat and tumors. Guggul (in Latin, *Commiphora mukul*), a tree resin, has stimulant, antispasmodic, and expectorant qualities, and is used in treating arthritis, rheumatism, gout, lumbago, nerve disorders, debility, obesity, and skin diseases. Taken internally, it disinfects and deodorizes the body.

Triphala churna, a balancing laxative powder, also available in Indian groceries, works particularly well with guggul. A pill combination, **Trifala Guggul,** can be ordered from Planetary Formulas (see Herbal Access appendix).

INFLAMMATORY JOINT PAIN

Caution: Strongly anti-inflammatory herbs such as the combinations that follow are not recommended during pregnancy. If the home-cooked brews cause diarrhea, reduce the dosage by half. Otherwise follow directions and consume them between meals.

Home remedies

I include the following two recipes in the home remedy section because you have to cook them yourself. They taste like medicine (or mud), not soup, so are better served cold. Eventually these cook-your-own remedies are cleansing and soothing. You may even get to like the flavor. The same batch of herbs can be boiled twice, in order to save money, and the resulting broth should be stored in the refrigerator when not used.

The first recipe is taken from a required course textbook of the Shanghai College of Traditional Medicine (Clinic of TCM, vol. II). The second comes from *A Barefoot Doctor's Manual* (Running Press). You can order the ingredients from any of the Chinese herb shops listed in the appendix. (Fax this recipe to them.)

AN ANTIBIOTIC REMEDY

For rheumatic arthritis with inflammatory symptoms that include fever, swollen painful joints, red, hot limbs, red tongue with yellow, greasy coating, and rapid pulse, simmer these herbs together in 1 gallon water for 45 minutes and drink several cups a day:

30 grams   honeysuckle
30 grams   dandelion
30 grams   viola (Chinese violet)
15 grams   wild chrysanthemum flower
9 grams   root of muskrootlike semiaquilegia (**Radix semiaquilegiae**)

12 grams   achyranthes root
24 grams   plantain herb
24 grams   fu ling

The antibiotic treatment of rheumatic arthritis combines herbs that normalize body temperature, replace fluids, and reestablish electrolyte balance. Such antibiotic herbs are said to clear *heat* and toxins from the blood and promote circulation. That stops the spread of bacteria.

The first several herbs are antibiotic, anti-inflammatory blood cleansers, the last three diuretic. Achyranthes is specifically added to guide the cleansing herbs to treat soreness and swollen joints in the lower body, especially the knees. The remedy's treatment principle is to kill germs and reduce fever, pain, and water retention in the most effective manner, through the urine.

A BAREFOOT DOCTOR'S BREW

This non-antibiotic herbal treatment for inflammatory joint pain clears fever, controls *wind* by reducing excess nerve irritation, and increases circulation. It is suitable for anyone with painful, red, swollen joints, rheumatoid arthritis, or aches due to food allergies or inadequate digestion. It is a decoction, to be cooked for 30 minutes. Use one handful each of three herbs in 1 gallon water. Drink two or three cups per day cold, between meals:

wu jia pi (**Cortex acanthopanacis**)
wei ling xian (**Radix clemetidis chinensis**)
mulberry twigs

These herbs are commonly used to "dispel wind damp" by increasing circulation and quieting nerve pain.

The All-In-One Super Whammy Arthritis Pill

It may be very well for some to stay home, adding spices to soups or cooking murky brews, but many people live with one foot out the door, eating on the run. They need an all-in-one pill for *hot* or *cold-wind-damp* pain. Here are some herbal combination pills that treat a variety of joint pains.

CHINESE PATENT REMEDIES

All of the following can be ordered from Chinatown shops.

Guan Jie Yan Wan, "Close Down Joint Inflammation Pills," is used for both *cold* and *hot-wind-dampness* leading to arthritis, rheumatism, cold limbs, and aching joints. One major ingredient, erythrinae bark, "expels *wind dampness* . . . for soreness and pain in the lower back and knees." Other ingredients, such as barley, ginger, cinnamon, and ephedra, reduce phlegm, while stephania and achyranthes "lead" the other herbs and reduce swelling in the legs and knees. The dosage is usually 8 pills, three times daily.

Wan Nian Chun Zi Pu Ziang, "Thousand Year Spring Nourishing Syrup," is a vegetarian herbal tonic for improving *chi* and blood, especially for the lung, liver, spleen, and kidneys. Used for general weakness, it improves such chronic illnesses as asthma, arthritis, and malnutrition. It is well suited for malabsorption problems in older persons, containing 80 percent royal jelly and other herbs to nourish blood and improve strength. Dosage is 10 cc daily, with water.

Xiao Luo Tong Pian, "Rheumatalgia Relieving Tablet," is recommended for *wind/dampness* arthritis and other rheumatic diseases. The dosage is 8 pills, three times daily.

HEALTH-FOOD STORE HERBAL REMEDIES

Arthritis herbs come as single herbs or as combination remedies. You'll find them not only in health-food stores, but frequently in pharmacies, supermarkets, and health clubs. Curative herbs are no longer a specialty item. Several of the largest American vitamin manufacturers are now making and distributing combinations that feature a wide variety of international herbs.

For painful knees

One of the best single herbs for painful knees I have found is yucca root, a relative of the century plant, native to the American Southwest. Many people eat the boiled root in place of potato, but a stronger dose is obtained from capsules. It contains saponin, a naturally occurring steroid.

The consistency of yucca root is slick,

like soap, so that yucca capsules, taken internally, make joints slip more easily and reduce swelling. You can take handfuls of yucca capsules between meals throughout the day. Only you can find the dose that makes you feel comfortable; the manufacturer hasn't a clue about the severity of your pain. A dozen or more capsules, taken for two or three days, is often enough of the dosage to unlock painful knees. That frees *chi* to move. Then reduce the dose to a comfortable number: for example, 4 to 6 daily.

Combination remedies

American-made combination herbal remedies for arthritis often contain both *cooling* and *warming* herbs along with others that increase circulation and support hormone production. This put-it-all-together approach has become popular because Western consumers are not expected to differentiate their symptoms as Asians do. The wisdom in such a combination is that combining a variety of such herbs can break apart stuck *chi*. These combinations are safe and recommended for long-term use, not acute attacks. As you will see, using Asian energetic principles, you can improve upon their approach.

For prevention and treatment of arthritic pain

Arth Plus is easy to find in supermarkets and pharmacies. It's made by Nature's Herbs, a Twin Labs company, the huge health conglomerate known for body-building and general health supplements. **Arth Plus** is a well-put-together combination of support and cleansing herbs that improve pain and mobility.

It combines black cohosh and sarsaparilla to help maintain hormone balance, along with many herbs such as yucca, devil's claw, prickly ash, and white bark to treat pain, and alfalfa and trace minerals to supplement nutrition. It presents a balanced diet of building and cleansing herbs necessary to ease sharp pain and swollen joints. This is a good remedy that covers many bases at once.

Using the genius of Asian medical principles, you can take such a baseline combination as this, and add a few other herbs to take its pain-relieving action to where it is most needed in the body. In other words, my herbal additions will make the baseline remedy work more specifically.

- For shoulder pain and stiffness, take 4 capsules of **Arth Plus** along with one cup of tea made from ⅛ teaspoon each of cinnamon and turmeric powder.
- For swollen, painful knees, take capsules of **Arth Plus** with a tea made by boiling a handful each of Chinese fu ling and stephania root. Boil the Asian herbs for 45 minutes in one quart of water, strain it, and drink 3 cups per day, each time also taking capsules of the baseline remedy.
- For painful lower back and lumbago, add a handful of eucommia bark to cook with the above two herbs.

For improved mobility

Crystal Star's **Ar-Ease Caps** (and tea) combine yucca, alfalfa, devil's claw, guggul, buckthorn bark, dandelion, bilberry, parsley, burdock, black cohosh, rose hips, slippery elm, Saint-John's-wort, yarrow, hydrangea, licorice, hawthorn, turmeric, pantothenic acid, ligusticum, fu ling, and DL-phenylalanine—herbs that help neutralize acid and increase mobility. In addition, black cohosh and yarrow (precursors of estrogen and progesterone) supplement hormones, while alfalfa and rose hips enhance nutrition.

Mobility 2 treats arthritic inflammation and pain of the lower body, such as gout, sciatica, lumbago, and numbness in the extremities that is more severe at night and that worsens in damp or cold conditions.

Mobility 3 treats *wind/dampness* anywhere in the body. Symptoms might include headache, numbness, pain, malaise, and fatigue. It is recommended for arthritic discomfort in persons over thirty years old, especially after exposure to *internal cold, wind,* or *dampness.*

Inflamed joints and skin rash

Sometimes joint inflammation becomes so intense that it spills onto the skin, leaving an exasperating itchy rash. In that case, anti-inflammatory cleansing must be augmented. You can use a health-food store arthritis remedy as a baseline and combine skin-cleansing herbs.

Ar-Ease is a strong liver cleanser, suited for long-term inflammatory pain, a red tongue with a coating, and swollen or deformed joints at the hands, wrists, or knees. It breaks apart toxins and cools *internal heat.* **Arth Plus** is gently cleansing, useful for weak or older persons with fragile bones.

You can combine either remedy with the following tea in order to treat painful itchy skin rash, or eczema. Make this laxative, antibiotic tea by boiling a handful each of dandelion herb and honeysuckle flowers (ordered from Chinatown) in 2 quarts of water for 45 minutes. Strain the tea and keep it in the refrigerator when not in use. Drink 2 cups daily of the tea, along with a dose of your baseline remedy. If the combination of tea and pills becomes too laxative, reduce the tea to 1 cup daily.

OTHER TYPES OF JOINT-PAIN REMEDIES

Homeopathics

The homeopathic remedy most suited for joint pain that improves with warmth and exercise is rhus tox 30c. A dose, usually 5 pills, can be melted under the tongue or added to drinking water between meals.

Rub-on remedies

Triflora Arthritis Gel, made by Boericke & Tafel, Inc., is available in health-food stores. It is recommended for pain and stiffness associated with arthritis, rheumatism, tendinitis, backache, and sprains. It contains a number of homeopathic remedies, including rhus tox and ledum. I use it to increase circulation in stiff shoulders.

If joints feel better with the application of heat, rub in **Tiger Balm;** one of the world's most widely available liniments, it can be found in health-food stores and Oriental food markets almost everywhere.

For inflammatory pain, apply real ice or a *cooling* cream. But be very careful where you put it! Ice on the back and neck can sedate vital internal organs more than ice on the fingers.

You may wish to rub painful joints or gout with a *cooling* oil; use sunflower or sandalwood oil. An acupuncture doctor in China might treat such symptoms with acupuncture of the red joints, pricking until slight bleeding occurs. That "lets out the steam" of excess acid collected at the joints. But I recommend using a loofah or a skin brush gently on painful joints and along the entire spine during a hot bath.

Special help for osteoporosis

We tend to think of osteoporosis as a disease of age, a menopausal complication. But it is also encouraged by blood deficiency that can occur at any time from cancer therapies, corticosteroids, blood diseases, severe blood loss, and weak adrenal strength. These contribute to malabsorption, fatigue, and poor immune response.

If you have osteoporosis or wish to prevent it, nutrition and blood-building are just as important in your health-care routine as cleansing. Certain tonic herbs enhance the body's ability to generate

what makes bones strong—blood and bone marrow.

One popular remedy in China is thinly sliced deer antler, now sold in Chinese pharmacies in the West as well as Asia. Deer antler is shed yearly. It is quite effective in rebuilding bone marrow depleted by harsh medical therapies or illness. If you ever go to the trouble of simmering sliced deer horn for hours in a double boiler, you will feel the benefits immediately. It feels as though your bone marrow is relaxing, taking a deep breath, and sighing from relief. Several types of deer horn are used. Cervus sika stag horn contains protein and collagen and is used as a tonic stimulant. Antelope horn contains calcium phosphate and is an antispasmodic, antipyretic (antifever) tonic.

Fortunately, a less expensive vegetarian substitute is now available: Simmer one handful each of epimedium leaves and lycium fruit in a quart of water for twenty minutes, strain, and drink two cups a day.

Pill treatments

For treatment of osteoporotic pain, Chinese traditional doctors recommend herbal combinations that nourish kidney/adrenal energy and generate blood production and at the same time build *chi*, help balance hormones, and prevent pain. This multifaceted approach requires combining one or two main herbal remedies along with others that deal with secondary complaints.

Start with two combinations by Seven Forests that nourish kidney and liver blood and bone marrow: **Antler 8** and **Restorative Tablets.** (Your health-food store can order them.)

The first of these contains 50 percent deer antler and less than 10 percent salvia, dendrobium, rehmannia, tortoiseshell, tang kuei, aquilaria, and cardamom. **Antler 8** provides nourishment and support for persons who have suffered immune depression from Western cancer therapies, corticosteroids, HIV, leukemia, severe blood loss, fatigue, kidney-related problems, and osteoporosis. It helps generate blood and bone marrow.

Combine this with **Restorative Tablets** for osteoporosis and osteoarthritis. **Restorative Tablets** reduce *heat* symptoms such as afternoon fever or hot flashes. Men or women can use it for prolonged feverish diseases and general weakness related to *internal heat.* It is *cooling* because it replaces moisture with 10 percent each of processed human placenta, tortoiseshell, and rehmannia. It contains antifever herbs such as anemarrhena and ophiopogonis as well as other blood-building herbs.

A vegetarian substitute for this remedy could be the less expensive Chinese patent remedy **Liu Wei Di Huang Wan,** which builds blood (and *yin*) for kidney and liver.

Antler 8 and **Restorative Tablets** or their equivalents ensure blood production and nutrition necessary to slow inflammatory and consumptive symptoms of a long-term inflammatory disease.

ADDITIONS FOR SPECIFIC PROBLEMS

Add to **Antler 8** and **Restorative Tablets** the following combination for specific problems: **Ganoderma 18** for fatigue and low immune strength.

Nature's Sunshine products, from Spanish Fork, Utah, offers two formulas used to balance the Water element: **Qu Shi** ("Remove Dampness") and **Jian Gu** ("Strengthen Bones"). The first, which treats edema in the legs, poor digestion, ascites, and joint swelling, is more for cleansing. The second, as its name implies, is more of a supportive remedy. **Jian Gu** is recommended for weak and sore back and legs, urinary dysfunction, recovery from broken bones, osteoporosis, exhaustion from work, and difficulty in hearing or breathing related to kidney (adrenal) weakness. Both formulas are vegetarian and are best taken between meals.

By merely reading the list of symptoms these herbal remedies treat, we clearly see that osteoporosis is more complicated than we thought. By the same token, there is much more we can do to prevent or treat it than lift weights and take calcium pills when we remember.

ARTHRITIS

What makes it worse?

nerve pain or *wind bi* (shifting pain, neuritis, neuralgia)	stimulants; exhaustion; *drying,* hot, or irritating foods; aggravation; worry; anger
Hot bi (inflammatory arthritis)	acidic foods; hot spices; alcohol; hot emotions (rage, jealousy)
Cold bi (rheumatism)	exposure to inclement weather; cold foods; iced drinks; anti-inflammatory drugs
Damp bi	humidity; *phlegm*-producing, low-nutrition diet; weakness; depression; hormone imbalance
Rheumatic arthritis	infection *wind-cold-damp* and *hot-damp*
Rheumatoid arthritis	*wind-cold-damp*; malnutrition; weakness
Osteoarthritis	malnutrition; exhaustion; chemotherapy; hormone imbalance; immune-threatening illness

What makes it better?

TYPE	EXAMPLE	TYPE OF HERB	EXAMPLE
Nerve pain *wind*	neuralgia	nervines, herb combinations for local relief	valerian
Inflammatory arthritis (*chill* stage) (*hot* stage)	early rheumatoid *cold-hot-wind-damp*	*drying/warming* nervine, increase circulation, antiphlegm	myrrh, **Mobility 3**
knees, pain, and stiffness		demulcent	yucca capsules
knees, lower-body joint pain, swelling	*hot-cold-wind-damp*		**Arth Plus, Guan Jie Yan Wan**
Osteoporosis		nutritive tonics, anti-inflammatory herbs	**Antler 8, Restorative Tablets, Eucommia 19**

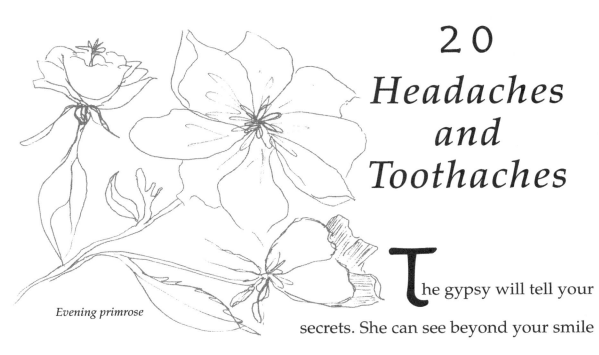

Evening primrose

20
Headaches and Toothaches

The gypsy will tell your secrets. She can see beyond your smile with her almond-shaped hazel eyes. Let me read your hand. Is it the square hand of one who loves Mother Earth? You have a sweet tooth. Life for you must be as mild as bread and honey. Have you been unlucky in love? When you have a headache, your brain is heavy, pounding, as though stuffed with cotton. You need the camphorated air of high peaks.

Do you have a hand lined like tree bark? A hand of Wood?

You have a quick mind, a keen memory. You remember every hurt. Your headache is a searing line of pain encircling your brain. Your eyes ache. You are allergic to everything mediocre. Keep your feet on the ground, mingle with the current of a cool river, and strive for balance.

Do you have the hand of Fire, your waving fingers festooned with rings? Your heartbeat is your signature. Wear it on your sleeve and you're bound to get a headache.

Everyone's headache is different. Your tension headache is not the same as his sinus ache or her trigeminal neuralgia or nauseating, liverish migraine. How could they be the same? You do not have the same stress, diet, or lifestyle. If the causes are different, why shouldn't the remedy also be? Asian herb cures are built to move *chi*, affecting several meridians at once, so they can treat a local area of pain quite effectively.

Types of Headaches and Remedies

Asian headache remedies fall into several large categories: those that clear *phlegm* or improve digestion, those that increase stuck circulation, and those that reduce inflammation, treat allergies, and build blood. Some herbal pain medicines serve several of those functions at once. Such a remedy might clear *toxic heat* (infection), *real fire* (inflammation), and *phlegm heat* (infected mucus) from eyes, ears, nose, and throat.

SINUS HEADACHES ARE POUNDING *PHLEGM*

- Does your headache make your sinuses feel stuffed?
- Does the top of your head hurt with a dull pain?
- Does your head pound?
- Does your headache make it hard to think clearly?
- Does it feel like your head is expanding or floating?
- Did your headache start after eating rich, oily, or sweet food?
- Does thinking of what you ate last make you feel sick?
- Do you wake up with a dull, heavy headache?

Many people recognize they have a pounding sinus headache because they have congestion from nasal polyps or a deviated septum. But other cases go unrecognized: A *phlegm* headache that obscures thinking and makes you feel groggy may accompany indigestion and constipation from a heavy, rich meal, even from the previous day.

Energetic origin

Have you ever wondered why certain foods lead to sinus congestion? The answer lies in the stomach and large intestine acupuncture meridians. The first meridian starts under the eyes and moves downward to speed the movement of food toward the intestines. The second one starts in the second finger of each hand and extends up to each side of the nose. Both meridians meet in the sinus area, so that what we eat has direct bearing on the sinuses. When we clear sinus passageways, we can breathe, think, and digest better.

The remedy: clear phlegm

Asian sinus remedies clear congestion, thereby relieving pressure. The simplest example of this is most suitable for a pounding headache that makes your head feel like it is full of cotton. It is a cure used in Ayurveda for headaches resulting from excess *phlegm*. Take one capsule of gotu kola, an herb normally taken orally to calm and balance nervous system and brain functions. This time, use the opened capsule like snuff. It clears sinus passages, relieves pressure, clears the senses, and stops a congestion headache immediately.

ALLERGIC SINUS HEADACHES

These headaches can drive you indoors during allergy seasons.

For headaches from allergic sinusitis, combine **Angelica 14** and **Xanthium 12**. Both Seven Forests products can be ordered by health-food stores. Directions are on the bottle (normally 3 to 5 between meals). The first remedy contains a large portion of *Angelica archangelica* to normalize digestive acid/alkaline balance, and chrysanthemum flower, an anti-inflammatory, to bring circulation to the head and eyes. They clear congestion while tang kuei and cordyalis increase circulation, and nardostachys, a

form of valerian, quiets the nerves. **Xanthium 12** is often used for hay fever and allergic asthma or skin rashes. These remedies' effectiveness in reducing sinus headache is proof of the important connection between adequate breath and reducing head pain.

Some other remedies for sinus and allergic headache go even further. They heal poor digestion resulting in *phlegm*, congestion, allergies, and "stuck *chi*."

INDIGESTION HEADACHES

- ℅ Does your head hurt after you eat raw, spicy, or fatty food?
- ℅ Do your eyes hurt or do you feel feverish with a headache?
- ℅ Do you have nausea or diarrhea with a headache?
- ℅ Is your tongue coated with green, brown, or yellow phlegm?
- ℅ Do you have hypoglycemia? Do you get a headache when hungry?
- ℅ Do you often feel anxious, nervous, or depressed with a headache?
- ℅ Is your diet poor? Do you eat on the run?

The indigestion headache is worse after eating foods that are rich, spicy, or too raw and cold. Digestive disturbance does not always accompany this kind of headache, but facial coloring may turn greenish or yellow from stuck bile. The headache is weakening, disorienting, and depressing. Aspirin will not relieve the pain because its origin is stuck bile.

Energetic origin

If headache accompanies nausea, vomiting, diarrhea, stomach cramps, dizziness and abdominal distension, it is related to poor functioning of digestive organs. That is the main problem to address. Dulling the nerves or the mind with a typical painkiller will not help. When bile becomes stuck in the bile duct, either as a result of repeated assaults from rich food or from emotional turmoil, the resulting chest and abdominal pain may refer upward to affect the sinuses, the back of the neck, the eyes, the temples, or the forehead. This is because acupuncture meridians related to digestion all pass through those areas on their way to the brain. Indigestion has stopped smooth circulation.

The remedy: ease digestion and circulation

Sometimes people get sick headaches from eating strange things they are not used to, or eating rich, spicy foods in a humid or polluted climate. This kind of indigestion headache often happens on the road.

Many world travelers swear by several Chinese patent remedies. **Po Chai** pills (also known as China **Po Chi Pills** or **Bao Ji Wan**) are the best known of this over-the-counter variety of "I-ate-the-wrong-thing-and-got-sick" pills. They treat sick headaches and have been known to stop the room from spinning. It is an acute remedy; usually one dose will do. These pills come in a box containing ten plastic tubes of little red pills. A dose consists of one tube of pills, the contents of which should be swallowed with warm water.

For digestive and circulatory problems of longer standing, **Xiao Yao Wan** is better. It treats headaches that are due to weak digestion, irregular and painful menstrual periods, PMS, food allergies, and depression. Both of these remedies work by building *chi* to strengthen the digestive center—the stomach, spleen, and pancreas—while encouraging bile to flow and freeing liver and gallbladder function. They contain antiphlegm ingredients such as fu ling and ginger. **Xiao Yao Wan** is a blood-building, balancing remedy that can be used long-term for a great number of digestive and pain problems. (See chapter 3 for a detailed description of **Xiao Yao Wan.**)

If you often get sinus headaches or allergies that impair breathing, digestion, and energy, refer to section I of chapter 13 for dietary recommendations that reduce excess *phlegm*.

LIVER HEADACHES

- ✐ Do you get eye-splitting headaches?
- ✐ Are you often constipated?
- ✐ Do you get so angry you feel as if your head will explode?
- ✐ Do you sometimes have pimples or cold sores with headaches?
- ✐ Are your headaches and mood swings worse before your period?

You know you have a liverish headache when you feel green, when you can't even look at that color because it makes you feel sick. That's because bile, which is green, is stuck. You have a bitter taste in your mouth; your head throbs and burns; your stomach is upset; the world seems like a terrible place. All noises are too loud and lights too bright. Your nerves are on edge, but you can't eat. This is the kind of headache that occurs when anger gets stuck in your throat, or when undigested fat gets stuck in the digestive tract. Or when you get stuck in a relationship you would rather destroy.

Energetic origin

This special category of indigestion headache results from poor circulation affecting the liver and gallbladder organ systems, especially "stuck liver *chi*." Some traditional Chinese medical texts describe such symptoms as "rising liver *chi* or rising liver fire," because inflammation from stuck *bile* can cause hot, pounding headaches. All Chinese herbal cures that treat liverish symptoms, such as red, dry eyes, facial flush, menopausal hot flashes, fever, and trigeminal neuralgia bring *internal heat* downward along the liver and gallbladder acupuncture meridians, relieving pressure in the temples, the eyes, or the entire head.

The remedy: anti-inflammatory cleansing

Many anti-inflammatory herbal medicines "bring inflammation down" by encouraging cleansing. For example, they are laxative. Other herbal painkillers contain natural steroids. The difference between liver headache cures and the other digestive remedies already mentioned is that liver headaches are emotional. They can give you a bitter taste in the mouth because of bitter things you would like to say. There are two approaches to treat it; one is long-term, the other acute.

The long-term approach requires clearing waste that impairs circulation. For example, nutritional acids from evening primrose and flaxseed oils can break up cholesterol that clogs blood vessels, leading to such headaches. These remedies are preventive in nature, as is the anti-inflammatory program in chapter 13. But when in the grips of severe pain, you need fast relief, not prevention.

Several Chinese patent remedies quash liver fire and fury fast—for instance, **Lung Tan Xie Gan Wan** ("Clean the Heat from the Blood of the Liver Pills"). Its main ingredients are bitter digestive tonics, such as gentian, which supports the pancreas, and bupleurum, which encourages healthy flow of bile. This remedy is recommended for bilious headaches, fever blisters on the mouth, constipation, urinary tract infections, thick yellow leukorrhea, and oral and genital herpes. The usual dosage is 6 pills twice a day, but a higher dose (15 pills twice daily) is used in China to curb violent behavior. (See chapter 35 for its uses in psychiatry.)

Combine **Lung Tan Xie Gan Wan** with **Xiao Yao Wan** for PMS headaches. In a later chapter we will learn how PMS headaches (and anger) can result from blood deficiency and stuck *chi*. The dosage for both would be 6 to 8 pills three times a day, but the dosage will vary depending upon the severity of the problem.

EARACHES AND *PHLEGM HEAT* HEADACHES

- Do you get headaches and sores in your mouth?
- Do your gums bleed or hurt?
- Do you get chronic ear infections or yellow ear phlegm?
- Do you get headaches with sore or infected throat?
- Do you get head or face pain from hot, spicy foods?
- Does your head feel stuffed and burning?

Some headaches are related to swelling and inflammation rising from liver, stomach, and heart. Congestion from this type of pain blocks sinus, head, and ears, and is called *phlegm heat*.

Energetic origin

The *phlegm heat* headache can be caused by indigestion, but it is sometimes accompanied by infection from illness or dental problems.

The remedy: cool inflammation

Remedies for this headache treat fever, inflamed throat and gums, irritated eyes, earache, swollen lymph glands, toothaches, headaches, dizziness, and oral sores.

One such remedy is **Niu Huang Chieh Tu Pien** ("Ox Gallstone Dispel Toxin Tablet"). Its main ingredients are rhubarb, gypsum, and skullcap. These are strongly anti-inflammatory, encouraging toxins to leave the liver and large intestine. Platycodon is added to clear phlegm, borneol opens the senses, and the 1-percent ox gallstone that gives the combination its name is extremely bitter and therefore anti-inflammatory.

BLOOD-DEFICIENCY HEADACHES

- Do you get a headache after your menstrual period?
- Are you listless with pale lips?
- Do you have thinning hair and bloodshot eyes?
- Do you have throbbing headache or vertigo?
- Do you feel depressed and have a poor appetite?
- Do you get headaches from boredom or nervous burnout?
- Do you have long-term insomnia or a drinking problem?

Some headache remedies treat a damaged liver by correcting a blood deficiency. When the liver has adequate blood to function well, it can detoxify the body and refresh the senses.

It's important to build blood to prevent chronic nervous headaches, because blood deficiency is a deep problem that affects many areas. Headache is only a symptom of something more serious. When the body is chronically blood-deficient, everything goes into high gear and burnout. But reversing blood deficiency with herbs stops pain, dizziness, and blurry vision, improves mental functions, and slows aging.

Energetic origin

Blood deficiency can result from feverish illness or injury. In these cases the acute problem, whether from infection, injury, or other causes, should be addressed first. The headache is a secondary symptom that will disappear easily with antibiotic or *cooling* herbs. But chronic blood deficiency leads to spasm, pain, or degeneration of tissue. Whether it's due to stress or aging, it can be treated with blood tonic herbs that reverse dehydration, hormone imbalances, and faded mental functions. They can also gradually eliminate headaches.

The remedy: herbs that build blood

I won't go into detail here, because other chapters treat blood production and supplements, but I'll mention a few headache remedies that nourish blood. When you take them to treat pain, you will notice they have a profound healing effect, because blood is the deepest source of our vitality. You may be surprised how much better you feel, aside from losing your headache.

As far as dosage is concerned, most blood tonics are very moistening, so the dosage must be adjusted to individual use. If your tongue is red, you can use larger and more frequent doses—for example, 5 pills three times daily. If the tongue is pale

or indicates *phlegm,* reduce the dose to a comfortable amount—for example, 3 pills twice daily. Take blood-building herbs daily for two weeks between menstrual periods, otherwise as directed on the box.

Tienma and Shou Wu is a Chinese patent remedy named for its two main herbs—the first one quiets spasms, the second builds blood. This general tonic for either sex treats vertigo, dizziness, headache, fatigue, poor appetite, and poor memory. As an added attraction, shou wu is reputed to reverse graying and thinning hair if used daily for one year. This is a fine remedy for victims of the Fast Track or those suffering menopausal headache and dizziness. Other Chinese patent blood elixirs include the following:

Shou Wu Pien (a.k.a. fo ti)
Eight Treasure Tea
Tang Kuei Tablets
Tang Kuei and Gastrodia (tienma)

The herbal combinations used in **Tienma and Shou Wu** as well as the pure **Shou Wu Pien** pills are *cooling,* moisturizing, and sedating for frayed nerves. They make a relaxing, nourishing headache remedy suited for those with a reddish, dry, and shaking tongue, indicating nervous exhaustion. A mere aspirin cannot rebuild damaged nerves as these can.

Those containing tang kuei are *warming,* which means they increase circulation and are recommended for weakness, pallor, and chronic chills (a pale tongue), not menopausal or feverish headaches. If you have been blood-deficient for a long time,

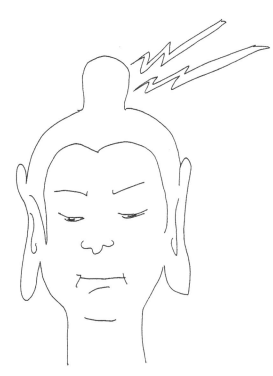

How did you get a headache?
Catch a cold? Work too hard? Eat a bad diet?

the first few doses of a *warming* blood-builder will calm you, not stimulate you, because it nourishes your real strength.

PMS AND INSOMNIA

Another popular remedy for headache and dizziness caused by blood deficiency is a Chinese patent remedy, **Ansenpunaw Tablets.** These are described on the box as a brain tonic and sedative medicine. They are suited for weak, tired persons with a pale tongue. The ingredients also treat in-

somnia because they are so nourishing that they help you rest when you've worked so hard you can't stop.

Ansenpunaw Tablets cure dull, throbbing headaches and vertigo and contain many blood-building herbs, including tang kuei, ligustrum, eclipta, and he shou wu, along with anti-inflammatory painkillers such as the herbs polygala and cinnabris.

The dosage on the bottle says 3 to 4 tablets three times daily, but I usually end up taking a handful of them when I can't sleep from too much thinking or worrying and my head is beating from overwork. The herbal ingredients offer more than a simple headache sedative. They rebuild damaged liver, kidney, and nerves.

The Headache Remedy for You

How can you know what headache remedy to take? A problem as well as an advantage of Asian medicine is that it offers many opportunities for treatment. Some people might say there are *too* many choices. But there's a solution. The advantage in studying all the possibilities for treatment is that someday you may need them. But how can you choose your headache cure for today? Here are some questions and answers to help you:

Is it better to take an aspirin for pain?

How aspirin works is not completely clear. Western doctors think it works by blocking the release of prostaglandins, substances se-

HEADACHE PAIN

TYPE OF PAIN	RELATED TO	TYPE OF REMEDY	EXAMPLE
eyes burning, bloodshot	liver, toxic chemicals	cleanser	aloe gel
eyes and head throbbing, anger	liver congestion	cleanser	**Lung Tan Xie Gan Wan**
top of head and sinus congestion	*phlegm*	decongestant	gotu kola snuff
headache with nausea	liver	digestive	**Xiao Yao Wan**
head, ear, or tooth, hot and throbbing, thick yellow phlegm	infection	*cooling,* cleansing	**Niu Huang Chieh Tu Pien**
headache, fever	colds, flu	*cooling* antibiotic	**Yinchiao Chieh Tu Pien** (see chapter 30)

creted by the cells that cause fever, swelling, and pain. Inhibiting them is, in effect, anti-inflammatory. Unfortunately, inflammation can be a very important warning signal that indicates congested circulation, infection, or toxins. Eliminating the fire alarm while ignoring the fire can be hazardous.

Sometimes aspirin seems more convenient than herbal treatment because it requires no diagnosis. When a headache is due to a change in the weather, or when the pain is only occasional, many people take aspirin. But we should also consider the reasons for the headache and work to eliminate them.

Problems arise when we take aspirin repeatedly. Since it's absorbed into the bloodstream through the stomach lining, the resulting irritation or ulcers often make aspirin more a problem than it's worth. Aspirin also thins the blood, which is not a good thing for weak, anemic people. Luckily, aspirin is not the only answer for pain.

Is there an aspirin alternative?

Many herbs are excellent, safe anti-inflammatories. For example, capsules of evening primrose oil also prevent inflammation by inhibiting prostaglandins, but without side effects.

Evening primrose oil has been recommended for the prevention of migraines, arthritis, menstrual pain, PMS, acne, and weight loss. It helps clear toxins as well as treat pain. The usual dosage for prevention is 2 or 3 capsules daily.

DIET AND HEADACHES

Indigestion is the underlying cause of many headaches. See which diet is the best for you to avoid stress and "sick" headaches.

TONGUE	AVOID
red, dry	hot spice, greasy, oily food, excess coffee, alcohol
phlegm coating	all of the above, also cream sauces and dairy foods
pale tongue	cold foods, salads, excess sour or sweet foods
phlegm coating	all of the above, also dairy foods, sprouts, grapefruit

When should you use herbs for prevention of headaches?

If headaches are recurrent, the underlying problems should be addressed. Stress shows up in a number of ways, including fatigue, blood deficiency, and high blood pressure. If medical problems such as cholesterol, injury, or seizures are not an issue, it pays to support nutritional and energetic weakness with herbs. Sometimes taking only a bottle of blood-building herbs will reverse many nervous exhaustion symptoms, including headache.

If you know your headaches are not a chronic problem, if you suddenly develop a severe headache, then you have to determine its type.

NON-PILL HEADACHE REMEDIES

Smear-on cures

My Hungarian grandmother used to tie sliced, raw hot pepper onto her forehead with a red bandanna. I don't recommend

it. Many people use **Tiger Balm** instead. This small jar of red or white salve is sold in all Asian vegetable stands.

The red type is *warming,* and the white type stimulates circulation through both *warming* and *cooling* action. Rub the red salve into painful areas, avoiding the eyes, only if the idea of applying heat sounds good. The remedy brings blood circulation to the pain the way massage or acupuncture might. That would work well for headaches resulting from stuck *chi.*

Another such remedy is a mildly camphorated oil called **White Flowers,** available in Chinese herb shops. Its pleasant, *cooling* aroma as well as its *warming* sensation eases tension.

INHALER REMEDIES

Everything that enters the nose directly affects blood vessels that nourish the brain. It's little wonder that irritants such as pollution, cigarette smoke, and cocaine compromise our concentration.

Indian and Tibetan doctors offer snuff

HEADACHES: THE TIME AND PLACE

❂ After meals (phlegm or sinus allergy): Possible remedies include ginger tea, **Xiao Yao Wan.**

❂ After your period: **Ansenpunaw Tablets.**

❂ On airplanes: Take valerian; it's grounding, useful for migraines.

❂ In smoke-filled rooms (allergic liverish headache): Drink lots of aloe juice or gel, **Lung Tan Xie Gan Wan.**

❂ During PMS (stuck liver *chi*): **Xiao Yao Wan.**

❂ From high blood pressure: **Angelica 14** and **Uncaria 6** (made by Seven Forests).

---

remedies for headaches. For sinus congestion, I've already mentioned powdered gotu kola capsules, available in herb shops and supermarkets. Indian groceries also offer pure *edible* camphor, a refreshing inhaler. The first is more *drying*, the second *cooling*, like the air on high mountains.

For liverish headaches accompanied by red, dry eyes, a bitter taste in the mouth, fever, and anger, sniff aloe vera gel with a dropper. It cools and restores normal nerve stimulation to the brain.

For nervous anxiety, fear, and resulting insomnia, try a drop of pure raw sesame oil into each nostril. It is a heavy, nutritious oil (used in cooking) that quiets nerves, treating spasms and seizures. Asian doctors say it settles *wind.*

sign of imbalance. Use the appropriate oil daily for a fifteen-minute massage, then wash it off.

Phlegm: Corn oil stimulates nerves and reduces *phlegm.*
Heat: Sunflower and olive oils are *cooling.*
Wind: Raw sesame oil is sedating and grounding; it slows digestion.

You may want to leave the oil on for a longer time. A good way to do that is to rub some oil onto the soles of your feet before bed, and wear socks. Of course, if you're a gypsy, you'll need to rub raw sesame oil on the soles of your feet before bed to sleep deeply and prevent you from traveling.

MASSAGE REMEDIES

Sometimes a relaxing body massage that eases tension can also cure underlying problems with the *humors* (see chapter 10). They can prevent recurrent headaches, a

Toothaches

I got my tooth problems from being a gypsy. It wasn't diet. I was raised on creamed chicken, dumplings, stuffed cabbage, and prune-filled sweets, although

I've not eaten that menu in years. It's the gypsy's way to search out the other side of the field. I visited tiny villages and grand, ancient ruins in jungles and mountains, traveling light and fasting when provisions were unsafe or unavailable, while feasting on exotic sights and sounds.

I once consulted a large, well-off-looking dentist in my Manhattan neighborhood. When he read me the list of things he wanted to do in my mouth, along with the considerable price, I bolted up in the chair and said, "I'd rather go to India." He looked indignant, whisked away the white paper covering me from my chin to my knees, and retorted, "Well, then, go to India!" So I did. It was wonderful! I came back changed, forever blessed. But I ignored my teeth. Eventually I got tooth pain and went to another dentist. If only the crowns for our heads were our only crowns!

Herbal remedies work better than aspirin for root canals, extractions, and local nerve irritation, that searing burn in the jaw or head after nerves have been inflamed by drilling. Nerve pain can also come from cold foods or cold air. Valerian, a nerve sedative, is best for that torture. I have taken as many as three capsules every four hours to control nerve pain. **Yunnan Paiyao** controls pain and bleeding quite well for gum surgery. **Niu Huang Chieh Tu Pien,** a local anti-inflammatory, reduces not only tooth pain, but also headache, earache, and sore throat.

These tooth remedies all work differently. **Niu Huang Chieh Tu Pien,** which we'll study in detail later, is an anti-inflammatory remedy. Use it when pain feels hot and throbbing. **Yunnan Paiyao** removes pain by increasing circulation. Use it when there is swelling, bruising, and bleeding. Valerian stops pain by sedating irritated nerves. It's perfect for pain after the dentist has been in your mouth with a drill. Use it for pain that is sharp, shooting, and electric. It quiets the nerves to let you sleep.

I finally got my dental work done in Vermont. It cost less, and the dentist was nicer. After many crowns, he gave me the royal treatment—thanked me and shook hands when I left. A Hungarian would have kissed my hand, but shaking hands was very good. I took a lot of valerian to ease the pain, and sent him a photo I'd taken of a street dentist in rural Yunnan. It showed a sign with big red Chinese characters announcing his trade, while he sat awaiting new clients. His tools were arranged in front of him: various sizes of horse pliers. Some things are better at home.

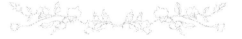

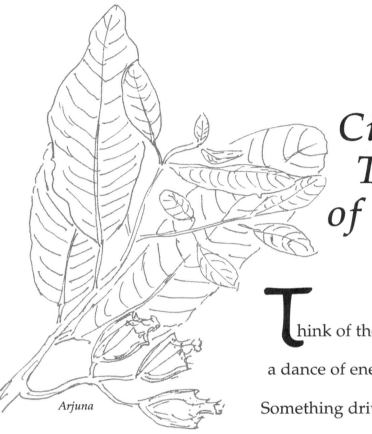

Arjuna

21
Circulation: The Heart of the Matter

Think of the human body as an atom, a dance of energy, movement, and light. Something drives its inner workings and motivates its change. Something keeps it going. That something is energy. Invisible, it is the source and direction for life.

When traditional Asian doctors refer to circulation, they describe the flow of that vital energy. Whether it is called *chi, prana,* or *rloong,* it is life force that moves through us like the wind. That force field has been charted by all Asian medical traditions. We can perceive energy circulating through the body the same way we perceive electricity: by its effects, which can be observed and measured.

The following two chapters cover an array of health questions related to circulation. The first deals with the upper body, describing complaints such as chest pain, high blood pressure, and bruises; the second, with the lower body, hemorrhoids, and sciatica. When the flow of energy is interrupted or reduced, life processes are impaired. We suffer pain and emotional "stuckness." The ebb and flow of health is not consistent but is shaped every day. The circulation of energy and blood is so fundamental to life that it influences the whole person—mentally, physically, and spiritually.

A key to resolving circulation problems, whether they result in a red complexion, pain, bruises, or emotional issues, is to reduce *chi* congestion from unhealthy diet. Fat and sweet foods combined with stress are a constant in urban life. It would be nice to be able to take three weeks off on a regular basis to cleanse, but most people don't take the time or trouble. Some others need immediate relief. Several of the remedies in this chapter will be of great use.

Digestive and Emotional Aspects of **Chi**

Poor circulation, and an extreme condition known as blood stasis, can lead to a breakdown of life functions. Without free-flowing *chi*, internal organs have no fuel. *Chi* has solid and nonsolid components. Enhanced by food and oxygen, it is also affected by the psyche. *Chi* is not blood or electricity moving through veins, but rather the movement of current. Pain from blocked *chi* results from weakness, injury, disease, or negative emotions. Circulation of *chi* and blood deteriorates from stress and diet because they involve the heart. In turn, the heart pumps blood while maintaining the smooth flow of *chi*.

Most people have experienced the temporary effects of poor *chi* circulation—sharp pain or numbness—but some people cultivate discomfort with extremist habits. Damaging actions and attitudes attenuate the ebb and flow of life.

For example, many persons have cold hands and feet because circulation is trapped in the digestive center. They may overindulge in hot pepper or garlic, overstimulating the liver, or oily and fried foods, congesting the liver. The person who eats garlic daily may enjoy its antibiotic properties even while suffering from *internal heat* complaints such as tachycardia, headache, anger, or skin rashes. Acid inflammation becomes trapped in the body when not eliminated in wastes—for example, at the joints, creating inflammatory arthritis. Or it directly affects the heart, provoking anxiety attacks. When we tie a knot of stuck circulation in the center, *chi* cannot smoothly reach the extremities.

Other people tie a knot in the center by eating too many sweets, compromising the digestive function of spleen/pancreas. Either knot damages the heart. The person addicted to sweets will be plagued by poor digestion, flatulence, bloating, or water retention in the middle, as well as low energy and cloudy thinking. When digestion is impeded, circulation for the rest of the body suffers. Eventually the heart suffers.

Emotions also cause *chi* circulation problems. We have all suffered a "broken heart." Feelings affect heart rhythm. Not only does stress encourage cholesterol, but the workings of internal organs are affected by attitudes. I have seen people in frustrating love affairs react with intense liver or heart pain. The *chi* is stuck. Whether it's due to digestion or purely emotional is an individual matter.

Diagnosis

Informal Asian diagnosis of the face and tongue offers a guide to reading deep imbalances. According to the *Nei Ching*, a red face denotes *heat* emanating from the heart. Purplish lips indicate stuck blood circulation. Whether they result from excess cholesterol or hormone or emotional imbalance, the effects of poor circulation can be temporary or long-term. As we shall see, in extreme cases, emotional stability can be rocked and even the elasticity of blood vessels can be damaged by a combination of factors. We'll study facial diagnosis in chapter 25, which covers herbs for skin problems.

What are other indicators of poor circulation? Aside from local pain or bruising caused by trauma, Asian tongue diagnosis identifies signs of chronic poor circulation. Long-term *internal heat* or *internal cold* conditions precipitate poor functioning of internal organs, a buildup of toxins, blood and energy deficiency, and damage to organs themselves. When poor circulation has allowed impurities and imbalances to remain unchecked, the tongue reveals signs of *stagnant chi*. The body of the tongue itself may be discolored with gray, dark red, or black inside, or dark spots will appear on the surface, indicating areas in the body where oxygenation and nourishment are hindered.

POOR CIRCULATION AND THE LIVER

Ancient Chinese doctors felt that internal organs had psychological as well as physical functions. According to them, the liver contained a "soul" that decided our desires. The scope of our wants, drives, and ambitions may be decided by the liver, but they are carried out only with the collaboration of both liver and gallbladder energies. Following are several stories of frustrated desires, liver pain, and bruised spirits.

EMOTIONAL STUCK LIVER *CHI*

I once treated two brothers from a well-to-do Long Island family. Both were lawyers with *internal heat* symptoms. Tim slept every night with his teeth and fists clenched. He kept his wife awake by grinding his teeth during sleep. Over the years, this gave him tremendous headaches and dental bills. He had a sharp pain in the right side at his liver, and a slight yellow cast, when I first saw him.

"I'm under stress," he said. "The doctors haven't helped a bit. I had $20,000 worth of tests run to tell me there is nothing wrong. I could kill them all!" His eyes bulged.

His *chi* circulation was stuck at the liver. When I touched the area, it was sensitive though not swollen. On my advice, Tim took a thermos of aloe vera juice, adding homeopathic natrum sulphate, the liver cleanser. Drinking this combination all day at work eliminated his chronic constipation and jaundiced color. The remedy encouraged his liver to work better, freeing the flow of bile.

Shu Gan Wan, the Chinese patent remedy, helped Tim's digestion, circulation, and mood. Its ingredients remove jaundice resulting from stuck bile because they smooth *chi* circulation in the center. The digestive center is also the center of our emotions, so that better circulation there helps calm depression and anxiety. **Shu Gan Wan** works well for chest pains and digestive or emotional disturbance caused by weakness and stuck *chi,* whereas cleansing remedies such as **Lung Tan Xie Gan Wan** reduce *internal heat* symptoms such as constipation, headache, and anger. The two remedies can be taken separately or together, depending on the discomfort. Tim took the recommended dose for both combinations at mealtime until all chest discomfort disappeared.

Tim's teeth-grinding also stopped after he took an herb before bed. **Essence of Tienchi Flowers** is a *cooling*, extremely sweet-tasting Chinese instant beverage. He used it daily as a sugar substitute at work, and one half package in warm water before bed. Tienchi is a form of ginseng used to dramatically increase blood circulation, heal wounds, and resolve bruises. The tienchi flower, which is the main ingredient of the instant crystals, cools inflammation from an overactive liver.

It worked in about a week: No more tension headaches, facial pimples, bad breath, grinding teeth, nervousness, dizziness, nausea, or palpitations. These symptoms are referred to as "bilious" symptoms, related to liver and gallbladder function. **Essence of Tienchi Flowers** reduces *internal heat* resulting from high blood pressure, rich diet, alcohol, and stress.

With better circulation and digestion, Tim relaxed somewhat. People at work wondered what had happened. His wife was overjoyed to get a good night's sleep at last, and sent me all their friends, including Tim's brother Jim.

I never understood why Tim had so many "liver symptoms" until I met Jim. He told me, "I'm allergic to everything— pollen, dust, trees, dogs, you name it. It started last year when I married Julianna."

The Long Island family had put the sons through Harvard, paid for their apartments, and bought them cars with the understanding that they would become lawyers, like all male members of the family, and grow up to be respectable company presidents. Tim gritted his teeth and tried to make a good show. He wore black suits, developed an ulcer at twenty, and at thirty was a junior executive.

Jim wore blue jeans and sneered, "When we were growing up, we'd drive to the country club and my parents would complain if the kid who parked the car wore dirty sneakers. Now they don't even talk to me. Dad said he'd take back my car and apartment after he heard about Julianna." His wife, a gorgeous Jamaican, had hoped to endear her relatives to her by pursuing her career as an artist.

Jim's allergies, a symptom of his rage, were caused by his overactive liver. The liver, a major detoxification organ, rids the body of irritants. When a person is under physical or emotional stress, it can overreact with unnecessary defenses. Jim's liver reacted as though he needed to defend himself against everything. Although we shall study allergies in chapter 23, I will bring up the point now that poor circulation and emotional stress can make allergies worse.

SPASMS, TICS, AND CALCIUM

When liver *chi* functions well, we have adequate absorption of calcium, so that muscles react in a smooth coordinated manner. When *chi* circulation is impaired, we are apt to have spasms, tics, pains, and "held-in feelings," which Chinese doctors recognize as symptoms of "stagnant liver *chi*." Stuck blood circulation causes severe pain, bruising, and, nervousness, or even feverish conditions because of hidden imbalances. After circulation improves, the deeper imbalance can surface. We often see this with massage or chiropractic adjustments, where patients respond with acute emotions after a stressed area becomes free.

INDIGESTION, STUCK *CHI*, AND ANXIETY

Rex walked in looking like a big sunbeam. Six feet three, suntanned, and freckled, you'd think he'd stepped off a billboard. He flashed a polite smile but then hunched over and, without breathing, went immediately into his list of complaints.

"I have indigestion all the time, with pain and flatulence. My knees hurt. I'm tired and nervous. And lately I have this." He showed me a rash on his arms. "I think it's cancer." He looked gloomy.

His bright red tongue and pulses indicated *internal heat*. The blood pulses were low from a deficiency of moisture, while the energy pulses were overly high. The beat was "stagnant," as though trying to push forward but stopped by a brick wall. Circulation in the chest was troubled. The skin rash did not look like cancer, but I advised him to check with a plastic surgeon .

As I gave Rex acupuncture, we chatted, and I learned he was an artist. He had enjoyed some success in SoHo galleries, but had not made the kind of money he wanted. He was presently painting apartments to make a living. He started by saying, "I am very intelligent and have an excellent education, much better than most people's." But he was not living up to the high goals he had set for himself, and now his wife was pregnant. "We can hardly pay the rent now," he gasped.

All this came out while I was giving him acupuncture to release stuck liver *chi,* using points on his feet, stomach, and back. Then Rex breathed deeper, and grinned. "It's working," he said. "I feel better."

Rex needed to shake off pent-up energy and emotions. When I recommended dance, he laughed. He had done paintings of dancers, but never danced himself. He decided to take a class in Haitian dance. After the acupuncture treatment, he lifted me off the floor with his hug. With smoother *chi* circulation, Rex was his happy self again. Now we had to maintain his high energy and enthusiasm with herbs.

Rex loved the name of the herbal combination I recommended: **Relaxed Wanderer.** It's a Jade Pharmacy formula made by East Earth Herbs (see Herbal Access) that treats "stagnant liver *chi.*" It combines tang kuei, paeonia, atractylodes, ligusticum root to nourish blood, and poria, bupleurum, mint, cyperus, moutan, gardenia fruit, and ginger to increase circulation. A small amount of licorice root is added to make the other herbs work smoothly.

Similar to the Chinese patent formula **Xiao Yao Wan, Relaxed Wanderer** is useful for nervousness, depression, chest pains, indigestion, distension, and stomachache. It has a stronger dose of blood-building herbs than the Chinese remedy, as well as gardenia to rid the body of *damp heat* (thick yellow phlegm discharges) and gastrodia to "settle wind," i.e., treat nerve irritation and spasm. The herbs combine in such a way as to bring down inflammation from the upper body, quiet nervousness, and nurture the digestive center.

In a week, many of Rex's nervous discomforts cleared up. He treated his stomach acid burn with one-half cup of aloe vera gel added to apple juice daily. That greatly reduced his skin rash. I hear he is adding aloe plants to his paintings. I'm sure he will become a great Haitian dancer.

ARJUNA

Arjuna is the Indian herb of choice for the prevention and treatment of heart disease. The powder or decoction of this bitter-sour tree bark is taken during and after an attack. For prevention, fill one empty capsule and take it on an empty stomach twice daily. For treatment, take four capsules daily according to your constitutional type.

WIND types who are weak, have poor circulation, and ache all over can take the capsules along with a nourishing broth made with warming spices and a little olive oil.

BILE types who have inflammatory symptoms can take the capsules with rice or soy milk, rice, and green vegetables, avoiding hot spices and fried foods.

PHLEGM types who are overweight or have excess congestion can take the capsules with barley soup and digestive spices.

Order Arjuna from Bheshaj Bhawan, A 24 Krishan Nagar extn., Delhi 110051.

HIGH BLOOD PRESSURE
AND CHEST PAINS

Hugh came in and nervously sat down. He wore a black suit and formal shoes—immaculate. His blond hair was thin and his face too pink, as though his tie were choking him. As usual, I was casual, squatting on a futon couch wearing jeans. We were quite a contrast. He stared for a minute at wooden masks from Ladakh and the Thai jungle, thangkas from Nepal, weavings from Guatemala. My "office" resembles a jungle camp.

A professor of pathology at a medical college where I had lectured, he had waited nearly a year to call me. He had high blood pressure, he said, and listed his medications. He stuttered when he said they made him sexually impotent.

His tongue was reddish with purple spots, and quivered, showing *stagnant* liver, lung, and heart circulation. I was not surprised. His thinning hair and red complexion were signs of *internal heat.* His cholesterol was high, and he occasionally experienced chest pain. He smoked two packs of cigarettes a day, and often consumed red meat and wine. He was forty-two and divorced. His father and two uncles had died of heart attacks. He would not have come to see me except that he wanted to get off the blood pressure medicine that was ruining his love life.

Blood circulation is a problem inherent in high blood pressure. *Stagnant chi* and partially blocked blood vessels result in chest pain and numbness of the hands. Heart valve problems and high cholesterol are often involved.

Hugh said he was willing to change his diet, but didn't know where to start. I recommended he read Dr. Vasant Lad's book, *Ayurveda: The Science of Self-Healing,* to get an idea of foods that are *heating* and *cooling.* After that, he could change his diet to include *cooling* foods such as oatmeal, green vegetables, white meat of chicken, and white basmati rice, slowly eliminating *heating* and congesting foods such as red meat, nuts, and cheese.

Anti-inflammatory, diuretic herbs

I recommended a Chinese remedy called **Blood Pressure Repressing Tablets** for Hugh. The combination contains skullcap and coptis, which is high in berberin, a natural anti-inflammatory, as well as diuretic herbs. It reduces headache and nervous insomnia while lowering blood pressure. The interesting thing about these herbs is they are anti-inflammatory for the head, but not for the sex life. Their overall effect is diuretic and *cooling,* but balancing. During our first meeting, I gave Hugh acupuncture in the feet and back of the neck, which quickly made him feel cool and relaxed as it brought down his blood pressure.

Chest pains

For prevention of chest pains, numb extremities, heart attack, and stroke, I recommended another Chinatown remedy, **Mao Dung Ching,** capsules of holly. Many Asian herbal remedies for high blood pressure work the way holly does, dilating blood vessels near the heart while increasing blood circulation. They give immediate relief from chest discomfort because of increased blood circulation.

Dan Shen Wan, another patent remedy for chest pain, works in the same way: Camphor dilates blood vessels, while sage increases circulation to reduce pain. It is recommended for angina, pain radiating down the left arm, palpitations, and chest pain. It reduces cholesterol and lipids. Both **Mao Dung Ching** and **Dan Shen Wan** are available with instructions in English from Chinese herb shops. Persons living far from Chinatown should consult Herbal Access for mail-order sources.

Other hypertension herbs

Uncaria 6 is a hypertension remedy made by Seven Forests. It reduces facial flushing, palpitations, headaches, and dizziness. It contains uncaria, prunellas, scute, eucommia, loranthus, and tang kuei. The first three herbs move inflammation downward, eucommia and loranthus energize the legs and back, and tang kuei, the blood tonic, increases circulation to free painful areas.

Uncaria 6 can be combined with other Seven Forests remedies such as **Salvia Shou Wu** to reduce pain and blood stasis from general cardiovascular disease; with **Angelica 14** for headaches due to hypertension; and **Ardisia 16** for hypertension associated with extreme stress.

Hugh continued with Chinese herbs, monitoring his own blood pressure at the same time each day for two months. It stabilized at a normal level. He cut back his Western medication and said he felt greatly improved. There was an additional, unexpected improvement: With less inflammation and congestion in the blood vessels, Hugh's vision improved. It was as though the anti-inflammatory acupuncture treatments, along with the *cooling* herbs, lifted a cloud from his eyes. He said he could see colors more clearly. He also seemed more calm and self-assured when he spoke.

His brother, also an M.D., called me from Michigan. He had the same lifestyle. He smoked, was overweight, and had high cholesterol. Other than that, he said he was very healthy and played tennis twice a week. He asked if there was an herb he could take for irregular heartbeat and high cholesterol.

I recommended Seven Forests' **Lotus Leaf Tablets,** which are slimming herbs for obesity that reduce blood lipids, cholesterol, and triglycerides. A main ingredient is hawthorn berries. Hawthorn tends to normalize a stressed heartbeat by strengthening muscles; sour and bitter, it also moves sluggish digestion. It can eventually eliminate congestion or even clear masses in the intestine.

BRUISES: A DEEP PROBLEM

Bruises involve a number of health issues in that they have both superficial and internal aspects. They appear on the skin, but are made worse from weakness, poor circulation, and deep imbalance. They are created by the spillover of blood from damaged vessels into the surrounding tissue after injury. Given good circulation, minor bruises go away in a few days with no help at all. Major ones require herbs that increase blood circulation. (See chapter 18, on **Yunnan Paiyao.**)

Bruises on the skin's surface are influenced by the Wood and Fire elements, the liver and heart organ systems. Important factors are poor circulation and toxic blood conditions. Digestion, the Earth element, is also involved. It is said that when the spleen/pancreas is not strong enough to facilitate absorption of protein and minerals, the "blood spills over the boundaries of the blood vessels." In other words, when digestion and absorption are inadequate, we have fragile blood vessels, bruises, and broken capillaries. To cure the underlying conditions, we must address digestive problems.

Nutritional supplements of vitamin P strengthen fragile capillaries. These include vitamin C complex, citrus bioflavonoids, rutin, hesperidin, and foods such as the white skin parts of citrus fruits—oranges, lemons, or grapefruits. Apricots, buckwheat, blackberries, cherries, rose hips, and green tea also contain vitamin P.

FALSE FIRE, BROKEN CAPILLARIES, AND ROSACEA

Some cases are more complicated because they involve internal imbalance, such as problems with metabolism or hormone balance. Bright red or purple broken capillaries can appear under the skin without injury, as though blood vessels were bursting from excess heat. Fragile capillaries play a part in what Chinese doctors call "false fire," inflammation caused by deficiency of blood and *yin,* especially as it concerns the liver and kidney organ systems. An example of this may be what dermatologists call acne rosacea, a ruddiness of the skin around the mouth and cheeks, which is believed to occur most frequently among blond women over forty. It may be related to menopause as much as to skin type. (Beauty problems affecting skin and hair will be covered in a later chapter. The present chapter deals with underlying problems involving circulation.)

Fragile capillaries are a deeper problem. They appear as "spider veins" anywhere on the face, arms, and legs. They can also occur in the brain. Exhaustion, diet, hormone imbalance, alcoholism, poor circulation, and conflicting emotions weaken *chi,* hindering circulation, detoxification, and metabolism. That makes broken capillaries more frequent. Here's an analogy: When making a pottery vase, the potter must be sure the clay is strong enough to support its shape. In the same way, digestion creates the body's strength. When the building material is rich from adequate nutrition, blood, and moisture, we have strong capillaries. But if the clay vase is filled with hot, corrosive liquid, it could wear thin, the way toxins or cholesterol damage blood vessels. And, finally, the vase has to be respected, protected on a shelf, or else it could be accidentally smashed.

The Asian herbal treatment of fragile

capillaries reduces inflammation and toxins from liver and blood, while supporting the function of spleen/pancreas to strengthen blood vessels. This improves circulation in general, and speeds healing time. Often the damage can be slowed; sometimes it can be reversed.

Capillaries and the heart: Circulation and emotions

Because the problem of fragile blood vessels can be profound and long-term, we must address the emotions. Ancient Chinese doctors believed the resilience of blood capillaries indicates the health of the heart. According to the Correspondences, a red face indicates *internal heat* troubling the heart (see chapter 9). That may be an oversimplification, but circulation is quite sensitive to emotions.

Western medical students are taught that the heart is only an elaborate pump, but to traditional Asian doctors, it does more than circulate blood. Through its smooth rhythmic movements, a healthy heart maintains the balance of hormones, brain chemicals, and emotions. I once knew a person whose fiery red capillaries were a result of calcium malabsorption combined with a hormone imbalance and frustrated rage come to the surface.

Kaye lived in an airtight New York apartment. You perspired the moment you walked in. Decorated with brown walls, hieroglyphic wallpaper, and gold-colored drapes, the place reeked of lily of the valley, a *heating* stimulant. Installed on a couch near a bust of Cleopatra, her haircut a helmet of curls, Kaye wore a purple toga and many rings, and had dagger-point fingernails. All she needed was a scepter. Her beet-red face and raspy, barking voice completed a picture of *internal heat* and *stagnant chi.* Her husband, Ralph, stayed out of the way while she crocheted tablecloths he called "webs."

The heat in their home made them boil over. During arguments, they yelled. Kaye kicked, scratched, bit, and jabbed with crocheting needles or kitchen knives. Books and vases flew through the air. Some hit their mark on both sides. Gallery owners, they were battered veterans of the New York Art–Scene Wars. Each consulted me for their health.

Ralph had high blood pressure and chronic toothaches. His headaches and dizziness cleared up quickly with herbs I recommended, **Blood Pressure Repressing Tablets** from Chinatown. For toothaches he took **Niu Huang Chieh Tu Pien,** a combination of ten *cooling* herbs including camphor, honeysuckle, mint, skullcap, blood-builders, and bovine gallstone, which clears sore throat, bleeding gums, mumps, earache, toothache, and nausea. Ralph said his symptoms also disappeared during separate vacations.

Kaye's problems were harder to solve. For one thing, her self-awareness was limited. Her house was afire, but she didn't know it. Her only complaint was broken capillaries on her arms and legs, even though her *stagnant heat* symptoms were many and long-standing.

Signs and symptoms of **stagnant heat**

Kaye's tongue was reddish black, with a thick coating of gray phlegm. That and many other signs pointed to an overheated liver. For example, her pulses were thin and very tight, indicating that *chi* circulation at the deepest levels (the internal organs) was troubled. Her eyes were cloudy, chronically bloodshot, and dry. Her thin, rippled fingernails had white spots that showed that her calcium absorption was faulty, from liver *heat*. In public she grimaced, and scratched or bit Ralph. The outcome of their debates was damaged liver *chi*.

A diet of fats and sweets

Aside from occasional fruits and vegetables, Kaye's diet consisted of *warming* grains, honey, tahini, lots of nuts, cheese, cookies, and large daily doses of chocolate —in other words, mostly sweet, oily, congesting foods that result in *phlegm*. When I met them, they both weighed over two hundred pounds.

Congestion caused by diet, combined with the scalding apartment—not to mention their fights—gave them both tempers. Kaye overheated herself further by smearing herself with heavy creams, hoping to reduce broken capillaries. Instead, the oil blocked her skin's breathing, and increased inflammation. Kaye rarely ventured into the sun or exercised vigorously. She complained bitterly that when she did, her capillaries left fine red spiderwebs on her skin. But merely addressing the fragile capillaries, while ignoring the underlying *heat* con-

dition, would have been like painting green leaves on a burning tree.

A cooling, *cleansing diet*

I recommended the *cooling* foods discussed in section II of chapter 13 and big doses of a Chinese liver-cleansing herbal combination, **Lung Tan Xie Gan Wan,** as many as 15 pills three times a day, until all *heat* symptoms cooled. That would have calmed her temper while clearing skin ruddiness and blemishes. After not taking my advice, Kaye consulted a battery of learned Asian physicians, including a famous Tibetan doctor and several Chinese ones, as well as one Ayurvedic healer. But three years later, Kaye's *internal heat,* bad temper, and broken capillaries remained a way of life. She took high doses of vitamin C and smeared herself with creams, avoiding all fresh air and light, but her problem was actually much deeper than the skin.

Appearance, circulation, and spirit

According to traditional Chinese medicine, our facial color and actions indicate the health of the *shen,* the spirit of the heart. It is that spirit which keeps us balanced and sane. When the heart *chi* is unstable, the *shen* becomes disturbed. The person may become hysterical, have nightmares, chatter excessively, or suffer anxiety attacks. Kaye had all of the above. *Internal heat* can start anywhere in the body. But when it penetrates the deepest levels, it reaches the heart and blood. *Internal heat* deranges not only circulation, but also the spirit.

So-called *heat* in the blood can have either physical or emotional repercussions. If purely physical, the result might be high fever, coma, or delirium. "Reckless blood" caused by *internal heat* can burst blood vessels, causing nosebleed, blood in the urine, broken capillaries, or hemorrhage. If the *heat* imbalance affects the *shen,* the results are psychological, with resulting anxiety or mania.

Compassionate Sage–Heart Spirit, an herbal pill, treats a number of such *heat* symptoms. Based on ancient recipes brought up to date by Jade Pharmacy, it is manufactured by East Earth Herbs (see Herbal Access). It is recommended for disturbed *shen* to "nurture heart blood and *yin,* invigorate blood to break *stagnation,* tonify heart energy and reduce heart fire." It regulates a variety of complaints, including restlessness, poor memory, palpitations, and anxiety. At the same time, it's useful for resolving fatty deposits in the heart and blood vessels.

Not more face powder, but less fat

After about four months, the recommended dose of **Compassionate Sage** pills and one teaspoon of raw tienchi ginseng powder, taken daily with cold water, helped cool Kaye's red face and removed some of the inflammation from broken capillaries. The herbs reduced *internal heat* and stuck circulation by reducing congestion surrounding the heart encouraged by cholesterol and stress.

Compassionate Sage contains fifteen herbs that build blood and immune strength, including ganoderma (reishi mushroom), a major Chinese health food used for prevention of cancer. Coptis, high in a natural anti-inflammatory agent, berberin, reduces *internal heat* and blood toxins. Zizyphus (Chinese red date) calms the heart. Polygala, longan, and tang kuei build blood and improve circulation. Sage provides vital energy (strengthens *chi*) and helps in the absorption of the other herbs.

Raw tienchi ginseng is a noted remedy for internal bleeding and chest pain, and is a natural corticosteroid that reduces inflammation. (See chapter 32.)

BALANCING BOTH MIND AND BODY

How could a circulation remedy treat both body and mind? In all traditional Asian medicines, internal organ systems have physical and emotional aspects. Our spirit indirectly reflects hormone and brain chemical balance as well as nerve stimulation, affected by blood and circulation. **Compassionate Sage** and other such balancing herbal combinations quiet the emotions while strengthening energy. Another way to look at it is that a compassionate heart is both calm and strong.

CIRCULATION AND THE EMOTIONS

A discussion of mental problems seems out of place in a chapter on circulation, but for Asian herbal medicine, it is not. Its holistic approach links heart energy with circulation and emotional balance. Many Chinese patent remedies for memory, concentration, mental clarity, or psychotic conditions work by clearing the heart area of obstructions, while calming the *shen.* These may include herbs that reduce atherosclerotic plaque (leading to hardening of the arteries), along with herbal sedatives for anxiety and palpitations. One example is the Chinese patent remedy known as **Cerebral Tonic Pills** (**Bu Nao Wan;** see page 448).

THE MIND AND THE FACE

What is more difficult to explain is the link between mental state and appearance. Do I mean to imply that persons with a red face or fragile capillaries are unbalanced? No, too many factors intervene. But we can observe chronic *internal heat* and poor circulation from appearance. The result of years of *internal heat* with poor circulation from plaque, chronic fever, biliousness, drugs, hormone irregularities, or emotional upheaval can take many forms. The capillaries are only one area of least resistance. Other consequences might include mental problems, high blood pressure, stroke, or cancer. They are all roads that twist through a burning forest.

In Asian medicine we seek the root cause of an illness, whether it manifests deeply or superficially. Facial appearance, gestures, and tone of voice can offer subtle signs of inner conflict. They are a way to view the *shen.* When *chi* circulation is smooth, body, mind, and spirit are at peace. People are compassionate when they have love in their hearts. Lacking love, calm sometimes helps. Tranquillity brings order, peace, and smooth circulation that strengthens the heart's spirit and blood vessels. This brings nourishment to the brain for mental clarity and good memory.

Signs of the heart's unrest—giddiness, a red face, broken blood vessels, fast chatter, or nightmares—can signal a deeper imbalance. They sometimes speak of hurt pride, swallowed rage, disappointed love, or failed ambition.

POOR CIRCULATION AFFECTING THE UPPER BODY

STAGNANT *LIVER* CHI

What makes it worse?

Oily, greasy, excessively hot or sour foods; alcohol, drugs, chemical toxins; disturbed emotions, especially anger, jealousy, and envy; hot, damp, and windy climate; environmental pollution.

What makes it better?

Nourishing foods; rest; herbs to smooth circulation; stimulant and cleansing herbs; blood tonics.

	HEAT SYMPTOMS	*COLD* SYMPTOMS	*PHLEGM*
TONGUE	mauve, black dots, dryness	pale, black dots, scalloped edges	coated green or brown
COMPLEXION	ruddy	greenish, pale	dull
SYMPTOMS	bitten fingernails, spasms, tics, irregular heartbeat, headaches, chest and abdominal pain, constipation, anger, jealousy, insomnia	weak muscles, irregular heartbeat, depression, indecision	lethargy, depression
HERBS AND FOODS	*cooling*, cleansing	*warming* stimulant	

STAGNANT *HEART* CHI

What makes it worse?

Caffeine, cigarettes, stress, jet lag, excitement, drugs, indigestion, overweight, hot, humid weather.

What makes it better?

Anticholesterol herbs, herbs that increase circulation, green tea.

	HEAT SYMPTOMS	*COLD* SYMPTOMS	*PHLEGM*
TONGUE	red, dry	pale, scalloped	coated
SYMPTOMS	palpitations, anxiety, hysteria, insomnia, chest pain, stuttering, mania	depression, poor memory, numb hands	insanity, poor concentration and mental clarity

REMEDIES

Abdominal pain and bloating: **Shu Gan Wan**

Anxiety, poor mental clarity, memory, mania, palpitations: **Cerebral Tonic Pills**

Bruising: **Yunnan Paiyao,** vitamin C, green tea

Chest pains: hawthorn, **Mao Dung Ching, Dan Shen Wan,** with high cholesterol: raw tienchi ginseng

Headache, shoulder pain: **Ansenpunaw Tablets**

High blood pressure: **Blood Pressure Repressing Tablets**

Indigestion, hiatal hernia, hypoglycemia: **Xiao Yao Wan**

Palpitations, restlessness: **Compassionate Sage–Heart Spirit**

氣爲血帥 氣爲血帥 氣爲血帥 氣爲血帥 氣爲血帥 氣爲血帥 氣爲血帥

[qì wéi xuè shuài] Vital energy is the "commander" of blood, for it serves as the dynamic force of blood flow, keeping the blood circulating.

22
Circulation: Why Do I Have Cold Feet?

Hawthorn berries

Weak circulation in the lower body is not an isolated problem related to sitting, stress, or bad luck. When *chi* is strengthened and lifted, varicose veins, pain, and stiffness improve, and hemorrhoids are eliminated. Watch a brook as it careens through a wood: Its nature is movement. When it is made shallow or twisted by curves, its current is suspended to form stagnant ponds. In the body, the nature of *chi* is movement. Stuck *chi* results in poor circulation. In this chapter we shall observe the flow of *chi* greatly enhanced by herbs.

Hemorrhoids

The Asian herbal treatment for hemorrhoids includes pills made of anti-inflammatory, antiseptic herbs and those that increase circulation and lift fallen *chi.* The pills reduce local pain and swelling very quickly. But improving circulation can have many long-term benefits, because *chi* becomes free to move. Healthy *chi* is the basis of all positive change.

Tom walked into the clinic one rainy afternoon. Thirty-two years old, with short black hair and steel blue eyes, he was handsome and shy. He smiled stiffly as he took off his gun, pointing it away from the birdcage, and laid it on the table.

"I've been a cop for five years, and all that time I've had this problem," he mumbled to the floor.

"How can I help you?" I smiled.

"Circulation."

The birds stirred uneasily as he looked in their direction. His voice was sweet. He seemed the kind of man who'd run into a burning building to save a child, but the birds sensed his tension.

"Circulation?" I repeated. "You mean varicose veins and cold feet?"

He nodded.

"And hemorrhoids?"

"How did you know?" He looked shocked.

It all fit together. Tom didn't get much exercise, and ate on the run. He was constipated and addicted to foods that didn't help. I showed Tom a section in *Acupuncture, A Comprehensive Text,* compiled by the Shanghai College of Traditional Medicine,

and published by Eastland Press. This large compendium recommends acupuncture treatments for everything from the common cold to leprosy. According to the text, hemorrhoids are attributed to "chronic constipation, irregular eating habits, alcoholism, overindulgence in spicy foods, sexual excess, and general weakness." The energetic problems associated with hemorrhoids—fatigue, bad circulation, and indigestion—concern not only the police but all those who work at desks.

Tom worked long, irregular hours in a patrol car. Since his beat was Manhattan, he enjoyed a diet that included not only hamburgers and French fries, but spicy Asian and Middle Eastern foods, at any hour of the day or night. Coffee kept him awake. Off duty, he drank beer. He was a little thick in the waistline, and I could see that his gait was stiff from a sore lower back. He did not need a diet high in protein and fat. Physical inactivity and constant stress created the weak *chi* underlying his poor circulation.

He needed to eat more fresh fruit and salads and fewer fried foods. Fat and oil, when heated, become extremely difficult to digest. When left to turn rancid, they become poisons, congesting circulation and increasing cholesterol. He continued flipping through my acupuncture text, examining charts showing meridians. He found a section for the back and hips, and turned white. "Are you going to give me acupuncture?"

"No." I smiled. "Don't even think about it. American-born acupuncturists, like myself, realize the large difference between our clients and the Asian populations that have used acupuncture as a healing modality for generations. Normally I use a cold laser rather than needles, because it's less invasive. Even so, some new clients have problems tolerating a method they do not understand. I gave him herbs instead. I handed him a small bottle from Chinatown. As he peered at the Chinese characters, I told him it was called **Fargelin.** It's for piles and hemorrhoids, I said. It contains pseudoginseng, which lifts prolapsed rectum; skullcap, an anti-inflammatory; corydalis, which stops pain; and fels ursi, which used to mean "bear's gallbladder . . ."

"A real bear?" His gasp momentarily interrupted the list of ingredients. Chinese pharmacies now substitute herbs or domestic animal ingredients for wild animals. He didn't want any sort of animal product. So I recommended that he drink aloe vera (either juice or gel), one quarter cup over the course of a day, in a thermos of green tea or added to apple juice. Aloe eliminates pimples, bad breath, constipation, and hemorrhoids. I told him to take it until his circulation problems cleared up, and to drop French fries and hot spices for now.

He could expect fast relief from constipation, because the aloe would reverse *internal heat* symptoms in the lower body. If it didn't improve in a couple of days, he could add a laxative, either homeopathic natrum sulphate or 10 drops of barberry extract, to the aloe. I suggested foods from section II of chapter 13, Achieving Balance, to reduce the inflammation, pain, and

poor circulation associated with a hot, spicy diet.

Tom asked about herbs for his uncle George, who had painful indigestion even though his gallbladder had been removed. Surgical removal of digestive organs does not eliminate problems related to their functioning, because *stagnant chi* is still trapped in the local acupuncture meridians.

Tom's uncle had hemorrhoids related to chronic diarrhea, not constipation. He had abdominal pain and bloating, and had previously had a hernia. He could not use the same laxative herbs as Tom. For hemorrhoids or prolapse symptoms associated with weakness and diarrhea, his uncle could mail-order **Bu Zhong Yi Qi Wan** from any American Chinatown. (Several addresses are listed in the Herbal Access appendix.)

Another possible remedy was **Zhi Wan** ("Hemorrhoid Pills"), which contain several powerful herbs that increase circulation: tang kuei, frankincense, myrrh, and anteater scales. It also contains anti-inflammatory, antiseptic herbs such as honeysuckle flower.

The last time I saw Tom, he said his hemorrhoids and other circulation problems were gone. I was happy to hear he enjoyed drinking green tea. He was getting Oriental massage each week to improve circulation. And he beamed. "I've started taking a kung fu class in Chinatown." His movements were more connected and graceful. He looked me straight in the eye and said, "Thanks."

Sciatica

Sciatica is a sharp pain that shoots down the leg like an electric jolt or that rivets the hip, a pain that makes you jump and walk with a limp. The discomfort comes and goes, and sometimes feels worse from cold weather or fatigue. It results from inflammation of the sciatic nerve.

Sciatica is often diet- or stress-related. I had one client, Gabriella, who one day limped up the stairs to my office. Her whole leg felt stiff, and a sharp, agonizing burn ran down her leg. Her pain followed exhaustion during a trip with extremes in hot and cold weather. The pain had started in Paris and followed her all the way to North Africa. While acting on tour, she'd eaten French fries and candy bars every day. Now, at home a month later, she still felt a twinge when she moved in the wrong way or lay flat in bed. The pain was debilitating and depressing.

I gave her acupuncture to get her blood circulating again, and to relieve the inflammation in her lower back and leg. She felt about 75 percent better after the first treatment. Then I recommended some herbs to keep her comfortable until the next treatment.

There are a number of Chinese herbal combinations for sciatica. Some are useful at the same time for arthritis and rheumatism because they ease joint pain that feels heavy and dull but shifts around in the legs, knees, or back. Such "traveling" pain, which shifts from one acupuncture meridian to the next, is called "evil *wind*" by tra-

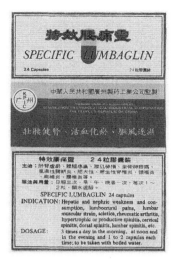

ditional Chinese doctors. The following remedies work by increasing blood and circulation in order to unlock stuck *chi*.

Specific Lumbaglin is a capsule used for sciatica, backache, and lumbago. The herbal painkiller loosens tight muscles and moves stuck *chi* along the whole spine. It relaxes tendons and relieves muscle strains, while strengthening the kidneys. The capsules contain eucommia bark for backache. Other herbs include morinda, ligusticum, shou wu, and tang kuei, which all build blood and circulation, while achyranthes and clematis roots help move stuck *chi.* Increasing blood flow to important internal organs in the area, in this case the liver and kidney, while easing circulation, gives much stronger, localized pain relief than any sedative.

Another combination, called **Guan Jie Yan Wan** ("Close Down Joint Inflammation Pills"), is used for a cold sensation in limbs, aching joints, inflammation of the sciatic nerve, and rheumatoid arthritis. It contains barley to reduce phlegm that can trouble the joints, as well as cinnamon, ginger, and erythrina bark for improved circulation (see chapter 19).

Gabriella used the above combinations at different times, and found them both quite effective. (She felt they worked because she switched from French fries to corn chips, but I was doubtful.) Once she called me from Cincinnati when she could not get to Chinatown to buy herbs. She got some relief from this soup I recommended:

1 cup barley
¼ teaspoon cinnamon
⅛ teaspoon dried ginger powder
⅛ teaspoon dried orange peel
6 drops gentian extract
10 drops myrrh extract
10 drops valerian extract
12 drops skullcap extract
2 cups water

Gabriella cooked the barley without salt or spices until it was tender, then added pinches of pungent spices and herbs to taste, including cinnamon, ginger, and a dash of dried orange peel. Then she added the bitter herbal extracts (gentian, myrrh, valerian, and skullcap) to a little water as a chaser. She ate a small bowl of soup several times a day. Its oddly sweet fragrance stirred comment from stagehands and makeup people also troubled by aches and pains.

When constipated, Gabriella took two capsules of cascara sagrada before bed. Her pain improved even faster when she added the *cooling* diet from section II of chapter 13 and stopped eating cheese, eggs, and nuts for two weeks.

SERIOUS SCIATICA AND "SILLY SCIATICA"

Mark, a therapist with a health practice in three separate offices, also limped up the stairs one day to see me. In addition to a booming practice, he taught a class in stress reduction at a community college. He was forty, thin, and a vegetarian, with dark circles under the eyes. He looked dreadfully tired. His strength was out of focus, blurry around the edges. He spoke with a sigh. He conducted his psychotherapy practice, first out of his home, then with partners, with no vacation for nine years. Then his wife announced they were having their sixth child.

The sciatica started two weeks later. He'd seen a chiropractor who told him the treatment would take a dozen visits. After two visits, there was a little improvement. Sciatica and muscle spasm pains are treated very quickly with acupuncture, often with one or two treatments with a cold laser, perhaps longer with needles. A cold laser does not penetrate the skin, so that none of the usual discomforts of acupuncture are a problem.

Mark moved with difficulty. He said he trapped tension from his health practice in his leg. It seemed an unlikely place, but pain and tension do go to our weak areas.

During the previous week, Mark had seen an M.D. who gave him a muscle relaxer. There had been no improvement. I reminded Mark that the heart is also a muscle, and that his circulation, energy, and mood might be dulled by such a medication. That day, when I released trapped pain with a session of acupuncture, he let go of some of the grief caused by his work. He cried.

Health practitioners get special illnesses. When not careful, they collect maladies from their patients. It's not voodoo or simple identification; healers acquire stress they need to unload. Too often, they're so busy taking care of everyone else that they forget about themselves. Herbs protect me. I take my own medicine, work out at the gym, or dance flamenco, so that when I begin to feel like the Great Universal Fix-it Mother, I can work it out. Mark didn't have any means of emotional clearing. In that way, Mark's sciatica problem was very deep. It had to be addressed on an emotional level.

I recommended that he take homeopathic ignatia, 30c potency (Saint Ignatius' bean), because it brings hidden emotions like worry and grief to the surface, then out of the body. The clearing process the remedy provides makes us relive troubling emotions on another level: It clears their physical aspects from the body. Homeopathic ignatia can resolve a lingering cold or joint aches associated with stress. It's a remedy for the person who is too busy— for the healer who does not take time to grieve, experience his own feelings, or ask for more time. It's for the person in shock after an accident, who assures you everything is okay. Mark decided to use the remedy periodically in his tea, allowing for the right time and place to air his feelings. This would prevent what he described as feelings getting stuck in his leg.

To increase circulation and resolve sciatic pain, I recommended a Chinese herbal formula, **Chen Pu Hu Chien Wan,** roughly translated as "Walk Vigorously Like a Stealthy Tiger Pills." It's used for pain affecting legs and knees and for sciatica as well as chronic arthritis and lumbago. It contains achyranthes root, used to invigorate blood circulation and strengthen joints, and for pain in lower back and knees caused by energy deficiency. It also improves dizziness and headache. Another ingredient in **Chen Pu Hu Chien** pills is Chaenomeles lagenaria, commonly called Chinese quince fruit, used for cramping, severe pain, and weakness in the lower back and lower extremities. Other well-known ingredients such as tang kuei get circulation moving.

This remedy is said to contain tiger bone. Perhaps the original formula at one time did use real tiger, but no longer. Other formulas, such as **Guan Jie Yan Wan,** do not contain animal ingredients and work well for sciatica and rheumatoid arthritis.

Mark got some relief from the above patent remedy. He said the pain localized more in his back, so we switched remedies to address the new location of pain. He took **Specific Lumbaglin** (in Chinese, **Te Xiao Yao Tong Ling**), which, according to the instructions, "strengthens waist and kidneys, invigorates blood circulation, removes blood stagnation, dispels wind and damp, relaxes tendons . . . to relieve inflammation, pain and achiness in back and treats sciatica." (See chapter 17 for a discussion of pain due to *wind* and *dampness*.) After he took **Specific Lumbaglin,** his pain went away quickly.

Mark also applied insights gained from the homeopathic remedy to his own healing practice. He said that never again would he let emotions lodge in his leg or anywhere else in his body. He would also recommend homeopathic ignatia for his clients to bring their worries and frustrations to the surface to speed their healing.

That same day, Ralph, Kaye's husband, limped up the stairs with what he called a "silly sciatica." His circulation was poor. He'd eaten rich food for years, and he was too heavy. The sciatica, he said, was due to cold weather. Cold temperatures constrict blood and energy circulation, but he'd also been out with friends, eating rich, spicy foods and ice cream and smoking cigarettes, which was rare for him. He'd noticed the pain soon after that. It traveled along the gallbladder meridian, down the right side of the chest, through the outer hip, and down the outside of the leg toward the little toe, all on the right side. Sometimes it was sharp, sometimes dull.

A Chinese doctor recommended **Tu Zhung Feng Shi Wan** ("Eucommia Bark *Wind-Damp* Pills") for aching joints and lower back, sciatica, and gout. He said the Chinese herbal remedy took away his back pain, but made the pain in his right side more noticeable. It may have uncovered deeper problems. I suspected he might have gallstones, but couldn't be certain without Western medical testing.

I've known many cases when a person does not actually have a stone, but pain is intense because of *stagnant chi* affecting the meridian. Chinese doctors sometimes use **Lidan Pills** to dissolve stones or congestion resulting from poor circulation. The pills treat acute and chronic gallstone inflammation, and are made of 30 percent skullcap, with honeysuckle flower to detoxify the body and quell inflammation, and bupleurum and rhubarb to move stuck energy in the gallbladder meridian. Ralph took the pills from me, offering me a candy. He winked and said all those years with Kaye had given him a refined taste for sweets.

Helpful Hints

In this and the preceding chapter we have covered an array of circulation discomforts from head to foot. In general, middle- and upper-body pains or circulation discomforts are made worse by stressful emotions. Lower-body circulation involves movement and physical stress. Any pain or circulation difficulty is augmented by an unwise diet.

Fat and sweet, rich foods encourage heavy and dull pains, swollen joints, and oozing, slow-healing wounds, because they slow circulation by congesting digestion. Hot, spicy, or sour, acidic foods increase sharp electric pain, red, inflamed joints, and muscle spasms. Pungent foods increase acid in joints and muscles. Long-term extremes in food temperature, either very spicy or cold and raw, interfere with the smooth circulation of *chi* controlled by the liver.

Spoiled or rancid foods and oils or honey, when cooked, congest the digestive process like toxins. When foods interfere with the smooth flow of *chi,* they cause pain and swelling.

Clearing Joint and Muscle Pain: An Activity

First observe your tongue. Make notes on its shape, color, and coating. Record the location and severity of joint and muscle pain, and also daily diet, during this activity. Mood, fatigue, and hormonal shifts may also affect pain. Use the herbal suggestions recommended below, and periodically check with a health specialist among those listed in the back of this book, to make sure everything is going well.

Persons with *internal heat* will tend to have a dry, red tongue. Joints or painful areas will feel warm, and may be swollen or red. There may be a skin rash or irritability. For three to five days, follow the routine to decrease inflammation outlined in section II of chapter 13. Add anti-inflammatory herbs for joint pain such as alfalfa or yucca. See the chapters on arthritis, headaches, and allergies (19, 20, and 23) as needed. Remedies

for joint pain should be taken between meals. Continue with the diet and herbs, while observing changes in the tongue. A red tongue will become less inflamed, dry, and yellow-coated with *cooling* cleansing herbs. If the diet and cleansing herbs you have chosen feel great, continue to watch pain and inflammation melt away as long as necessary.

If you have joint pain from weakness, *internal cold, dampness,* or long-term debility, the tongue will tend to be large, pale, and puffy. Pain will feel worse in cold weather or from fatigue. Arthritic pains will improve with herbs that warm joints, such as myrrh. Follow the diet and healing practices in sections I and III of chapter 13. One or the other of those sections may feel more appropriate. Also see the chapters on arthritis, fatigue, and depression (19, 31, and 35). Pay special attention to preventing and treating colds and flu quickly with remedies from chapter 30. As you make your diet more warming, nourishing, and strengthening, as you fight to keep colds and depression away, you will start to feel better than you have in years.

Pains are only fixed emotions, immobile weakness, and fatigue. As you move stuck circulation with remedies like myrrh or **Yunnan Paiyao,** new doors will open in your energy, new opportunities for growth, joy, and change.

WEAK *CHI* CIRCULATION AFFECTING THE LOWER BODY

What makes it worse?

Weak *chi* from fatigue, overwork, lack of sleep, excess sexual activity (weak adrenal *chi*); poor diet (rich, greasy, congesting foods, sweets, alcohol, coffee, cigarettes); constipation, stress, sedentary habits.

What makes it better?

Vitamin C, flavonoids, antioxidants, rest, herbs that clear toxins, encourage bile, and stimulate circulation.

	HEAT SYMPTOMS	*COLD* SYMPTOMS	*PHLEGM*
TONGUE	reddish dots or dark spots	pale dots	coated yellow, green, brown
SYMPTOMS	sharp pain, joint stiffness, difficulty walking, hemorrhoids, sciatica, lumbago, bad breath, kidney and gallbladder stones, varicose veins	dull pain, chills, weakness, paralysis, numbness	dull pain, swollen joints

REMEDIES

Hemorrhoids: aloe vera gel, **Zhi Wan**

Painful walking: **Guan Jie Yan Wan, Chen Pu Hu Chien Wan**

Sciatica: **Specific Lumbaglin, Guan Jie Yan Wan, Chen Pu Hu Chien Wan, Tu Zhung Feng Shi Wan**

Stones: **Lidan Pills**

Weakness, chronic diarrhea, prolapsed rectum or uterus: **Bu Zhong Yi Qi Wan**

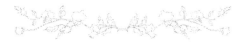

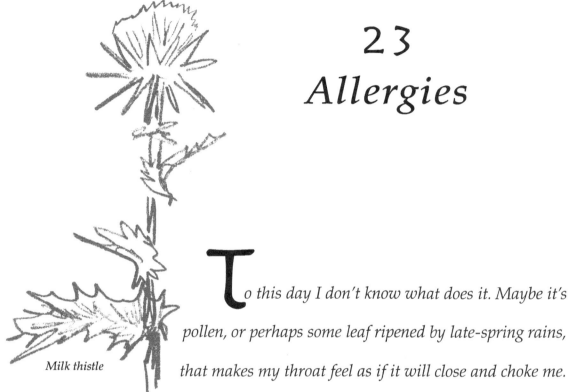

Milk thistle

23
Allergies

To this day I don't know what does it. Maybe it's pollen, or perhaps some leaf ripened by late-spring rains, that makes my throat feel as if it will close and choke me.

It has only happened two or three times: once in a restaurant and once when one of my students wore an acrid scented hair spray. I was teaching a class outdoors, guiding a crowd of people through a maze of streets, weaving past food vendors and dodging delivery boys on bicycles. We'd stopped in an alcove near a stand where boys were selling fireworks.

Suddenly I started a coughing fit. I grabbed my throat because it felt *sandy and dry. As I spoke, it got worse. I have a few friends who have allergic asthma. When they breathe a particular allergen, they gasp and rush to the hospital, feeling that their throat is swollen shut. One friend has the same allergic reaction when she eats peaches or shellfish. It feels like your throat is a tube of toothpaste being squeezed.*

I know that my strangling cough is an allergic reaction because it happens in late spring, when the Wood element is in full bloom. That's when the liver organ system becomes hypersensitive, making some people react with spasms, headaches, runny nose, watery eyes, or convulsive sneezing and coughing. I realize I should do my spring cleansing each year to prevent allergies. But on that occasion on the street it was too late for prevention: What I needed to stop choking in that alcove was a remedy for acute allergic swelling, homeopathic apis 30c. That homeopathic dose of honeybee would have eliminated all the symptoms of a sting: redness, swelling, pain, and throbbing heat. But there was no health-food store in sight.

The moral of this story is: Be prepared. In this chapter I will present a five-day prevention plan for allergies, explaining several wonderfully useful natural medicines so that you will no longer need to suffer the weakening effects of allergic reactions to foods and environmental irritants. This chapter concerns primarily indigestion symptoms and head and sinus problems; other allergic reactions, such as hives, rashes, and eczema, will be discussed in chapter 25, on cleansing and rejuvenating the skin.

An Energetic Definition of Allergies

Think of an allergy as an over-reaction, a defense that is unnecessary. Allergic symptoms result from a hyperactive state of the body's detoxification and protection mechanisms that causes imbalances.

Allergy Prevention

Allergies are predictable. People know they're sensitive to an allergen because, confronted with it, they always react the same way: They get indigestion, pains, fatigue, or eye or sinus problems. One way to deal with allergies is to avoid allergens. I've known people who have gone to great lengths to duck certain foods, or to avoid ducks, cats, dust, pollen, or molds. I've known others who've bought second homes in the Caribbean because conifers do not irritate their allergies as deciduous trees do. But for those of us who do not wish to spend on expensive allergy shots, and cannot (alas!) move to the beach, there is another answer: We can reduce allergic reactions by lowering the irritability of the body. This is done by reducing acid wastes that underlie the over-defensive state required for allergies to happen.

The routine summarized on page 274 is best done for five days *before* allergy season arrives. Do not wait for irritants to be in full bloom or for your body to be most sensitive. For most people, that will be in very early spring, before plants start to bud. If you smoke or have *internal heat* symptoms, or if you're weak and nervous, it's best to repeat this routine again in early fall. The following prevention plan will reduce both food and environmental allergies.

A Five-Day Allergy Prevention Plan

Our approach to allergy prevention is to remove excess acidity and increase natural processes of cleansing in the body. In that way, our toxins and hyper-reactions are reduced in time to avoid the crippling struggle between our bodies and allergens. This will be accomplished with a daily cup of anti-acid tea after breakfast and digestive supplements after meals. By bringing the digestive process into balance, many food- and stress-related allergies will be reduced. Also by cutting down the by-products of poor digestion, such as excess phlegm, sinus allergies will be improved.

Acidic foods, cigarettes, and environmental allergens cause irritation, which can affect the lungs and also the digestive and urinary tracts. But *cooling* digestive and diuretic herbs reduce burning, itchy symptoms. For that purpose, we have a cleansing tea made with kitchen spices.

A cooling *tea of cumin, coriander, and fennel*

In chapter 7 we learned that herbs and spices vary according to their type, taste, and temperature. The following tea is made from three spices that free the body of excess acid caused by diet, hot climate, and stress.

1/8 teaspoon cumin powder
1/8 teaspoon coriander powder
1/8 teaspoon fennel seed powder
1 cup water

You can find these ingredients in most supermarkets. Do not boil them, but steep them five minutes as a tea if you like the taste. Otherwise, add just enough lukewarm water to swallow them comfortably. The best time to have it is after breakfast, because it is strongly cleansing. I do not recommend drinking it on an empty stomach or when you have a cold.

How often you drink this tea depends on your internal acid/alkaline balance, which you can observe on your tongue.

REDDISH TONGUE

If you have a reddish tongue and other signs of *internal heat*, such as dark yellow or odorous urine, bad breath, red skin rash, bloodshot eyes, or nervous irritability, you can drink this *cooling* tea once each day for five consecutive days.

PALE TONGUE

Persons with a pale tongue tend to have slow digestion and might have excess alkaline conditions. The real test of acid/alkaline balance is in the tongue's coating. A thick yellow, green, or brown coating indicates digestive weakness and toxins. If your tongue has such a coating, you can follow the instructions for a reddish tongue, drinking the tea for five days.

But if you have a pale tongue with no coating or a thin white coating, then you do not need to cleanse acids as much as someone with *internal heat;* therefore, drink the tea after breakfast for no more than two days, unless you have *internal heat* symptoms other than a red tongue. For example, if you've spent time in a very hot climate, if you have chronic fever or menopausal hot flashes, or if you are very angry at something or insomniac from nervousness, then treat your condition as *internal heat.* If you are overheated for those reasons, then you can drink between 2 and 5 cups of tea as it feels comfortable.

What to expect

The results of this anti-acid tea might surprise you. After a cup or two, you will have lost much of your nervous and aggressive hype. It is not a sedative tea, but it reduces enervating toxins. Be forewarned that acid wastes burn as they are excreted. Urine and bowel movements will feel hot and look orange for a day. That is because dangerous excess acid is leaving your body. The discomfort will stop in a short time.

How cumin/coriander/fennel tea works

Each of the ingredients is an anti-inflammatory cleanser that works on a different part of the body.

Cumin reduces excess stomach acid and appetite, which makes it the ideal spice for ulcers and weight loss. We are using it in the anti-allergy tea because excess acid collects in the digestive tract to cause problems throughout the body.

Coriander (seed and leaf) is a fine home remedy for burning urine, cystitis, acid indigestion, food allergies, and hay fever. The fresh juice of cilantro (coriander leaf) actually works best for hay fever. Some people take one teaspoon three times a day between meals. But I have recommended the powder because it's easier to find year-round.

Fennel seeds are digestive and slightly laxative, which encourages cleansing.

AN ACID-REDUCING DIET

Persons with long-term allergies and *internal heat* are advised to follow the inflammation-reducing diet in section II of chapter 13. Steamed green vegetables, white basmati rice, and green tea are especially soothing. Since this *cooling* diet will be maintained for two to five days, significant cleansing, and possibly weight loss, can take place.

Weakness is also an underlying cause of allergies. Make sure to get enough protein by adding tofu or fish to your diet. Also continue taking your usual daily vitamin and mineral supplements. Zinc is important to avoid stress-related allergies, as are vitamin C, antioxidants, and beta-carotene.

DIGESTION-RELATED ALLERGIES

Many times, poor digestion leads to weakness and stuck circulation. This results in a clogged-feeling head, poor concentration, and a sinus condition. Please answer the following questions to find out whether your digestion affects your allergies:

✤ Do you get headaches or dizziness after eating certain foods?

✤ Do you frequently suffer from stuffed sinuses after meals?

✤ Do you get hiccups, burping, or nausea after eating richly?

✤ Do you perspire profusely after meals?

✤ Can you identify the foods that trouble you?

✤ Do you avoid eating some foods because you are "allergic" to them?

Certain foods may, in themselves, be too hard to digest. For example, combinations such as fruit eaten with dairy products and meat cause indigestion and parasites. If you often suffer discomfort after eating even simple foods, the real problem is that your digestion is weak. Chinese doctors say that to reverse this condition, we need adequate digestive *chi*. The best way to build *chi* is with herbs.

STRENGTHENING DIGESTIVE WEAKNESS

The Five-Day Allergy Prevention Plan includes herbal digestive supplements that reduce stuck *chi*. This eliminates excess acid, indigestion, and pain. It ensures that toxins are removed and that fewer allergens will irritate. When we begin the allergy season in balance, there is a better chance we can remain strong and healthy.

Each day of the Five-Day Plan, take either **Xiao Yao Wan** or **Relaxed Wanderer** after meals. The usual dose is 6 pills each

time, but the actual dosage depends on your acid/alkaline balance. If your tongue is pale, you can use 6 to 10 pills each time. But if your tongue is reddish, use 6 pills and add up to one half cup of aloe vera juice daily in apple juice or tea. There is a direct relation between digestion and certain allergies. These balancing herbs will increase your vitality and resistance.

Xiao Yao Wan (also spelled **Hsiao Yao Wan**) is an excellent all-around digestive panacea for indigestion, bloating, hiccups, food allergies, and hypoglycemia. Its blend of *warming* and *cooling* digestive herbs treats *stagnant* liver *chi*. That means it helps digestion and circulation work more smoothly, especially in the liver organ system. It contains herbs that regulate liver and galbladder, such as bupleurum and mint, which ease redness, blurry vision, or pain in the eyes, distension or lumps in the chest, and irritability.

This digestive remedy has many functions because digestion has many effects. Smooth digestion enables us to have strong, steady energy, adequate blood production, and comfortable circulation. Balancing the center of vitality, the digestive center, helps prevent chronic weakness, blood-sugar instability, and hay fever.

Xiao Yao Wan treats both food and sinus problems, including hay fever. Hay fever is an over-reaction of the body to normal stimulus. We may not be able to move to the mountains to avoid spores, grasses, or trees that make us sneeze and our eyes itch, but **Xiao Yao Wan** will help moderate the body's reactions to such irritants.

Other cures for food allergies include

YOUR FIVE-DAY ALLERGY PREVENTION PLAN

You can use this menu as a rough guide to your Anti-Allergy Program. Make sure to avoid dairy products, hot spices, alcohol, coffee, cigarettes, and pastry. They cause inflammation and phlegm.

MONDAY

8:00 A.M. hot green tea, oatmeal with pumpkin seeds, ½ cup cumin/coriander/fennel tea

10:00 A.M. **Xiao Yao Wan,** hot tea (optional lemon)

12:00 noon salad and sandwich or fish and salad, **Xiao Yao Wan**

2:00 P.M. apple juice and ¼ cup aloe vera juice

6:00 P.M. tofu, vegetables, nondairy dessert, **Xiao Yao Wan**

11:00 P.M. an apple

TUESDAY

8:00 A.M. hot green tea, fresh fruit or rye toast, poached eggs, ½ to 1 cup cumin/coriander/fennel tea

10:00 A.M. **Xiao Yao Wan,** green tea

12:00 noon chicken breast, rice, vegetables, **Xiao Yao Wan**

2:00 P.M. half vegetable juice, half aloe juice

6:00 P.M. green salad, sandwich with hummus and vegetables, **Xiao Yao Wan**

11:00 P.M. dried apricots, hot tea

WEDNESDAY

8:00 A.M. coffee substitute, bran cereal, apple juice, toast, 1 cup cumin/coriander/fennel tea

10:00 A.M. **Xiao Yao Wan,** green tea

12:00 noon soup and salad or rice and vegetables, **Xiao Yao Wan**

2:00 P.M. fresh fruit or vegetables, tea (optional aloe juice)

6:00 P.M. mushroom omelette, steamed vegetables, ginger tea

11:00 P.M. fresh applesauce or low-fat cookie, mint tea

THURSDAY

8:00 A.M. hot green or oolong tea, canned sardines, rice cakes, 1 cup cumin/coriander/fennel tea

10:00 A.M. **Xaio Yao Wan,** raw carrots, cucumber

12:00 noon pasta, vegetarian marinara sauce, salad, **Xiao Yao Wan**

2:00 P.M. celery, radish, carrots, ginger tea (optional aloe juice)

6:00 P.M. sushi or fish, pineapple, tea, **Xiao Yao Wan**

11:00 P.M. warm Almond Milk (see page 184)

FRIDAY

8:00 A.M. coffee substitute, cooked cereal, toast, 1 cup cumin/coriander/fennel tea (optional)

10:00 A.M. fresh fruit, **Xiao Yao Wan,** green tea

12:00 noon tabouli salad, hummus, stuffed grape leaves, pita, **Xiao Yao Wan**

2:00 P.M. carrots, cucumber, cherry tomatoes, tea (optional aloe juice)

6:00 P.M. candlelight dinner with friends (aloe juice and **Xiao Yao Wan** at home)

11:00 P.M. nondairy rice pudding (optional)

new herbal combinations based on the above patent remedy—for example, **Relaxed Wanderer,** a Jade Pharmacy combination. This formula combines additional herbs with the original **Xiao Yao Wan.** For example, cyperus is added to increase blood circulation, gardenia bud to clear phlegm, and gastrodia to reduce nerve irritation and excitability.

Relaxed Wanderer treats many of the same conditions that **Xiao Yao Wan** does, such as stomachache, belching, water retention, or loose stools. It strengthens the stomach and spleen while moving *stagnant* liver *chi.* What that means in plain English is that **Relaxed Wanderer** treats physical or emotional discomfort from eating on the run, eating poor food combinations, or eating unwisely or when under stress. It reduces food allergies because it makes digestion stronger.

Now that you understand how digestive weakness leads to toxins that invariably make allergy season worse, you can add the three parts of your Allergy-Prevention Plan together: an anti-allergy tea, a cooling, cleansing diet, and digestive supplements.

Sinus Allergies

Sinus allergies are a special problem augmented by weak digestion, but also independent of it. Weather conditions, animal fur, pollen, trees, or grasses can also irritate eyes and cause sinus congestion and inflammation. In extreme cases, they lead to allergic asthma.

If allergies are complicated by excess phlegm or digestive parasites, follow the Five-Day Allergy Prevention Plan, substituting barley for rice and oatmeal. Also follow the regimen outlined in section I of chapter 13. Phlegm is the sticky, clogging part of our allergies. By cleansing it, we lower sinus congestion, bloating, and fatigue. Please answer the following questions to decide whether your allergies depend on phlegm:

- Does allergy season knock out your energy and concentration?
- Do you crave oily and sweet foods or alcohol very often?
- Do you crave grapefruit or other sour foods daily?
- Do you tend to digest slowly or with difficulty?
- Do you feel sleepy in humid weather, after eating?
- Do your joints feel stiff and sore with allergies?
- Do you often get sinus headaches or feel congested?
- Does your sinus allergy feel better when you breathe natural edible camphor or gotu kola powder?
- Do you feel better outdoors in fresh air?
- Do you get depressed when you experience sinus allergies?

Although digestive phlegm increases all head and sinus allergies, hay fever requires additional help. You may need both kinds of remedies if you have indigestion along with sinus problems. Most herbs that treat hay fever, facial congestion, and sinus pain work differently from herbs for digestive weakness. They dry mucus while increasing circulation in the head and neck. Because sinus remedies are not designed to strengthen digestion, they should be taken between meals.

A Word to the Wise (But Tired Out by the Fast Track)

If poor habits, rich foods, and high stress are your lifestyle, it's wise to take **Xiao Yao Wan** with meals and one of the following sinus allergy remedies three times daily, about an hour after meals. You may need to continue this routine long after completing the Five-Day Allergy Prevention Plan. All these pills are available in Chinese groceries or by mail order.

POLLENS, SEAFOOD, AND DUST ALLERGIES

Bi Yan Pian ("Nose Inflammation Pills") contains philodendron bark, forsythia fruit, and anemarrhena to reduce inflammation and feverish head symptoms such as red, itchy eyes and sinus pain. It combines platycodon with schisandra fruit, which dries phlegm while quieting cough, and schizonepeta, which alleviates itching. This phlegm-clearing action is focused to affect the sinus area by adding magnolia and chrysanthemum flowers.

Bi Yan Pian treats sneezing, itchy eyes, facial congestion and pain, and typical discomforts of rhinitis, sinusitis, hay fever, and nasal allergies. For chronic mucus congestion of the face, this remedy can be combined with **Xiao Yao Wan.** Any problem involving phlegm that has been around for a long time involves poor digestion and *stagnant chi.* Take both remedies together one half hour after meals.

Pollen Allergy Pills treat allergic reactions to seafood, dust, and most pollens. The formula contains magnolia, ma huang (ephedra), mint, anemarrhena, centipede, mouton, xanthium, and a few other items such as fels ursi (I am assured by Chinese herbalist friends that this traditional Latin name no longer refers to bear's gallbladder, but to a synthetic product with similar bitter qualities).

Pe Min Kan Wan treats allergic rhinitis, chronic and acute sinusitis, rubella, and skin rashes. It is used primarily for hay fever, sneezing, runny nose, and itchy eyes. Its ingredients include the antibiotic honeysuckle, also wild chrysanthemum, angelica, and xanthium fruit. Directions for these remedies are in English.

Chronic Rhinitis

Chronic rhinitis can be very weakening. After a while, explosive sneezing will be accompanied by tiredness, difficult breathing, chills, and frequent urination from weakness. Then the best remedy must do more than stop the allergy. It must build strength as well as remove congestion. What a different approach from Western sedative drugs used for allergies!

Your herbalist can advise you on treatment for chronic breathing and allergy problems that result in exhaustion, but here is a suggestion for chronic rhinitis from *Clinic of Traditional Chinese Medicine,* vol. II (published by the Shanghai College of TCM). Cook these herbs as a decoction (at least one half hour) in order to "strengthen spleen, replenish *chi* and remove obstruction from the upper orifices":

astragalus root	18 grams
ginseng	9 grams
tang kuei	9 grams
xanthium (*Fructus xanthii*)	9 grams
magnolia flower	9 grams
peppermint	9 grams
cimifuga	9 grams
tangerine peel	9 grams
atractylodes	9 grams
licorice	9 grams
bupleurum	9 grams
dahurian angelica	15 grams

You can fax a copy of this recipe to your favorite Chinese herb shop. It's gratifying to cook such herbal brews at home. You'll relish their energy as they pervade your space, lending a pungent aroma therapy, a powerful curative presence.

Take milk thistle for long-term treatment of chronic allergies, including rebuilding the health of your stressed liver. Milk thistle (in capsules or liquid extract) has been used to treat cirrhosis, jaundice, hepatitis, and liver poisoning from chemicals or drug and alcohol abuse. The young leaves (with spines removed) are eaten as a vegetable.

Acute Allergy Cures

Homeopathic medicines work particularly well for acute illnesses because the dosage depends on your needs. The pills melt in your mouth and are immediately absorbed into the blood, no matter how weak you may be. They offer quick, effective relief for allergic discomforts, and leave no trace or side effects in your body.

Typically, homeopathic allergy medicines contain tiny doses of allergens specific to seasonal allergies such as ragweed, goldenrod, and onion for relief of sinus headaches. They may also contain ingredients that dry watery eyes and nose, such as pulsatilla and natrum muriate. When you take a homeopathic dose of an allergen, your body reacts by strengthening your natural immune responses, and you can better tolerate the allergen.

The best strength of homeopathic remedy to take for acute problems is 30c, which refers to the number of times the original substance has been diluted. The remedies come in small pills, pellets, or liquid extracts that are easy to carry with you. When you know your allergen is present and your resistance is low, you will need to carry a bottle of these tiny pills in your pocket. For instance, I have a friend who is deathly allergic to bee stings. One more sting and she'd end up in a hospital. I recommended that she keep homeopathic apis 30c, a remedy for bee stings and allergic swelling of all kinds, in a locket around her neck when she gardens. The following homeopathic medicines are often available in supermarkets and pharmacies:

ALLERGIC SWELLING, INSECT BITES

Homeopathic apis 30c eases swelling, pain, allergic asthma with swollen throat. (See also chapter 18.)

SEASONAL ALLERGIES

Allergy Relief, distributed by SunSource in Maui, cures sneezing, runny nose, watery eyes, headaches, hay fever.

Sinus Relief, also by SunSource, is used for sinus headache.

Allergy, made by Medicine from Nature in Utah, treats allergies and rash.

Three useful homeopathic remedies manufactured by Boericke & Tafel:

Alpha SH treats sinus headaches.

Alpha HF treats hay fever and allergies to trees, grass, and pollens.

Alleraide treats allergies to dust, pets, and molds.

SEASONAL AND FOOD ALLERGIES

What makes it worse?

Dairy products; oily, rich, and sweet foods; hot spices; fatigue; complicated food combinations; allergens.

What makes it better?

Cleansing diet and anti-acid herbs; cumin/coriander/fennel tea; aloe vera; simple food combinations. (Do not mix fruit or dairy with meat and fish.) Keep the house free of dust and mold.

HEAT SYMPTOMS	*COLD* SYMPTOMS	*PHLEGM*
red eyes, sore throat, sinus and head pain, sneezing, dry cough, sinusitis, rhinitis	watery eyes, runny nose	congestion, moodiness, poor concentration, nausea

REMEDIES

Indigestion: **Xiao Yao Wan, Relaxed Wanderer**

Sinuses: **Xiao Yao Wan, Relaxed Wanderer, Bi Yan Pian, Pe Min Kan,** and **Alpha SH**

Anti-sinus-congestion tea: Boil one handful each of magnolia buds and Chinese chrysanthemum flowers in 1 quart water for 5 minutes and drink as hot tea, 1 cup two or three times daily, between meals.

(Also see pages 263–266 on sciatica.)

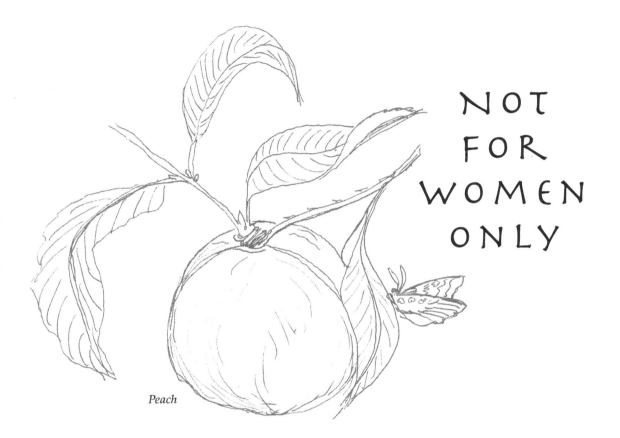

NOT FOR WOMEN ONLY

Peach

The following section concerns the health of our blood as both an energetic phenomenon and a vital body fluid. Blood helps to determine our beauty, the ebb and flow of our reproductive life, and our immune strength. For that reason, the subject of blood cleansing and tonic herbs is not meant for women only. The following chapters will determine the herbs you require for anemia. At the same time, these herbs will protect your skin, hair, and fertility, and help with problems associated with menstruation and menopause.

24
Beauty and the Blood

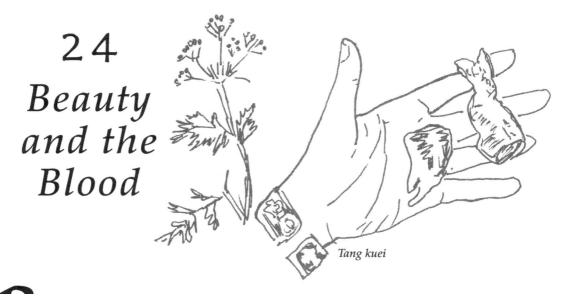

Tang kuei

Beauty is renewed each day with healthy meals, oxygen, and loving thoughts. Our blood and body fluids are the deepest source of nourishment and defense against aging. The Chinese medical attitude toward blood-building herbs has changed. It used to be that you'd walk into an herbal pharmacy and find a venerable Chinese man with a stringy beard, wearing a wrinkled white coat, eating rice with chopsticks as he eyed you suspiciously. No matter whether you asked for herbs to improve energy, looks, or circulation, he'd squint and give the same answer: "Men need energy, women need blood." He'd explain that women need blood because of menstruation, and that men need to improve vigor. He'd go on to say that tang kuei was the best herb for women and ginseng for men. That advice is now both sexist and obsolete.

Nowadays, when you walk into a sparkling modern herb shop, you may find a young Chinese American eating a bagel. She doesn't eye you at all. She's reading a magazine. When you ask for an herbal blood-builder—for example, tang kuei, because you've been reading Asian herb books—she rolls her eyes and says, "Awesome!"

The truth is, we all need to build blood, not just women. The new generation of Asian health practitioners, many of whom are youthful Western or Asian women, practice medicine differently from the way their forebears did. They recognize that times have changed, and so must our remedies. Both sexes need energy tonics and blood-building herbs to protect us from burnout and weak immunity to illness. Nowadays, tang kuei is not just for "women's problems." Blood-builders are necessary for everybody.

Beautiful skin and hair require herbs that support internal organs which produce, store, and circulate blood. If you need blood, you may or may not be considered anemic, but you have predictable signs and symptoms that can be classified as *internal cold* or *internal heat*.

Internal cold symptoms related to blood deficiency leave us feeling tired and listless. You may be pallid and have colorless lips, which are typical signs of anemia recognized by Western medicine. Asian doctors also check to see whether the flesh under your fingernails, inner eyelids, and gums is healthy pink. Signs of blood deficiency in those areas, such as paleness, can be corrected with blood-builders that increase *chi* or *yang: warming* herbs such as tang kuei.

On the contrary, *internal heat* symptoms related to blood deficiency are inflammatory, including chronic fever, night sweats, hot flashes, or emotional problems not usually recognized in the West as signs of blood deficiency. An Asian doctor will also pay more attention to bloodshot eyes, thinning hair, and ruddy complexion as a sign of *internal heat* anemia.

A Western-trained doctor may ignore an underlying blood-deficiency problem to treat many illnesses with strong anti-inflammatory drugs such as cortisone or sedatives, although many times *heat* symptoms are cleared up by *cooling,* blood-building herbs.

The "temperature" of an herb is extremely important. Increased inflammation or dehydration results from using *warming* herbs when we're already too *hot.* Weakness and lethargy are increased by *cooling* herbs when we're too *cold.* Blood-building herbs can bring us into balance, ensuring improvement in all aspects of health and beauty, because they affect metabolism and body fluids. You can find out whether you exhibit signs of blood deficiency by answering the following questionnaire.

Blood Questionnaire

COOLING, MOISTURIZING FORMULAS

HAN LIAN CAO (POWDERED HERB)

—— My hair is very thin, prematurely gray, or falling out.

—— My bones and teeth are weak.

—— I've had drinking problems, hepatitis, or cirrhosis of the liver.

—— I've had chemotherapy or other drugs harmful to the liver, blood, or bone marrow.

—— I'm hot-tempered.

—— It's hard for me to sleep. My mind races.

—— My fingernails are very thin and brittle.

—— I have bloodshot eyes.

—— My tongue is reddish.

—— I have a red complexion or broken capillaries on the face.

LIU WEI DI HUANG WAN

—— I have diabetes.

—— I'm often thirsty.

—— I wake up at night to urinate.

—— I perspire at night when I sleep.

—— I often have a ringing sound in my ears.

—— I feel tight in my lower back and behind the knees.

—— I have a ruddy complexion and dry skin.

SHOU WU PIAN

—— The bottoms of my feet feel hot.

—— My hair is prematurely white or gray.

—— I'm always dry and thirsty.

—— I lack sexual fluid (semen or vaginal).

—— I stay up late and drive my energy so hard that I overheat.

—— I get eye aches, headaches, and lower-back pain.

SUGAR-COATED PLACENTA TABLETS

—— I've lost a lot of blood.

—— I recently had surgery or gave birth.

—— I feel feverish but weak, and have a reddish tongue.

—— I'm infertile or impotent.

—— I have a dry cough and need body fluids.

—— I have vertigo or ringing in the ears.

CATARACT VISION-IMPROVING PILLS (NEI ZHANG MING YAN WAN)

—— I have itchy, painful eyes.

—— I have symptoms of cataracts or glaucoma.

—— My night vision is cloudy.

—— My eyes are tired, sore, and dry.

RESTORATIVE PILLS (A.K.A. RESTORATIVE TABLETS)

—— I have fever, thirst, night sweats, or heat flashes.

—— The soles of my feet burn.

—— I am restless and have insomnia.

—— I have a dry cough or am often thirsty.

—— I am experiencing peri-menopause or menopause.

—— I feel hot or feverish in the afternoon.
—— I have exhausted everything: blood, *chi*, and moisture.
—— I feel and look dry all over.

WARMING FORMULAS

WU CHI PAI FENG WAN

—— I have menstrual cramps and irregular periods.
—— I have dry wrinkled skin. I look emaciated.

EIGHT TREASURE TEA OR WOMEN'S PRECIOUS PILLS

—— I'm fatigued, dizzy, and have low appetite.
—— My menstrual period is scanty.
—— I feel weak and have palpitations.
—— I need a pick-me-up tonic after my periods.
—— I feel cold, weak, and anemic.
—— My joints hurt in cold, damp weather.

ESSENCE OF CHICKEN WITH TANG KUEI

—— I need nourishment and energy because I've been sick.
—— I'm weak and dizzy, and have a poor appetite.
—— My digestion and immune strength are weak.
—— My circulation could be better.
—— I need a boost to my energy and nutrition.

TANG KUEI GIN

—— I'm blood-deficient.
—— I'm tired following illness, surgery, or trauma.
—— I need a tonic to improve the quality of my blood, vitality, and mood.

STRONGLY WARMING FORMULAS

TZEPAO SANPIEN WAN OR EXTRACT

—— I've exhausted all my strength, and I ache.
—— My back hurts.
—— I'm so tired and weak that I can't think.
—— I sweat too much, for no apparent reason.
—— I'm very pale and have no appetite.
—— I have chronic asthma, wheezing, and weakness.
—— My sexual strength is very low.
—— My tongue is big, white, and puffy.
—— My hands and feet are cold and weak.

YANG RONG WAN OR GINSENG TONIC PILLS

—— I need strengthening and calming.
—— I'm weak from chronic illness.
—— I need to build and lift my energy and spirits.
—— I want a longevity tonic.
—— I feel tired, cold, and weak, and have a very pale tongue.

Note: The patent remedies listed above are given in Pinyin Chinese transliterations. They can be found in Chinatowns throughout the West or mail-ordered (see the Herbal Access appendix).

Understanding the Questionnaire

The Blood Questionnaire is actually a teaching device for blood-deficient men and women. By answering such questions, we can observe signs of blood deficiency. More than that, the items represent the notion of *temperature* as it relates to blood-building herbs. Blood-builders vary from *cooling* and moisturizing to *warming*. By now you've read enough of this book that you should never again answer a simple question such as "What's a good herb for blood-building?" without looking at someone's tongue. The answer varies according to individual energetic needs.

The questionnaire's herbal remedies are useful for both men and women because the herbs build energy and blood without directly affecting hormones. Chinese patent formulas were developed long before anyone ever heard of hormones; they're safe for men, who do not need estrogen, or for women, who are afraid of producing more. This can be an important consideration for menopausal problems, which we will discuss later.

The Blood Questionnaire offers herbal recommendations for problems related to metabolism. For example, the first section of *cooling* formulas contains individual herbs and patent remedies for *internal heat* conditions that arise from blood deficiency. These traditional formulas not only build blood for anemia, but also treat inflammatory symptoms resulting from inadequate body fluid. The herbs are *cooling* and moisturizing. *Internal heat* symptoms are diverse, depending upon where the body needs help. These time-tested remedies were formulated to ensure smooth action and adequate absorption.

Notice the sections of the questionnaire that caught your attention. Do you have inflammatory symptoms? Then you probably marked more responses in the *cooling* formulas section. If you have chronic weakness or slow metabolism, you require both blood- and *chi*-building herbs. You probably marked more responses in the two other sections of the questionnaire. The questionnaire follows a continuum progressing from *internal heat* and dryness symptoms to *internal coldness*, weakness, or deficiency of *chi* and *yang*. Chapter 8, on *internal heat* and *internal cold* symptoms, will help you understand how these imbalances came about.

Be sure to watch how your tongue changes while taking these herbs. *Cooling* remedies will eventually make a red, dry tongue moister and pinker. *Warming* and *chi*-tonifying herbs will help a pale, puffy tongue become more normal. You may want to check periodically with an herbalist from among those listed at the back of this book. They are expert in observing subtle signs indicating imbalance. You may have to vary the formulas, sometimes using *warming* ones and other times using *cooling* ones, depending on your energy level and the season.

If you catch a cold, stop taking cooling, *moisturizing herbs, because they increase phlegm.* Remember when choosing a remedy that observation of your tongue will always be your best guide.

Blood Deficiency and Diagnosis

Blood production and circulation are so important that they affect nearly everything we notice in diagnosis. Everything about us that can be seen, heard, touched, or otherwise perceived is affected by blood. It's safe to assume that everyone needs blood-building herbs occasionally. We can decide which ones to choose by determining whether the appropriate ones for now are *warming* or *cooling*. This simplifies everything.

INTERNAL HEAT, DEHYDRATION, AND BLOOD DEFICIENCY

If you suffer from *internal heat* symptoms, indicated by a reddish, dry tongue and a rapid pulse, you may also experience menopausal hot flashes, rashes, nervousness, dry skin, insomnia, or other problems listed in the *cooling* herbs section of the Blood Questionnaire.

No matter whether you are a man or woman, whether you have AIDS, diabetes, menopausal complaints, or excessively dry skin and hair, *internal heat* problems involve the same underlying condition: blood deficiency with inflammation or dehydration.

You must replenish your blood supply with *cooling,* moisturizing, blood-building herbs. It will also help if you eliminate hot spices from your diet and stop smoking (see section II of chapter 13).

INTERNAL COLD AND BLOOD DEFICIENCY

If you suffer from *internal cold* symptoms, you will feel typical blood deficiency symptoms that even your Western doctor will recognize: paleness, fatigue, and weakness. You should take *warming,* blood-building formulas, and generally follow the diet suggestions listed in section III of chapter 13 that reduce nervous exhaustion.

Why is an educated understanding of *warming* and *cooling* herbs better than simply taking an iron pill? Because if you don't know how to balance metabolism with appropriate blood-building herbs, you might do yourself harm. Continuing to eat unhealthy foods, smoking, or taking inappropriate herbs will affect metabolism. It could make problems worse. It could affect blood production itself. The health of our blood affects us on all levels. In the next section you will learn how to use herbs that beautify the skin by bringing about a harmonious balance of blood and energy.

BLOOD DEFICIENCY

What makes it worse?

Chronic illness, blood loss, imbalances in metabolism, stimulants, drugs, chemotherapy, grief, worry, and depression.

What makes it better?

Nourishing foods, good digestion and metabolism, blood tonic herbs, rest, and mountainous climate and altitude are said to increase red blood cells.

	HEAT SYMPTOMS	*COLD* SYMPTOMS	*PHLEGM*
TONGUE	dry, reddish	pale, scalloped	coated
LIPS	pale, dry	pale, dry	pale, dry
APPEARANCE	flushed	pale, sallow	
	thirst, dry cough	excess saliva, nausea, poor appetite	indigestion infertility
	fever symptoms	weakness, chills	overweight
	insomnia	insomnia	depression
	nervousness, anxiety	lethargy, depression	poor memory
	irritability	poor concentration	

REMEDIES

For chronic inflammation and blood deficiency, hot flashes, fever, dry skin:

    Cooling herbal combinations: **Liu Wei Di Huang Wan**

For chronic blood deficiency and weakness, chills, deficiency asthma, sexual weakness, and urinary incontinence:

    Warming herbal combinations: **Sexoton**

    Strongly *warming:* **Tzepao Sanpien Wan**

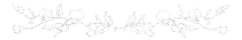

腎，其華在髮　腎，其華在髮　腎，其華在髮　　氣色　氣色　氣色　氣色　氣色

[shèn, qí huá zài fà] The kidney has its manifestation in the hair of the head.

[qìsè] Complexion is the outward manifestation of vital energy.

25

Herbs for Beautiful Skin and Hair

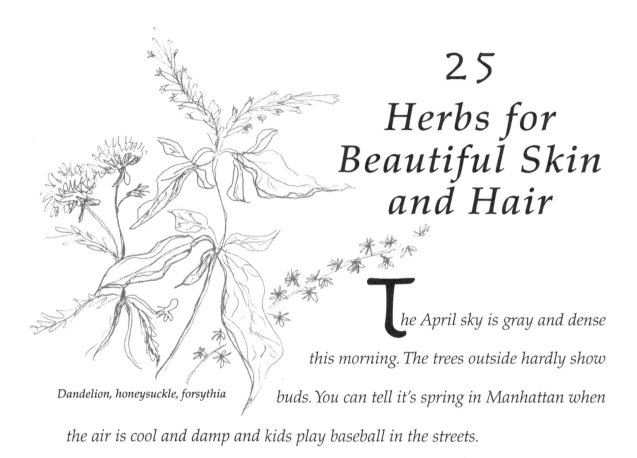

Dandelion, honeysuckle, forsythia

The April sky is gray and dense this morning. The trees outside hardly show buds. You can tell it's spring in Manhattan when the air is cool and damp and kids play baseball in the streets.

I've brewed a bunch of herbs to clear my skin of blemishes after rich holiday meals. Blood-cleansing and laxative teas first thing in the morning make me feel light and clear the skin. Mixing handfuls of honeysuckle flowers, gardenia buds, forsythia pods, dandelion leaf, Chinese violet, and mai men dong ("lush winter wheat"), I put them into a ceramic-coated pot. All the *flowers clear impurities, ensuring oxygen and nourishment for the cells. The winter wheat moisturizes the skin from the inside out.*

After simmering this in springwater for fifteen minutes, I strain the tea into a beautiful teapot from Chinatown. The aroma of the flower tea is springtime fresh. This morning as I sipped the cleansing elixir, I felt thankful for knowing the garden's secrets. Herbs have kept me young a long time.

Your Face Is a Map of Your Energy and Emotions

Beauty problems that show on the skin originate internally. Asian doctors observe specific areas of the face that indicate internal health.

Beautiful skin begins with healthy blood and good circulation. Ancient Chinese doctors knew that beauty problems were more than skin deep. Blemishes and facial flushing are explained as signs of *internal heat* in this quote from *The Yellow Emperor's Classic of Internal Medicine:*

The symptom of the sickness of heat, when it is located in the liver, is that the left side of the jaw turns red. The symptom of the hot sickness, when . . . located in the heart, is that the complexion (entire face) turns red. The symptom of the hot sickness, when it is located in the spleen, is that the nose first turns red. The symptom of hot sickness . . . in the lungs, is that the right side of the jaw first turns red. The symptoms of the hot sickness . . . located in the kidney, is that the chin first turns red.

Short-term and Long-term Approaches

If you have occasional breakouts from rich diet, PMS, or anxiety, you should consider making the temporary diet changes I recommend in the next few pages. They include restricting congesting foods and adding several cleansing herbs and teas. For added cleansing power, add pills from the listed Chinese patent remedies.

These remedies are not meant to be used for long periods. They will do their job, as long as you make the necessary diet changes, in two weeks to a month. Use these pills and teas with caution if you are chilled, very weak, or pregnant, or if you have chronic diarrhea. In all cases, use a dose that is comfortable, and observe changes on your tongue. After cleansing, you may notice that your spotted and reddish tongue becomes more pale and clear.

If, after a week or two, you begin to feel too chilled from these anti-inflammatory herbs, make sure to eat warm cooked foods. Depending on your tongue, you may also wish to add 1 or 2 capsules daily of myrrh to increase circulation. It works especially well for weak persons who have a very pale tongue with dots or gray areas showing *stagnation.*

LONG-TERM USE

The sections that I've called Cleanser/ Rejuvenator Herbs, Beautifying Herbs that Strengthen Weakness, and Wrinkles high-

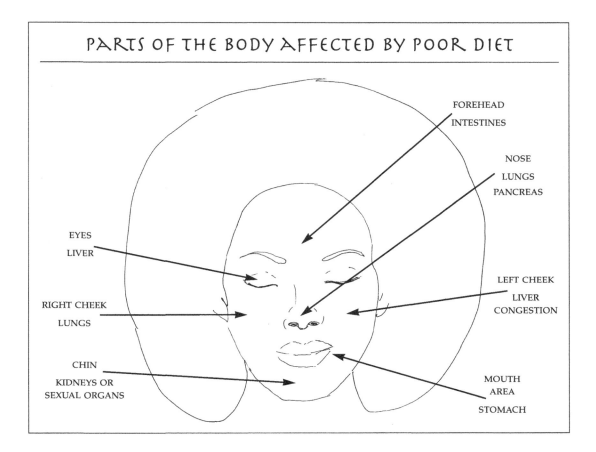

PARTS OF THE BODY AFFECTED BY POOR DIET

FOREHEAD
INTESTINES

NOSE
LUNGS
PANCREAS

EYES
LIVER

LEFT CHEEK
LIVER
CONGESTION

RIGHT CHEEK
LUNGS

CHIN
KIDNEYS OR
SEXUAL ORGANS

MOUTH
AREA
STOMACH

light remedies containing valuable vitamins and minerals that can be taken daily for long periods. They include herbs that build blood and increase vitality.

Diet and Skin Blemishes

Throughout this book I've referred to the cleansing diets in chapter 13, Achieving Balance, but their healing effects are most dramatic when focused on the skin. That chapter addresses the issues of cleansing excess acid and phlegm. Following the diet and herbal recommendations from sections I and II improves the skin's chances of attaining health and beauty from its primary sources, food and oxygen. Section III focuses on restoring the nerves and clearing the emotions through meditation. This cultivates an inner calm that leads to beauty. Have you ever seen an edgy Buddha, or one with wrinkles?

FATS, SWEETS, AND BLEMISHES

A diet rich in fat and sweet food causes skin problems because of resulting acid

TO AVOID BLEMISHES

Avoid Irritating Foods

Acidic and Heating Foods

Tomatoes, pepper, cayenne, onion, garlic, ginger, chili, sugar, pastries, oranges, pineapple, candy, sugar

Foods That Make You Perspire

Honey, cinnamon, basil, ginger, constipating foods

Add Bitter Cleansing Herbs

Try to add one of these cleansing routines to your diet for at least one month. You may wish to use a combination of several of the following herbs, depending on individual problems such as hypertension or blood deficiency:

dandelion and honeysuckle flower
    tea—red, itchy blemishes
burdock root—also treats
    hypertension
yellow dock—anemia, pale complex-
    ion, fatigue
sarsaparilla—herpes, urinary
    infection
aloe vera—PMS pimples, food aller-
    gies, nervous acidity

buildup, inflammation, and poor circulation. Congesting foods weaken digestion and elimination. Fat and sweet foods reduce digestive *chi*.

Fat foods result in sluggish digestion, cloudy thinking, and blemishes. A diet high in fried foods, butter, cheese, nuts, or tahini congests the Wood element (the liver and gallbladder organ systems), making it harder for the body to clear wastes. To make things worse, even certain healthy foods become harmful if misused. Heated oils or rancid fats are also clogging (i.e., they create *stagnant chi*).

Sweets give rise to acid impurities in the blood. Tibetan doctors call these impurities "organisms," and Ayurvedic doctors call them "parasites," in the blood. Certain nerve-related rashes, including herpes and shingles, are made worse from sugar, sweet fruits, and chocolate.

YOUR ADDICTIONS
AND YOUR SKIN

Nervous or depressed people are frequently addicted to foods that do harm to the skin. They reach for fats and sweets, in an effort to calm themselves, or for coffee and chocolate, to try and boost their energy level. Addictions signal the presence of an imbalance trying to maintain itself. We must break the cycle of nervousness, depression, and addictions that lead to low energy, poor digestion, and more addictions (see also chapter 35).

Cut your addictions in half

If you crave sweets, cut your pastries in half. I mean literally eat half of the Danish or doughnut. If it's cigarettes, cut them in half. No matter whether it's carbohydrates, cream sauce, or chocolate—cut them in half. Then fill in the rest with one of the following skin cleansers.

Bitter cleansing herbs to reduce addictions and clear the skin

Bitter cleansing herbs reduce sweet cravings and reduce impurities because they cleanse the liver and blood. When your body is cleaner, you crave cleaner food. That's how addictions work: They maintain our balance or imbalance. The trick is to develop healthy habits.

The best herbs for clearing the skin are diuretic, laxative, anti-inflammatory, antibiotic, and blood- and lymph-cleansing. Diuretics and laxatives work well because impurities leave the body through the best route of exit. If diaphoretic herbs and foods are used—for example, echinacea or honey—a rash will get worse. These sweat-increasing foods make acidic impurities leave the body through the skin. You can prevent or treat rashes by eliminating irritating foods and by adding herbal cleansers.

Dandelion is a wonderful cleanser for the skin, blood, and lymph system. An especially good combination for cleansing the skin is honeysuckle (an antibiotic herb) along with capsules of dandelion twice a day.

Make the tea by simmering a handful of dried honeysuckle flower for ten minutes. For each cup of honeysuckle tea, take 4 capsules of dandelion. Adjust the dosage to avoid diarrhea. Be sure to take capsules of acidophilus or eat yogurt anytime you take antibiotic herbs.

I've recommended this combination for red, irritated blemishes as well as itchy rashes such as eczema. When you take these herbs twice daily and limit sweets in the diet, the problem usually clears up in two to five days.

Burdock root is a blood cleanser, useful for hypertension. You can take 4 to 6 capsules a day of this *cooling* herb, or more if you are troubled by headache, dizziness, or irritability.

Yellow dock is an excellent source of organic iron for weakness, anemia, poor blood circulation affecting the head, or skin problems made worse after blood loss—for example, around your period. Iron-rich blood brings oxygen to the skin for a beautiful, glowing complexion. You'll also feel better and stronger after taking this herb.

Sarsaparilla is a diuretic usually recommended for simple urinary infections. It reduces the itch of herpes because it is antiseptic and *cooling*. You should take sarsaparilla capsules anytime your urine burns, is dark-colored, or seems thick and cloudy. You can take 6 capsules or more daily until the urine turns clear, pale yellow with no offensive odor.

If you have herpes, make sure to eliminate your intake of sugar, and take 6 capsules of sarsaparilla and up to 20 pills of **Lung Tan Xie Gan Wan** daily to prevent or treat outbreaks (see pages 238, 348).

Aloe vera is a favorite of mine. Aloe

juice or gel can be added to tea or apple juice as a laxative cleanser. It's useful for blemishes, menstrual cramps, and bad breath, a perfect addition to any PMS prevention plan.

For external use: Pour a little of the gel into your hand and add a tiny pinch of turmeric powder, an antibiotic from your kitchen. Mix well, and apply it to red itchy skin rash or sunburn overnight. By morning the problem will have cooled and practically gone.

Skin Allergies

For eczema, carbuncles, boils, and itchy allergies, Chinese herbalists sometimes recommend "counter-poison" pills or individual recipes that contain plants and anything from anteater scales, dried vipers, beetle skins, and gallbladders or horns from various creatures. The combinations work by stimulating a strong cleansing response.

I prefer plant remedies: a handful of honeysuckle flowers (jin yin hwa) sim-

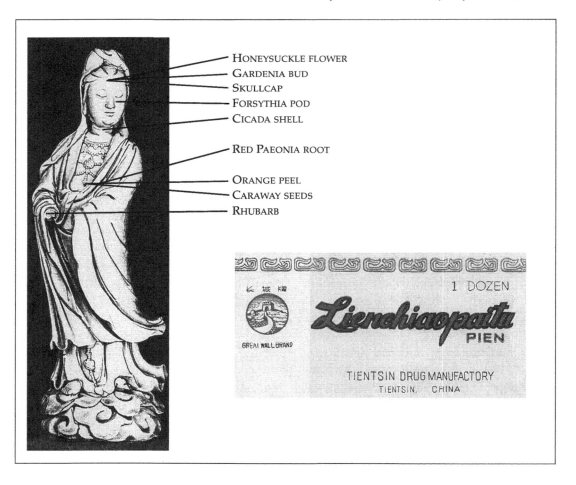

HONEYSUCKLE FLOWER
GARDENIA BUD
SKULLCAP
FORSYTHIA POD
CICADA SHELL

RED PAEONIA ROOT

ORANGE PEEL
CARAWAY SEEDS
RHUBARB

长城牌

GREAT WALL BRAND

Lienchiaopaitu
PIEN

1 DOZEN

TIENTSIN DRUG MANUFACTORY
TIENTSIN, CHINA

mered fifteen minutes for a cup of tea, taken along with four dandelion capsules several times a day, varying the frequency according to individual needs. To this basic recipe you can add other antibiotic herbs from the two pill remedies that follow.

For chronic skin allergies, take one cup of honeysuckle tea and 4 capsules dandelion along with 4 pills of either **Yinchiao Chieh Tu Pien** or **Lien Chiao Pai Tu Pien** twice daily for one week. Make sure to supplement your diet with acidophilus or yogurt. After stopping the cleansing for one day, observe the improvements and continue as needed for up to one more week. Adjust the dose to avoid getting too chilled or developing diarrhea.

ALLERGIC RASHES, INCLUDING HIVES

Yinchiao Chieh Tu Pien is known primarily as a cold and flu remedy. It's useful for the first signs of a cold, such as swollen lymph glands, stiff neck, and body aches. But its antibiotic ingredients, such as honeysuckle flower, also reduce redness and swelling of hives and allergic rashes. If you have *internal heat* (red tongue and hot red blemishes), you can take up to 6 pills daily, but stop them if they give you chills.

Lien Chiao Pai Tu Pien ("Forsythia Defeat Toxin Tablets") is a skin cleanser that treats abscesses—carbuncles with pus and fever from local or systemic infections—and red, itchy skin. The main ingredients cool and cleanse the liver, and are laxative. All ingredients are vegetarian except for ci-

cada beetle skins, used to reduce inflammation. Directions on the box recommend 8 pills per day. Rhubarb in these pills may increase movements, which is cleansing. But if you have diarrhea, take only these pills or one cup of honeysuckle tea and dandelion daily—don't mix both remedies.

Caution: Strongly cleansing potions should always be used with attention to individual differences. If a *cooling* remedy causes weakness and diarrhea, it should be taken less frequently or in smaller amounts. It might be best to start with one dose per day, then adjust the dosage to no more than two. Stop the remedy when the skin clears.

CLEANSER/REJUVENATOR HERBS

These herbs cleanse the blood and internal organs as well as build new skin. Some are high in vitamins and minerals that the body accepts more easily than pills. Plant sources of minerals such as calcium and potassium perform a *yang* function, speeding the turnover of dead cells and production of new cells. Others, sources of vitamins A and E, nourish and moisten the skin, a *yin* function. Plants also contain nutrients that build immunity. The herbs listed below have been traditionally recommended not only for clearing the skin, but also for protection against immune-threatening illnesses. The usual dosage is 6 capsules each daily, but a high-stress lifestyle may warrant more.

Red clover flower is high in protein, trace minerals, and highly absorbable calcium and magnesium. It makes the body more alkaline because it is diuretic, and its mild action makes it suitable for long-term use.

Alfalfa is rich in vitamins and minerals, including calcium, magnesium, phosphorus, and potassium, as well as chlorophyll. It's extremely useful for people with edema or inflammatory arthritis. It can also help soothe ulcers. Alfalfa, along with such other natural vitamin/mineral supplements as nettle, horsetail, parsley, and dandelion, makes the support of health and beauty a simple everyday pleasure.

Nettle's high mineral and chlorophyll content makes it an excellent tonic for the hormonal system. It has a special ability to strengthen the kidneys and adrenal glands, the source of our energy, enthusiasm, and vibrant good looks. You especially need nettle if you have dark circles under the eyes, drink coffee, often suffer jet lag, or have late nights or a weakening illness.

Comfrey and gotu kola are both *cooling*, rejuvenating herbs that rebuild injured tissue, though they work in different ways. Comfrey moistens the lungs, which is good for smokers who want pretty skin. When the lungs are moisturized, the skin can be fresh and glowing from oxygen. Comfrey promotes tissue growth when mucous membranes are inflamed, bleeding, and wasting away. That sounds like emphysema, but can also be the result of diabetes or sores anywhere in the gastrointestinal tract.

Gotu kola heals the nervous system, improves memory, and rebuilds the adrenal glands. It's great for super-stressed city dwellers who live on nerves and stimulants. For that reason it prevents such chronic rashes as eczema, or the zits and cold sores you get when nervous.

Beautifying Herbs That Strengthen Weakness

Some people react to stress with a breakout of pimples, while others are worn out by their lifestyle or hormonal imbalance. If you are one of them, you need special help.

- Do you smoke?
- Do you eat poorly?
- Does your skin look dull or sallow?
- Does your skin look dry or lifeless?
- Are you pale or have dry lips or brittle fingernails?
- Do you have poor circulation with cold hands and feet?
- Are you often weak and light-headed?
- Do you notice these effects more after your menstrual period?
- Does your skin break out after stress or a long gym workout?
- Are you a vegetarian?

If you answered "yes" to these questions, you need a beautifying, blood-building tonic. See the Blood Questionnaire in chapter 24 to see whether you require a *cooling* or a *warming* blood tonic. Many health and beauty problems clear up almost immediately after you take a blood tonic for only a few days. Many herbs are required to make a beauty tonic, because we are made of blood, muscles, and bones fed by energy, breath, and circulation. Asian health tonics address all those needs.

HEALTH-FOOD STORE AND MAIL-ORDER REMEDIES

There are a number of herbal health tonics available in health-food stores or by mail order. (All the blood tonics in the Blood Questionnaire are available from sources listed in the Herbal Access appendix at the end of this book.) Here are a few more to help your skin.

Restore, made by Health Concerns, tonifies *chi* and blood while improving circulation. Such a formula improves overall energy because it contains both blood and energy tonics, including codonopsis (a form of ginseng), atractylodes, fu ling, and ginger to strengthen digestion; rehmannia, peony, tang kuei, and other blood-builders that increase circulation. It combines *warming* herbs and moistening ones for dry skin and brittle nails and hair.

Restore's therapeutic actions address fatigue, pale complexion, reduced appetite, spots floating before the eyes, shortness of breath, vertigo, anemia from chronic illness, irregular menstruation, and depression. Such a tonic helps those exhausted by caffeine, athletics, illness, or a poor diet.

Restore can be combined with other Health Concerns products, such as the following:

Astra 8, which helps boost energy for frequent weakness, lethargy, muscle aches, and poor concentration

Women's Harmony, for dry skin and menstrual problems

Digestive Harmony, for building additional vitality for vegetarians

Other beauty and blood tonics available from Health Concerns are available under the guidance of professional herbalists. For example, **Eight Treasures** treats sallow complexion, reduced appetite, cold limbs, shortness of breath, and vertigo. It repairs anemia and irregular menstruation as well as dry skin and hair.

Tang Kuei 18, made by Seven Forests, treats anemia; fatigue; chronic menstrual problems such as PMS, irregularity, and pain; menopausal symptoms; chronic hepatitis; and eczema. We will study several of these important blood-builders again when we address the problems concerning menstruation.

Your herbalist can advise you on when and how to take such tonic formulas. If you don't already have an Asian herbalist, you can call one of the sources listed in the Herbal Access appendix for professional referrals in your area.

Wrinkles

According to *The Yellow Emperor's Classic of Internal Medicine,*

When the woman reaches the age of thirty-five, the pulse indicating the region of the sunlight [yang ming acupuncture meridian] deteriorates, her face begins to wrinkle, and her hair begins to fall. When she reaches the age of forty-two, the pulse of the three regions of Yang

deteriorates in the upper body, her entire face is wrinkled, and her hair begins to turn white.

When she reaches the age of forty-nine she can no longer become pregnant and the circulation of the great thoroughfare pulse [Conception Vessel acupuncture meridian] is decreased. Her menstruation is exhausted, and the gates of menstruation are no longer open; her body deteriorates and she is no longer able to bear children.

What do I say about that venerable old Chinese text, required reading for all Chinese doctors? "Hah!" That's what I say. Reverse the aging process! Were you ever content with the expected, the ordinary? No! Restore what you've lost. Prevent wrinkles, stay young and beautiful with blood- and *chi*-building herbs!

Why Do Facial Muscles and Skin Tone Sag?

Wrinkles begin from inside due to weak *chi*, originating from poor digestion and circulation. The Chinese medical text explains this energetically. The deterioration of the "upper Yang" refers to weak *chi* in certain acupuncture meridians located on the dorsal sides of both arms and hands. They naturally flow upward to lift the face. Wrinkles develop because those meridians become weak (i.e., they lack *chi*). The meridians are associated with the intestines and with the Triple Heater, an organ system that regulates body temperature and metabolism. An acupuncturist can give you a natural face-lift by strengthening those meridians, but you can also do a lot at home with herbs.

The Remedy: Lift Your Chi

Chi is the invisible envelope that lifts your energy. You can lift your face by lifting *chi*. This is done with good nutrition and herbs. Without proper nutrition, no amount of facial creams can feed the skin or increase circulation to prevent wrinkles.

Wrinkles need vitamin C, which maintains the production of collagen. Collagen, a connective tissue, holds your skin tone in place. Most dermatologists agree it does little good to smear on collagen creams because it's very difficult to absorb that way. Doctors give injections of bovine collagen, which works for some people, while others can develop such allergic symptoms as temporary red welts from cow collagen.

A safer approach is to increase collagen by increasing intake of vitamin C. That increases *chi*. You can take vitamin C pills, but in doing so you lose an important advantage: Herbal vitamin C cleanses the liver, which ensures healthy calcium absorption and circulation. Herbs can do many things at once because they combine natural vitamin C with important minerals that work to maintain healthy collagen and circulation. In addition, the body accepts herbs better than it accepts pills and injections, because herbs are foods.

HERBAL BEAUTY POTIONS

Tonic herbs work internally to create *chi* to tone your muscles and lift your face. The following teas are best used daily. They stimulate *chi* and move it toward the skin.

When to take herbs for the skin

Digestive or cleansing herbs such as dandelion can be taken after meals. But other skin herbs, including those in the following vitamin C tea, affect peripheral circulation and should be taken between meals. Here's the main thing to remember: At mealtimes, energy should strengthen digestive organs, not the skin. Otherwise you may get an itch, a rash, or poor digestion. Take these herbs when the stomach will be empty for a long time—for example, before bed. Reduce the dosage if you are weak or feel spacey.

A VITAMIN C FACE-LIFT

If you drink a daily tea made from one or more of these herbs, you will soon see the difference in improved skin tone and brilliance. They are all herbal sources of vitamin C. Use a handful of herbs per cup, and cook as directed. Then add ⅛ teaspoon of cinnamon or one of the other diaphoretic herbs to steep in the hot tea.

SPECIAL HELP FOR SMOKER'S SKIN

Smoker's skin is dry, dull, thick, and aged from abuse. Close up, it looks like cooked meat. Anything that irritates the lungs also dries the skin. But herbs that moisturize lung tissue will improve skin quality; so will eating soaked almonds, asparagus, and cooked oatmeal.

NATURAL SOURCES OF VITAMIN C

SIMMER DRIED HERBS FOR 5 MINUTES, STRAIN, AND DRINK:

elderberries
chicory root (1 tablespoon)
burdock root
red clover flowers
comfrey
coltsfoot
rose hips (2 tea bags)
nettle (2 tea bags)

STEEP FRESH HERBS AS TEA FOR 5 MINUTES:

dandelion greens
parsley
watercress with a pinch of paprika

THEN SEND VITAMINS, MINERALS, AND MOISTURE TO THE SKIN:

To the cup of tea you make with the above vitamin C herbs, add one of the following diaphoretic herbs. Steep it for five minutes with the tea.

⅛ teaspoon cinnamon powder **or**
1 teaspoon Chinese chrysanthemum (ju hwa), a **cooling** *diaphoretic herb, suitable for persons with internal heat*

If you smoke or have exceptionally dry skin, add one of these sweeteners to the vitamin C face-lift tea. They are sold in Chinese groceries.

Lo han kuo (momordica fruit) is a Chinese herb that looks like a hollow brown tennis ball. You can buy it, crack it, and simmer it for half an hour in water. But I prefer the instant form—a convenient sugar cube that's easier to take to work than a tennis ball. It's sweet enough to add half a cube to one cup of tea. The cube is called **Lo Han Kuo Instant Beverage,** an abbreviation (thank goodness) of **Luo-hanguozhikechongji.**

Another delicious cough remedy is **Fritillaria Loquat Syrup.** These two herbal alternatives to sugar are healthy sweets. Loquat leaf is moisturizing, and fritillaria is an expectorant. Why not heal a smoker's cough with morning tea? Cooling the lungs can help break a nasty habit. With healthier lungs, you'll crave fewer cigarettes and have pretty skin.

PEELING THE SKIN

Peeling is another approach to giving the skin fine texture and color. There are chemical peels, of course, but some have been known to burn the skin or, in time, dry body fluids. I question using chemicals because we breathe with the skin. We also absorb substances through the skin (for example, with estrogen patches, or those used to stop smoking). Are you sure you want to take chemical peels internally?

Several natural alternatives containing alpha-hydroxy complex from fruits are interesting. But I prefer to make fresh beauty potions from the kitchen.

Fresh papaya is a gentle skin refiner. It's delicious to eat or use on your skin, and contains many vitamins. If you can't find the fresh fruit, crush 10 papaya pills, add a little water, and put the paste on the skin for about five minutes, long enough to stimulate the surface without feeling a burning sensation. Papaya enzyme dissolves dead cells at the surface of the skin. Heavy creams only clog pores, starving the skin of needed oxygen.

BEAUTY CREAMS THAT LET YOUR SKIN BREATHE

A lot of moisture creams use animal products like lanolin that cannot be absorbed and eventually clog the pores. But plant oils and moisturizers are easily absorbed.

Jojoba oil actually dissolves sebum that clogs pores. These dead cells cause dandruff and flaky skin. Jojoba is much like natural skin oil. It's light, and stays fresh a long time. Most important, jojoba oil lets skin breathe and therefore make new cells.

I make a soothing, moisturizing cream that can be used at any time of day to protect the skin from dryness and harsh climate. Wash the skin, then place 1 drop of jojoba oil in the palm of your hand. Add aloe vera gel (either fresh or from a tube). Use a squirt the size of a dime. Mix them and spread the mixture onto your face and into your hairline. All the dyes, stabilizers, perfumes, preservatives, and whatnot in cosmetics we put on the skin eventually end up in our blood. Why not use something healthy enough to eat?

BLEACHING FRECKLES AND DISCOLORATIONS

Freckles and discolorations are a problem for some people, especially those who worship the sun. Some beauty experts recommend skin bleaches that contain peroxide or other chemicals . . . ouch! Asian medicine provides several alternatives.

Pills that clear moles and discoloration

A well-known Chinese herbal patent formula works from the inside out for lustrous skin with fewer discolorations aggravated by hormone changes, pregnancy, or birth-control pills. The herbs build blood and ensure good circulation. Follow the directions on the box.

Chinese Patch Removing Pills contain major blood-building herbs that not only moisturize the skin but help rebuild the liver. The formula is so moisturizing that three bottles of the pills, taken as directed, are considered a full treatment. More could create excess phlegm.

A person with a very coated tongue might develop temporary indigestion or head cold symptoms from too many mois-

turizing herbs. So I recommend capsules of myrrh as needed along with the **Patch Removing Pills** for persons with a white coated tongue.

If you develop blemishes while taking this formula, it's because impurities are coming to the surface. You can use one of the cleansing formulas discussed earlier in this chapter, alternating remedies, taking four days of **Patch Removing Pills,** then four days of the cleanser. If you want to attack all fronts at once, take a dose of **Patch Removing Pills** with 3 dandelion capsules and 1 myrrh capsule internally twice daily, and use papaya or pearl cream externally.

Chinese pearl cream

Chinese pearl creams are fun to use. One contains 15 percent powdered pearl (valuable for sea minerals) along with moisturizers and fine-grade paraffin. Others contain human placenta, which is nourishing, or pientzehuang, an herbal antibiotic, for clarifying while moisturizing the skin.

Two forms of **Beanne Extra Pearl Cream,** from Taiwan, are recommended for pimples and blotches. Directions inside the box read, "After applying one week, you will look younger and much charming."

The one packaged in a yellow box is for blemishes, and is made from ginseng, honey, pearl, and bird's nest. Cleaned and processed swallow's nests are used because the saliva the birds use to make the nest is medicinal. The formula also contains apple, vitamins, and unmentioned et ceteras.

The other one, in a green box, recom-

mended for bleaching the skin, lists powdered "pearl, lanolin, aloe vera, spice and
etc." as ingredients. Since recent increases
in U.S. governmental scrutiny, Chinese
manufacturers have become so shy in listing ingredients that sometimes the "et
ceteras" are the most interesting ones.

Both are pale cover creams that, when
applied, make you look like someone from
the Beijing Opera. You can wear either one
around the house to scare your pets. Meanwhile, you'll rid your skin of freckles and
last summer's faded suntan. I use them
under the eyes to refine the skin.

Hair Care

You can do your hair a favor if you take
good care of your scalp. Let it breathe. Aloe
vera makes the hair thick, its fibers strong
and resistant. It adds body and shine without harmful chemicals. Aloe and jojoba let
the pores breathe.

Mix a few drops each of jojoba and
aloe gel, and lightly massage them into
your scalp and hair daily.

HERBAL SHAMPOOS

Many shampoos now contain herbal moisturizers such as nettle, burdock, and comfrey. Chinese herbal shampoos, called **Cutie**
or **Meibo,** contain extracts of the blood-
builders tang kuei and he shou wu, along
with ginseng, which nourish hair and scalp
while improving blood circulation.

For sparkling hair, a favorite trick of
mine is to rinse off soap film, harsh chemi-

cals, and toxic metals from old water pipes
with a final rinse of springwater.

HAIR LOSS

Hair loss can be hereditary or a result of
blood deficiency, hormone or thyroid irregularities, or chemotherapy. Asian hair-
growth formulas work by nourishing
blood deficiency internally, while liniments
stimulate circulation at the scalp.

When hair loss is accompanied by *internal heat* symptoms such as dry skin, insomnia, red eyes, and irritability, it
indicates *yin* deficiency—dehydration of
blood and body fluids, hormone imbalance, or other causes. Blood-building herbs
can have good effects when they nourish
the source of the hair—blood, bone marrow, the liver and kidneys—especially
combined with herbs that increase circulation in the head.

Chinese herbs for hair growth and
prevention of premature graying include
he shou wu (known as fo-ti in health-food
stores) and han lien cao. He shou wu
comes in pills, called **Shou Wu Pien,** or in
liquid form, called **Shou Wu Chih.** It is a
nourishing, moistening blood tonic best
taken between meals because it slows digestion. Persons with slow metabolism can
combine moistening herbs such as this one
with stimulant tonic herbs such as Chinese
ginseng in order to speed digestion.

Over the years I've recommended
Shou Wu Pien for replenishing body fluids. Its *cooling,* moistening effects can offer
relief from a burning sensation on the soles

of your feet. In time, your hair and skin can gain new luster. Several gray-haired clients have enjoyed drinking a tablespoon or more of the liquid with water in the evenings to relax. After several months they noticed that the new hair growth near their temples was dark.

Han lian cao rebuilds the liver and bone marrow. It's recommended for thinning hair related to blood deficiency or liver damage. You can have han lian cao powdered and fill several capsules a day. It's very *cooling* and best taken during summer, when it feels comfortable. If you have a reddish or dry tongue, you can easily take up to 6 capsules daily until you see a difference in your hair. When a *cooling* herb gives you chills, it's time to stop it or add a *warming* one.

Cooling, blood-building herbs can be relaxing for some people and stimulating for others. If internal tissue is scorched by *internal heat* from cigarettes, cocaine, or chronic fevers (a dry, reddish tongue), moisture creates energy and provides fuel for an engine that is nearly incinerated. But for people with too much moisture and phlegm (a thickly coated tongue), more moisture could slow digestion and heartbeat to produce fatigue.

Persons with a thickly coated tongue are advised to take moistening herbs such as those discussed here with precautions, neither with meals nor during humid weather or when they have a head cold. I often combine a capsule of myrrh or a cup of cinnamon tea with moisturing or phlegm-producing herbs in order to help assimilation.

Sheng Fa pills also help prevent hair loss associated with blood and moisture deficiency. They contain herbs that not only build blood but strengthen the spleen and pancreas, which ensures healthy blood production.

HAIR AND CHEMOTHERAPY

Herbal treatments greatly improve recovery from chemotherapy. Frequent complaints during and after chemotherapy include nausea, dizziness, weakness, hair loss, and slow recovery from illness and wounds. The first step in finding balance after damaging drugs is to reestablish the health of the digestive center. This ensures absorption of other blood-building herbs. *Warming*, strengthening formulas such as **Xiao Yao Wan** or **Bu Zhong Yi Qi Wan** are most helpful. **Curing Pills** is another Chinese patent remedy useful for nausea and chronic diarrhea. They all help indigestion. Of the three, **Xiao Yao Wan** works best for depression, **Bu Zhong Yi Qi Wan** for extreme weakness, and **Curing Pills** for nausea.

Herbs for hair loss are an important part of recovery from chemotherapy, but they must be suited to individual needs and taken at the right time. Do not take *cooling*, blood-building herbs when medicines have left you exhausted with chills and a pale tongue; they might encourage *phlegm* conditions and weakness. After taking a digestive remedy such as those I mentioned, when your herbalist says you are ready, proceed with blood-building herbs for the hair.

THINNING HAIR

What makes it worse?

Internal heat; spicy diet; *drying* herbs and medications; hormone and thyroid imbalances; pregnancy; color and curl processing; cocaine; cigarettes.

What makes it better?

Nourishing, *cooling,* moistening diet; blood-building, *cooling,* moistening herbs; frequent gentle shampoos and massage with aloe vera and jojoba oil.

	INTERNAL HEAT	*INTERNAL COLD*	*PHLEGM*
TONGUE	dry, reddish	pale, scalloped	coated
SYMPTOMS	dry, brittle hair, dandruff bloodshot eyes blemishes insomnia, irritability hunger or bad breath		dandruff, clogged pores oily hair

REMEDIES

For *internal heat:* **Sheng Fa,** aloe vera gel (¼ cup daily internally) and gentle massage externally with jojoba oil and aloe gel.

One combination recommended for hair loss from chemotherapy is **Alopecia Areata Pills.** They contain polygoni multiflori, rehmannia, tang kuei, salvia, paeonia, schizandra, codonopsis, chaenomelis, and notopterygi to nourish the blood of liver and kidneys, build *chi,* and increase hair growth. They're useful for anemia, baldness, itchy scalp, and dandruff.

851 is the name given to an expensive (forty-five dollars for 60 pills) combination of amino acids, vitamins E, B_2, pp, and polysaccharides from soybean. They increase nutrition to promote hair growth. Talking about this remedy reminds me of the first time I drank protein powder made from pure egg white. After adding the vanilla-flavored powder to pineapple juice thinned with water, I drank it and my hair smelled of the drink. The protein went straight to the hair, where it was needed.

Hair creams have also been used traditionally to stimulate new hair growth. Western folk remedies have included peppers or hot spices to get blood flow to the head. Several Asian hair tonics offer their equivalent to pepper juice that clears pores and stimulates hair roots. **Formula 101,** from Zhongguang Hair Regrowth Liniment of China, is an alcohol-based liquid that stimulates circulation of the scalp,

SKIN BLEMISHES

What makes it worse?

Fats, oils, hot spices, sugar, alcohol, drugs, stress, hormone imbalances, inflammatory herbs or medicines, pollution, smoking, stress.

What makes it better?

Laxative and diuretic salad greens; minerals; herbs such as bitter cleansers, herbal antibiotics, nervines, and blood-builders; rest; fresh air.

	INTERNAL HEAT	*INTERNAL COLD*	*PHLEGM*
TONGUE	reddish, yellow coating	pale	coated
SYMPTOMS	red, itchy rashes	oozing liquid	pus
	dry skin		slow-healing pimples
	carbuncles, pimples		yellow scabs
	shingles, herpes	nasal congestion	nasal congestion
	irritability, PMS		
	bad breath, cramps	depression	depression
	constipation		

REMEDIES

All blemishes and boils: **Lien Chiao Pai Tu Pien**

With headache and cramps: aloe vera (½ cup in apple juice or water)

Chronic blemishes with nervous disorders: gotu kola

containing American ginseng, Angelica archangelica, salvia, Carya alba, corthamis, Anatherum muricata, lovage, ginger, and capsicum.

Another approach is to cool the head instead of peppering it, which is better for hot types, who don't appreciate smelling like a Szechuan dish. Indian grocery stores sell several chartreuse-colored oils to "cool the head and have luscious thick black hair." Amla, a fruit rich in vitamin C, is often a major ingredient. Brahmi (which is gotu kola), another possible ingredient, is a rejuvenating herb that nourishes the nervous system.

Blondes prefer jojoba oil, which doesn't darken hair as green oil does. Jojoba moisturizes and lets the scalp breathe.

Too often we forget that what we put on the skin eventually ends up in the blood. The body is in every way connected. The outer envelope of skin is an extension of the lungs. Our breath is a vapor of our energy; our eyes, the light of the soul.

天癸 天癸 天癸 天癸 天癸 天癸 天癸 天癸 天癸 天癸 天癸 天癸 天癸

[tiānguǐ] (1) Sex-stimulating essence of the kidney in both sexes; (2) menstruation

26
Phases of the Moon: Our Menstrual Life

P hases of the moon have been

used to describe women's menstrual

cycles. Both recount a period of waiting,

Cherries sweet

about 28 days. The metaphor has come to stand for changeability. But has

the sun been less capricious because it heralds the day? Was it fear of

night and its pleasures that led some to call the moon variable and

women fickle? Was it fear of changing? The moon has always been with

us, ever since our beginning. Crystal clear or veiled by clouds, it rotates on

its axis, slightly tilted to get a better view of earth.

This chapter concerns our cycles and how they can make us either sensitive and loving or miserable. Those aspects of life will always be with us, whether we have a period or not. When we keep them in balance, all is well with our health and happiness. We will study menstruation, both its normal process and possible problems, including amenorrhea and pain. The chapter is not written for women alone. Men also bathe in the light of the moon.

A Visualization for Building Blood

Before you read anything technical about menstruation, let's imagine something together. It will help bring mind and body into balance so that your period will become easier. Do this visualization now and then again during the week before your period, as often as you can. Also avoid extremes in diet, including hot, spicy, or cold, raw dishes, as well as physical exhaustion and cold showers. Even if you have passed menopause, or if you are a man, you will benefit from this visualization because it creates harmony.

We affect our *chi* and hormone balance with thoughts. *Chi* becomes smoother with deep breathing as muscles relax. Perhaps we can even derive some benefit from the blood-building foods we imagine.

Sit in a chair or lie on your back in a relaxed manner, breathing slowly, quietly, and deeply into the lower abdomen. If you usually have pain and muscle tension with your periods, press deeply with both palms along your inner thighs, gently relaxing that area. This may be painful, but continue until the tension releases, while breathing deeply.

Imagine you are surrounded by clear, dark blue sky. There is a glowing full moon above as you walk through a garden. The air is warm and fresh. The grass is covered with dew as you gather berries from many bushes all around the garden. There are ripe raspberries, sweet cherries, strawberries, and blackberries. Plums and apricots have fallen to the ground. Gather all the fruit you want. A breeze fills the air with sweet clover and honeysuckle blossoms. There is a bubbling stream full of lively fishes running through the garden. As you hear the sound, it helps you relax and breathe deeper. Remain, eating the ripe fruit as long as you like. It's your garden. Feel free and light, wearing no clothes. Feel the soft earth between your toes.

Your Period and Your Health

The menstrual cycle is a good indication of general health. When the flow is adequate, on time, and without discomfort, blood production and circulation are in order. Stressful lifestyle, poor eating habits, and emotional upset encourage blood deficiency and *stagnant chi*, leading to irregularity and pain. It is always better to take an herbal combination for pain than an aspirin. Curing underlying conditions leading to menstrual discomfort or blood deficiency with herbs can avert any number of serious problems, including infertility, tumors, or emotional imbalances. Because *chi* and blood are major determinants of health, taking herbs that regulate your periods will help you look and feel better.

All the herbal combinations we'll study in this chapter are for either sex, because they improve the glow of health and beauty without directly affecting hormones. For women, they will help normalize menstrual cycles and ensure well-being after menopause. The herbs I recommend here create adequate blood, moisture, energy, and circulation. We remain young, beautiful, fruitful, and strong by observing a healthy diet and lifestyle, while taking herbs that keep the menstrual cycle normal for as long as possible.

Observe Your Menstrual Cycle

What is a healthy cycle? Unlike Western-trained physicians, Asian doctors do not feel that a normal cycle is "whatever is normal for you." We watch for subtle signs of imbalance because we know they can indicate future illness. Studying the energetic imbalances that lead to these conditions helps to determine the herbs necessary to correct them. Please take a moment to observe your menstrual history and energetic profile.

Determine Your Menstrual Profile

The Menstrual Cycle Questionnaire will help you analyze the effects of your lifestyle upon your vitality, mood, and fertility. You can make sense of your habits by determining how they affect your *chi*. After filling out the questionnaire, note the words that come to your mind when describing your menstrual cycle. They might be "early, painful, anxious, and depressed." Or "scanty, late, and irregular." List them on a sheet of paper. On the same paper, create four columns headed *Heat, Cold, Phlegm,* and *Stagnation.* As you read the energetic analysis of menstrual cycles that follows here, note how your symptoms fall into these four categories. Later you'll choose herbal remedies that address your worst menstrual discomforts, and in so doing, you'll liberate and enhance your *chi.*

INTERNAL HEAT, INTERNAL COLD, STAGNATION, AND PHLEGM

Problem periods tend to be either hot and heavy or cold and watery. The hot and heavy ones (*internal heat*) have clots, pain, and sometimes fever, and tend to come early, whereas the periods that make you feel cold and empty (deficient *chi* or *internal cold*) tend to come late, last a long time, or disappear for a few days, only to return with fatigue or stress.

Although *internal heat* and *internal cold* underlie all menstrual and hormonal difficulties, such imbalances are always held in place by *stagnation.* In other words, there can be no illness without an interruption in the flow of *chi.*

Menstrual Cycle Questionnaire

DIETARY HABITS

I smoke:
—— a few cigarettes a day
—— up to a pack daily
—— more
—— I eat a lot of hot spicy foods.
I eat dairy foods:
—— once a day
—— more
I enjoy cheese, pasta, and creamy foods:
—— weekly
—— daily
I eat red meats:
—— weekly
—— daily
I eat chicken and fish:
—— weekly
—— daily
I eat fried foods:
—— weekly
—— daily
—— I drink coffee daily.
I often eat chocolate:
—— for its taste
—— when I am upset
—— I drink alcohol weekly. If so, how much? _____ .
—— I am overweight or under weight.

HISTORY

—— My periods last ____ days.
—— My periods are regular.
—— My periods come early.
—— My periods come late.

—— My periods are so irregular I can't predict them.
—— I never got my period.
—— My period stopped when _____ . (Explain what happened.)
—— Menopause is/was easy.
—— Menopause is/was troublesome. (Explain how.)

DISCOMFORTS

I usually have pain with periods:
—— slight
—— severe
—— I often have clots.
—— I get fever or headaches with periods.
—— I bleed between periods.
I have fibroids or cysts:
—— in breasts
—— in uterus

ILLNESS

—— I have frequently had kidney infections.
—— I have had abnormal Pap smear exams.
—— I have endometriosis.
—— I have had cancer. (If so, explain what kind and when.)
—— I have had chemotherapy or radiation.
—— I am under chemotherapy or radiation treatment now.
—— The cancer recurred after medical intervention.

EMOTIONAL

—— I often have PMS.
During PMS I feel:
—— angry
—— sad
—— nervous
—— anxious
—— other (Explain.)

—— I have children.
—— I have breastfed my children.

—— I am happy and satisfied in my love
   life.
—— I am not happy in my love life.
—— My love life has not been happy in
   years. (Explain.)
Lately I feel:
—— fine
—— tired
—— tense
—— sad
—— anxious
—— fearful

STAGNANT CHI: **PAIN AND THE PURPLE TONGUE**

You can expect *stagnant chi* with painful, difficult periods, fibroids, and endometriosis if you smoke, take drugs, or indulge in excess liquor, coffee, chocolate, hot spices, and oily foods, and also if you're often angry, frustrated, or sad. Herbal treatment is aimed at moving stuck *chi* with detoxifying herbs.

Tongue symptoms for stuck *chi* are a purple color that can vary from light to dark, or a tongue with dark discolorations inside the body of the tongue or dots on the surface. Menstrual symptoms of *stagnant chi* are most often noticed as *internal heat* or *internal cold,* so those are the most important factors to notice when choosing a remedy.

INTERNAL HEAT: **THE RED TONGUE**

Internal heat can cause bleeding between periods, clots, digestive upset, headaches, fever, pimples, and extreme mood swings.

The tongue will appear reddish and dry or yellow-coated. The *cooling* diet in section II of chapter 13 will reduce *heat* symptoms while helping move stuck *chi.* Seriously stuck *chi* may require both *chi*-building and *chi*-moving herbs.

INTERNAL COLD OR **DEFICIENCY: THE PALE, PUFFY TONGUE**

Deficient *chi* or *internal cold* can make you look sallow and feel cold, weak, tired, and depressed. The tongue will be large, pale, and puffy. The period may come early and leave you feeling empty. You must build adequate *chi* with a nourishing diet, rest, and tonic herbs. Long-term deficiency requires both blood- and *chi*-building herbs along with herbs that facilitate digestion. The best diet may be one to prevent nervous exhaustion (section III of chapter 13) or excess *phlegm* (section I of chapter 13), depending on your tongue diagnosis.

PHLEGM, OBESITY, AND THE COATED TONGUE

Phlegm (the *humor*) causes irregularity because digestion and metabolism are impaired so that periods may disappear for weeks or months. A rich or mucus-producing diet, a sedentary lifestyle, hormone imbalances, humid climate, and emotions such as worry, depression, and grief, all make *phlegm* worse. This causes cramps, bloating, and weight gain. It also gives you a phlegm-coated tongue.

Menstrual flow can be light in color, and scant. There may be continuous leukorrhea (vaginal discharge), bloating, profuse phlegm, listlessness, facial swelling, and chest discomfort. If you have a slow metabolism, you will have a thick phlegm coating on your tongue and phlegm in the throat, or lungs, along with abdominal bloating or possibly heavy and dull aches and pain. You'll feel stuffed up everywhere: in the sinuses, the head, and the whole body. The best herbs for you will increase circulation and speed digestion. If your discharge is yellow, indicating *internal heat*, you will feel best with a *cooling* antiphlegm remedy. The antiphlegm diet in chapter 13 will help reduce those symptoms because digestion and circulation will be improved, but so will exercise.

HOW TO START

Around your period, are you:
Hot and irritable?
Cold and weak?
Phlegmy and sad?

DIET, BLOOD TONICS, AND PILL REMEDIES FOR IRREGULAR PERIODS

First, start by following the diet that feels best from among those listed in chapter 13. Many of your symptoms will disappear immediately with improved digestion. Then, if necessary, add a blood tonic from the questionnaire in chapter 24, a pill remedy from the section in this chapter concerning menstrual pain, or one from the chapter on PMS. When choosing your herbal remedy, you must decide whether you feel more hot, or cold and weak. Looking at your tongue will help you decide. For stuck circulation, see the section on PMS.

Take the blood tonic you require for three weeks between your periods, and the appropriate pill remedy, treating pain or menstrual difficulties, during the week before and during your period. Even if you have not had a period for several months (assuming you are not pregnant), try this same approach for two months. If that fails to produce your period, see the Amenorrhea section of this chapter.

Cooling *remedies for early periods, sharp pains, and fever*

Some of the herbs used to treat this condition are *cooling* blood-builders, anti-inflammatory cleansing herbs, and antimalarial herbs. For example, **Qing**

Jing San contains moutan bark, atractylodes, raw rehmannia, lycii radicis, fu ling, phellodenri, and chinghao. Phellodenri "drains heat downward" (i.e., it reduces inflammation and water retention in the lower body) and Artemisia chinghao, sweet wormwood, is an anti-inflammatory antiseptic used for treating malaria.

Another patent remedy useful for clearing excess *heat* resulting in early or excessive menstruation is **Qing Lian Si Wu Tang,** which contains tang kuei, Ligusticum chuanxiong, radix paeoniae albae, radix rehmanniae, scutellariae, and coptidis. The first two herbs are *warming* blood-builders; the second two are *cooling.* Herbs used to "cool the blood" in this combination are scutellariae (skullcap) and coptidis (golden thread). They are strongly anti-inflammatory for liver and blood.

Warming *remedies for weakness, pallor, and long or late periods*

When you have deficient *chi,* you will look pale and feel tired, feverish, and thirsty. I recommend a combination called **Si Wu Tang,** which contains these *warming* and *cooling* blood-building herbs: rehmanniae, tang kuei, Ligusticum chuanxiong, Paeoniae albae, codonopsis, atractylodes, astragalus, schizandrae, and chen pi. The last five herbs are added in order to build strength and help digestion, thereby tonifying *chi.*

Another popular women's remedy used to normalize the period is a *warming*

chi- and blood-building combination of herbs called **Women's Precious Pills.** (See the Blood Questionnaire in chapter 24.) There are a number of variants of this combination. Your local Chinese herb shop can make up a similar combination of blood- and energy-builders.

Remedies for irregular periods related to excess phlegm and obesity

Xiong Gui Er Chen Tang contains ligusticum and tang kuei, which increase blood circulation. The formula also contains fu ling, citrus peel, pinelliae, and licorice, which are traditionally used to reduce water retention. (See Earth Slimming Soup Stock, page 194.)

Do-it-yourself soups

If you cannot find your appropriate herbal combination in pill form, you can take a handful of each of the ingredients in the remedies I've listed above, and simmer them in a quart of water for one hour. Chinese doctors call these "soups," although they're not the kind of thing you want to serve to guests.

Drink three cups a day until all inflammatory symptoms are better, and pain and water retention subside. After taking it for the time required to bring energy and hormone production into balance, the period will come on time again. For men, or for women who do not have periods, take the remedy until your tongue symptoms improve.

Amenorrhea

Amenorrhea refers to a condition in which a woman has either never had a period, or it has stopped for more than three months even though she is not pregnant, breast-feeding, or in menopause. Traditional Chinese doctors say the most frequent causes of amenorrhea are "blood stagnation due to emotional factors and blood exhaustion from a diet of excess sour and cold foods or exposure to cold temperatures during menstruation." This usually leads first to dysmenorrhea (painful period), then eventually to amenorrhea. In practice it becomes more complicated than that. Here are a couple of examples:

BLOOD *STAGNATION*

Ellie, an artist, walked in wearing tight jeans spotted with paint. At thirty, she had short-cropped hair and wonderful muscle tone that made her look like she lived in a gym. I thought she might be a dancer when she said that she had no menstrual period. Often, dancers start so young that their hormones become imbalanced. But Ellie had other reasons for her amenorrhea. Her period had stopped when her father died. Ellie is short for Electra. Ellie was in her teens when it happened. She still had many complicated feelings about her father that she could not discuss.

Blood *stagnation*, according to the Chinese, is caused by "stuck *chi* from excessive anxiety and anger or fright and grief." Ellie did not have the usual physical symptoms associated with stuck *chi* and deficiency. Normally there is dizziness, headache, chest pain, anorexia, lumbar pain, and leukorrhea. The tongue coating is whitish from *internal cold.*

"Congealed blood"

Ellie looked flushed. In fact her cheeks were overly red from tiny broken blood vessels, possibly resulting from poor circulation and blood deficiency. Her tongue was dark purple red, and her pulse was excessive, slow, and hesitant. She was tied in knots with *stagnant chi* from *internal cold.* Chinese doctors describe extreme blood and *chi* stuckness as "congealed blood." Imagine blood circulation that is so bad the blood actually becomes thick.

Normally a person's tongue is pale when she is weak and cold. But Ellie's was purple because her energy and circulation were *stagnant.* Her emotions were "stuck" in melancholy. After she took herbs for several months to build blood and circulate stuck *chi,* she said she was finally able to visit her father's grave and make peace with him.

She also changed her diet, which for years had been exclusively raw fruits and vegetables. That was how she got what Chinese doctors describe as *"stagnation* from exposure to cold." Does this mean you should never eat salad again? No! Most of us do not eat only raw food. But if you often do, you will benefit from taking myrrh capsules or from adding a pinch of turmeric or cinnamon to your cooking or teas. They increase blood circulation. Traditional Chinese doctors say they move stuck *chi.*

AMENORRHEA FROM MEDICATIONS

We can easily develop weakness or *chi* circulation problems after taking medical or street drugs because their "energy" is unnatural and their effects are so intense. Here's an example of how medication, poor digestion, and exhaustion lead to irregular menstruation.

Sheila came to see me because she'd lost her period after taking antibiotics. Thirty-four years old, she was bone-thin. Her hair hung limp and her skin was dull. There were black circles under her eyes. Exhausted, she spoke in a whisper. The kidney and adrenal pulses at the wrist were hard to find. She complained that she felt weak and spacey most of the time, and her pale, puffy tongue indicated deficient *chi.*

Her two-year-old son ran circles around her in my apartment. He jumped on her lap and tore into her purse to find crayons. I held my breath as he eyed my antiques. He ran up to my parakeets, screeching and flapping his arms, then, not pausing a moment, chased the cats. I imagined Sheila collapsing evenings after putting him to bed. What enjoyment could she have left for herself or her husband? She complained of having no sex drive. She said her period had stopped after a bout with pneumonia and antibiotics that had knocked out her energy.

Sheila got candida, a yeast problem in the digestive tract, after taking the antibiotics. The medication killed pneumonia germs while destroying bacteria necessary for digestion. She suffered from gas pain, bloating, irregular bowel movements, depression, and finally amenorrhea. She could not complain to her doctor about it because he would never link digestive distress, mood swings, and blood deficiency to irregular periods. In fact, he might think she was crazy to suggest such a connection. I'll describe the herbal cure for her yeast condition in chapter 34. For now, I'll address her periods. She needed a lot of help in building kidney *chi.*

Sheila's amenorrhea was not from the usual sources—from eating cold raw foods or from emotional imbalance—but from what traditional Chinese doctors call "spleen and kidney deficiency." Because fatigue is a major factor in that condition, the kidney organ system is always treated with herbs for adrenal exhaustion as well as blood-building herbs.

To increase adrenal and sexual strength, Sheila added ⅛ teaspoon of clove powder to one cup of hot water daily for afternoon tea. Clove is an extremely *heating* herb, affecting the *chi* of adrenal glands and lungs. It's an important strengthening herb that will be discussed in chapter 34. She used cloves for weeks until her nearly white tongue turned healthy pink, her urine turned from clear water to pale yellow, and her backache disappeared. Cloves improved Sheila's breathing because the adrenal glands and lungs finally had enough *chi.* After a month of herbs and improved nutrition, Sheila's period came back. She smilingly reported better vitality and less fatigue.

CHINESE PATENT REMEDIES FOR AMENORRHEA

The following patent remedies treat a variety of amenorrhea symptoms and are usually taken between periods to replace blood and help vitality.

To Jing Wan treats blood and *chi stagnation* for periods with clots, sharp cramps, or amenorrhea. Look for a purplish or black spotted tongue.

Xiang Sha Yang Wei Wan treats weak digestion, *phlegm*-related abdominal bloating, nausea, and amenorrhea. Look for a thickly coated tongue.

Butiao Tablets (Bu Xue Tiao Jing Pian) builds blood, stimulates circulation, and strengthens spleen and kidney energies. It helps fatigue, cramps, and irregular bleeding (excessive or deficient) caused by "stagnation of blood." Look for a pale, oversized tongue with dark spots.

Wu Chi Pai Feng Wan is packaged in a blue box with a picture of a black chicken on it, or in a pink box without the chicken ingredient. Each individual dose comes wrapped in its own plastic "egg" container. Discard the egg and eat the contents, one dose a day, or add it to soup stock. The blue box contains black rooster, a *yin* or moisture-building food, along with other herbs that stimulate the circulation. Both formulas are slightly *warming* but balanced enough for most women. This popular remedy, also called **White Phoenix Pills,**

treats many menstrual problems, including cramps and amenorrhea.

Menstrual Pains

Menstrual cramps, called *dysmenorrhea*, deserve special attention because pain can be very severe and can indicate other imbalances at the same time. The origin of this discomfort is said to be obstructed circulation of *chi* and blood. It can result from emotional stuckness. Have you ever been caught in an emotional impasse during your period and gotten cramps? Other factors are eating too many spicy or cold, raw, and sour foods, weak *chi*, blood deficiency, or irregular circulation of *chi*. Do a quick check:

- Is your period pain worse before or after menstruation?
- Does warmth and pressure make it feel better or worse?
- Does it hurt constantly?
- Is the pain sharp or dull?

Normally, premenstrual pain is a result of poor circulation. If it's aggravated by pressure or massage, it's from stuck *chi*. You need to take *chi*-moving herbs. They also help relieve depression. If the pain is worse after the period and feels better with pressure, it is from deficient energy. Take *chi*-building herbs. (See the Blood Questionnaire in chapter 24.)

If you feel better putting a heating pad on the pain, you have *internal cold*, so use *warming* herbs. If pain is sharp, and even the idea of heat makes you feel worse, you are

FEMALE REMEDIES

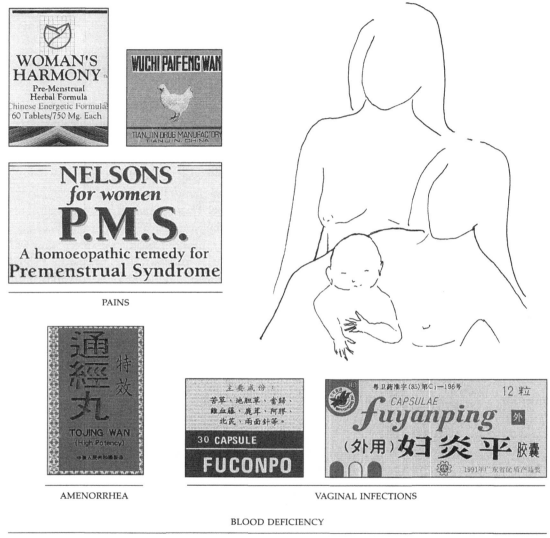

PAINS

AMENORRHEA

VAGINAL INFECTIONS

BLOOD DEFICIENCY

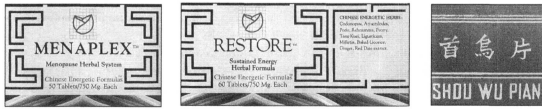

already too hot, so use *cooling* herbs. If the pain is insidious or constant, it most likely results from blood and energy deficiency. You'll have to change your diet and take tonifying herbs before you can feel better. Here are a couple of examples to help you:

INTERNAL COLD

Janet, pale and out of breath, looked slightly green. She immediately sat down, hunching over to protect her painful abdomen. She wore black pants and a dark blue shirt, and had unkempt hair. Her hands and feet were ice-cold in thin socks and wet sneakers. Stuffing a half-eaten white-flour bagel into her purse, she seemed depressed. She spoke in a nasal whine that made her sound clogged.

Without taking Janet's pulse or looking at her tongue, I knew she had an *internal cold* condition. She was too wan and listless to be otherwise. Perhaps she ate too much salad, ice water, or ice cream. Or when she walked out in the cold and got wet feet, her body reacted with a spasm in the uterine area.

Perhaps her *internal cold* had become chronic to the point where she was blood-deficient, another cause for menstrual pain. In that case her blood flow would be sparse and light-colored. Perhaps she was so weak that she craved sweets (weak spleen) or salt (weak adrenal glands). She suffered from water retention in the legs, a sign of deficient "kidney" energy.

The woman with *internal cold* may feel despondent and weepy. She may be hypoglycemic and have poor concentration. Her tongue is pale, her pulse deep, slow, and stagnant. She needs *warming* herbs, such as cinnamon, that break up *stagnant chi* and make her sweat. She can add a big pinch of cinnamon to hot water as a tea. Cinnamon increases blood circulation in the uterus; it also helps sweat out the cold. With cinnamon, menstruation will flow more smoothly because the body temperature will become more normal and muscles can relax.

Myrrh is another *heating* herb that strongly increases blood circulation to heal wounds. Taken in capsules, it can normalize menstrual flow that is thin and watery and has clots from *internal cold*. It treats chronic *stagnant chi* that shows on the tongue as tiny purple dots.

Myrrh rids the uterus of clots that could form other problems such as fibroids. Taking myrrh during the period or the rest of the month may make the flow increase temporarily. How many capsules should you take? Start conservatively with one at a time, then notice how you feel. If the increased circulation helps your pain, you are on the right track. Take 2 to 4 capsules daily, as they are comfortable. Watch what happens to your *chi* by observing changes on your tongue.

INTERNAL HEAT

Jerry walked in wearing a chic designer green and purple suit and high heels. She was a picture of *internal heat.* She looked flushed, and spoke and moved in a hurried, nervous manner. Her black hair was thinning on top. She wore glasses for near-sightedness. She had dry, lusterless skin with red pimples on cheeks and chin. She put her bag in the middle of the room and waited for me, arms folded impatiently, ready to tap her foot. Friendly but speedy, she spoke with a tight jaw. She looked ready to jump straight up. *Chi* was stuck in her middle, chest, and shoulders, squeezing her like a tube of toothpaste.

Internal heat menstrual pain does not feel better with pressure or heat. You may experience fever, headache with dizziness, and nausea. You may have a bitter taste in the mouth from poor digestion. The menstrual flow itself might feel warm or have a foul odor. There may be intense cramping. If there is stagnation of blood circulation, there will be clots with very dark blood, or endometriosis.

This is usually caused by a variety of factors, including liver inflammation. Perhaps Jerry frequently ate hot, spicy foods such as garlic, onions, and chilies. Perhaps she smoked or drank too much, or stayed up late, working or partying too frequently. Perhaps she ate lots of oily foods such as nuts, cheese, beef, or tahini. The body always reacts to extremes in temperature with spasms, whether caused by chili peppers or iced drinks. Oily and hot foods inhibit smooth circulation through the neck, chest, and abdomen.

Internal heat affecting the Wood element leads to anger, frustration, nervousness, or anxiety. At some point it becomes impossible to know whether the physical symptoms lead to or are caused by personal relationships. *Internal heat* symptoms may become so chronic that you may feel, "That's just the way I am, jumpy and irritable at period time."

If you suffer from *internal heat* symptoms, you need *cooling*, bitter cleansers such as aloe vera gel, added to tea or apple juice. Available in health-food stores, it resolves pimples, bad breath, nervousness, headache, and pounding menstrual cramps associated with *heat*. Aloe is relaxing to the muscles and slightly laxative. Drink aloe vera gel or juice all day until the pain subsides.

Sarsaparilla is a wonderful rejuvenator herb for women. It is antiseptic and anti-inflammatory, useful in urinary tract infection and inflammation in the urogenital tract. Use it for burning urine and throbbing pain.

Valerian treats uterine pain because it quiets the nerves leading to the uterus. If menstrual pain is so severe it keeps you awake, take 1 or 2 capsules of valerian before bed. It is a useful herb for anxiety, ungroundedness, dizziness, migraine, and menstrual pain due to nervous tension.

As your menstrual discomforts disappear, your emotions will even out, your tongue will become clear of inflammation, phlegm, or watery puffiness, and your period will become more regular. Watching the ebb and flow of your cycles can show you the balance and wealth of your internal garden, the fertile earth in your center, the richness and depth of your compassion.

MENSTRUAL PAINS

TYPE OF PAIN	INTERNAL HEAT	INTERNAL COLD	STAGNANT CHI	HERB REMEDY
pounding, sharp (red tongue)	*internal heat*			See *cooling* formulas (chapter 24) **Xuan Yu Tong Jing Tang** liver and blood cleansers and lots of aloe
dull, heavy (pale tongue)		*internal cold*		See *warming* formulas (chapter 24) **Wu Zhu Yu Tang** **Wen Jing Tang**
sore back, lumbago			*stagnant chi*	**Tiao Gan Tang**
rib pain and indigestion, constant cramps with emotional upset			*stagnant chi*	**Xiao Yao Wan**

INGREDIENTS

Xuan Yu Tong Jing Tang: radix angelicae sinensis, fried radix paeoniae albae, cortex moutan radicis, fructus gardeniae, prepared semen sinapis albae, radix bupleuri, rhizoma cyperi, radix curcumae, scutellariae, and raw radix glycyrrhizae.

Wu Zhu Yu Tang: fructus evodiae rutaescarpae, radix angelicae sinensis, radix platycodi grandiflori, herba asari cum radice, radix ledebouriellae sesloidis, dried rhizoma zingiberis, radix rehmanniae conqitae, and prepared radix glycyrrhizae.

Wen Jing Tang: radix angelicae sinensis, rhizome ligustici chuanxiong, radix paeoniae, rhizoma zedoariae, panacis ginseng, radix achyranthis, corex cinnamomi, cortex moutan, and radix glycyrrhizae.

Tiao Gan Tang: radix angelicae sinensis, paeoniae albae, rhizoma dioscoreae, gelatinum asini, fructus corni, radix morindae off. prepared with salt solution and radix glycyrrhizae.

Xiao Yao Wan: radix bupleuri, paeonia, angelicae sinensis, atractylodes, zingiberis, poria (fu ling), licorice, and mint.

To order, circle one and fax to one of the distributors found in Herbal Access.

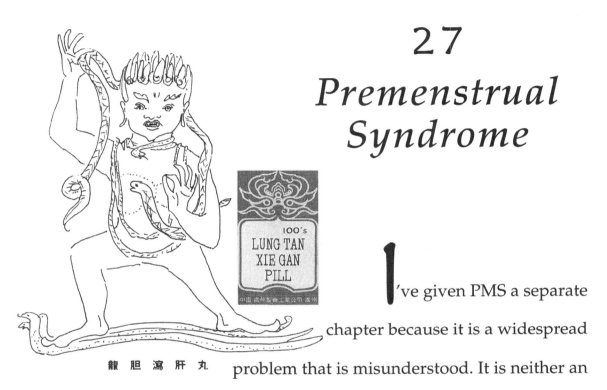

27
Premenstrual Syndrome

I've given PMS a separate chapter because it is a widespread problem that is misunderstood. It is neither an illness you catch monthly nor one you inherit. And it certainly is not the price of admission for being fertile. PMS is a crippling nuisance that you can eliminate with herbs but, hopefully, not before learning from it. PMS mirrors your deep feelings, the emotions you don't like to reveal, because it also embodies your deepest energetic and spiritual needs. It can change your life when you comprehend it.

PMS: WHERE DO YOU FEEL IT?

WEAK EARTH ELEMENT

Before my period:
- I crave sweets.
- I get very spacey if I don't eat often.
- I get moody and depressed.
- I obsess about old griefs and annoyances.
- I have water retention around my waist, hips, and thighs.
- My energy is low.
- I look pale and washed out.
- I can't seem to focus; I'm mentally foggy.
- I don't feel grounded or centered; my emotions carry me away.
- I call all my friends on the phone and feel needy.

TROUBLED WOOD ELEMENT

Before my period:
- I can't seem to make up my mind or think clearly.
- I feel weak and chilled.
- My coordination is troubled; I bump into furniture.
- I get nauseous or look jaundiced.
- I get headaches, facial pimples, or fever.
- I cannot control my anger.
- My muscles cramp and spasm.
- I become very nervous.
- I can't sleep well.
- I get upset over the silliest things.
- My rage could become dangerous.

Luckily, a new generation of herbal doctors has broadened the commonly accepted definition of premenstrual discomfort in order to formulate remedies that treat more than physical symptoms such as pain and bloating. This chapter covers an Asian energetic approach to PMS and describes some time-honored treatment as well as newly formulated ones widely available to the general public.

PMS: An Energetic View

The assortment of complaints we designate PMS can make life miserable from a few days to several weeks each month. This roller coaster of energetic and hormonal shifts typically entails fatigue, irritability, depression, water retention, constipation, breast tenderness, or disorientation, depending upon which of the Five Elements and the three *humors* are involved. First we'll consider the underlying factors that precede all aspects of premenstrual syndrome, then look more closely into three forms it can take, which we'll call "weepy," "angry," and "crazy" PMS.

PMS: Where Do You Feel It?

According to Five Element theory, Earth and Wood elements must work together in a coordinated manner to ensure proper digestion, circulation, and mental clarity. Problems develop when either element becomes troubled; then one unbalances the other. The most typical problems of PMS involve weak *chi* affecting Earth, and inflammation unbalancing Wood. If you suffer from chronic PMS, you can expect problems stemming from weak or ungrounded Earth and troubled Wood every month. Since Earth and Wood constitute your digestive and emotional center, problems there tend to be quite complicated and unsettling. In fact, they can knock you completely off your rocker.

UNGROUNDED EARTH AND RAGING LIVER FIRE

Imagine standing on quicksand, while holding a flaming torch that threatens to engulf you. That feeling of instability parallels the energetic problems that underlie PMS. In my analogy, quicksand is Earth that's not strong enough to support you, while the fire that threatens to engulf you monthly results from acidic toxins that are not adequately cleansed from the nervous system.

What this means, in terms of Chinese medicine, is that PMS symptoms are indicative of excess *phlegm*, weakening the Earth element, along with inflammation from stuck *chi,* affecting the Wood element.

Weak Earth element

Phlegm (the *humor*) is said to weaken the spleen and pancreas so that problems arising from excess *phlegm* lead to poor digestion and assimilation, water retention, and weak *chi*. That, in turn, leads to inadequate energy, blood production, and mental clarity. When that happens, because of poor diet, emotional turmoil, or hormonal changes, your digestive center in the Earth element is not strong enough to support you. Blood-sugar imbalances and yeast infections (also related to *phlegm*) can make you feel spacey, as though you were standing on quicksand.

Stagnant chi *affecting Wood*

Another factor in PMS imbalances is related indirectly to the Wood element. For two weeks preceding menstruation, blood calcium drops to half its normal level, precipitating backaches, nervous jitters, insomnia, and anger. This calcium deficiency can be explained as the inability of the liver to produce enzymes that enhance absorption. Inadequate calcium also reduces muscle strength, often resulting in palpitations or constipation, which can leave you feeling anxious and full of poisons.

Such imbalances involving Earth and Wood are frequently long-term, so that you may become accustomed to them, losing track of when you feel better or worse. Often they become the basis of addictions that perpetuate the imbalance. You may feel spacey, weak, nervous, and irritable, so that you crave sweets, stimulants, or medicines that further weaken Earth and Wood. You can see how taking a simple painkiller will not do the trick because it will not help your addictions.

The Advantage of an Asian Energetic Approach to PMS

By freeing ourselves from a purely medical —i.e., hormonal—explanation of PMS, we realize that its problems are energetic. They affect our mood, vitality, and relationships, and involve issues that influence both men and women equally.

You can get in touch with your health by noticing your energy, not your hormonal quirks. For example, it is practically impossible to perceive when your estrogen or progesterone level is up or down. But you can cure discomforts that you experience with herbs. Bloating, depression, and fatigue are what make you feel miserable, not your hormones.

WHAT HERBS FOR PMS DO

By treating premenstrual discomforts, you will ultimately reach their cause. Herbs for PMS improve digestion, blood production, and circulation; they also bring mental clarity into focus so that by creating balance, your hormone levels improve.

The chart on page 322 summarizes problems of *phlegm, internal heat,* and *internal cold* of the Earth and Wood elements as they apply to PMS.

PMS Prevention Diet

A good diet to prevent PMS is nourishing and easy to digest, consisting mainly of cooked vegetables and grains. (See the diets in sections I and II of chapter 13.) Also supplement healthy fats by taking a tablespoon of olive, sunflower, or flaxseed oil daily.

Iodine is essential to the health of the thyroid gland and normal estrogen levels. If you don't get enough natural iodine, the thyroid can become sluggish, and estrogen will build up. (*Phlegm* imbalances will also occur.) One way to take iodine is by eating 2 tablespoons or at least 4 capsules daily from among these: kombu, kelp, dulse, alfalfa, spirulina, Irish moss, watercress, or nettle.

Some teas that are most useful for preventing PMS pain and restlessness will also help balance hormones. Crystal Star makes some tasty herbal teas that combine antispasmodic herbs with those that supplement needed minerals. Two of these are **Female Harmony Tea** and **Flow Ease Tea.**

Teas you can make for premenstrual edema provide a diuretic action that does not reduce potassium. These include combinations containing uva ursi, cornsilk, parsley, dandelion, sarsaparilla, buchu leaves, queen of the meadow, juniper berries, kelp, unsweetened cranberries, or watermelon seeds.

ELIMINATE CONGESTION AND IRRITATION

Since *phlegm* and inflammation exacerbate PMS, the most sensible diet for prevention is one that increases neither congestion nor irritation.

PREMENSTRUAL SYNDROME

EARTH ELEMENT (stomach/spleen)	IMBALANCED BY	SYMPTOMS
	phlegm	indigestion, bloating, water retention
	fat, sweet foods	depression
	stimulants	
	hormones	irregular periods
	internal cold	nausea, chronic diarrhea
	weak *chi*	poor concentration and memory, spaceyness, out-of-body feelings, worry, grief, depression
Periods		late, slow, long, accompanied by anemia
PMS emotions		weepy, dependent
	internal heat	hunger, sweet tooth, skin blemishes, bad breath, mania, hysteria, out-of-body feelings, panic, auditory hallucinations
Periods		early, heavy, with hemorrhage or amenorrhea
PMS emotions		paranoia, exhibitionism

WOOD ELEMENT (liver/gallbladder)	IMBALANCED BY	SYMPTOMS
	wind	nervousness, seizures, dizziness, shooting pains
	internal heat	headaches, fever, cramps, spasms, constipation, skin blemishes, insomnia, anxiety, anger, rage
Periods		early, heavy, painful
PMS emotions		irritability to violent rage
	internal cold	pallor, anemia, weakness, poor mental functioning, difficulty in making and carrying through plans, clumsy coordination, numb extremities
Periods		sparse, pale-colored
PMS emotions		depression, indecision

Avoid oily and fried foods, dairy products, wheat, and sweets because they increase *phlegm* conditions. Instead, add their opposite: radish, barley, parsley, caraway seeds, fennel seeds, and other antiphlegm foods (especially if your tongue is coated).

Also avoid hot, spicy foods (like garlic!) and strong stimulants (coffee and black tea), because they're inflammatory. Instead, add cumin, coriander, and mint as spices, and drink roasted chicory with a dash of cardamom instead of coffee.

Alcohol can increase both *phlegm* and inflammation. Avoid it completely, or take one glass of wine with 2 capsules of **Yunnan Paiyao** to treat cramps and excessive bleeding (see chapter 18).

SUPPLEMENTS

You will need to take the following supplements for at least two months before they will have changed your hormones and energy enough for you to feel their effects. Choose the ones that seem the most appropriate to your needs.

Evening primrose oil has already been mentioned in chapter 20 as a treatment for headaches, but taking 3 capsules daily will also reduce pain and congestion associated with menstrual flow. This supplement releases the flow of prostaglandins, which are hormone-type compounds that regulate all body functions electrically.

Vitex Extract (chaste tree berries) is recommended for hormone imbalances and menstrual irregularities; it affects estrogen-progesterone balance, and reduces PMS symptoms such as water retention and fibroids.

If you prefer a diuretic pill or liquid extract, Nature's Herbs makes **Diurtab**, and Crystal Star makes **BLD-K Extract**. Both contain many of the diuretic herbs listed above. In addition, **BLD-K Extract** contains goldenseal, an antibiotic, and is 55 percent alcohol; therefore, take yogurt or acidophilus when using it.

ADDICTIONS AND PMS

Understandably, certain foods are more likely to become addictions at PMS time, when the body is unbalanced. Chocolate is a common one. It is a sweet and congesting stimulant—everything we need for an imbalance. Some people reach for it, not realizing the craving is a sign of problems to come. Food addictions are damaging because they seem harmless, while they increase indigestion and malabsorption leading to blood and energy deficiency.

Cravings show us the nature of an imbalance. Cravings for sweets indicate trouble with the Earth element or weak *chi* in general that can develop indigestion, excess *phlegm*, blood-sugar oscillation, and depression. Hot spices generate inflammation in the Wood element, affecting liver and gallbladder. We often crave heat when we're already hot enough. *Stagnation* or overactivity of the Wood element results in anger, insomnia, and increased sexual appetite, not to mention nervousness.

If you have a red tongue or crave chocolate or hot spices, you need to cleanse excess acid by taking *cooling* cleansing herbs such as ¼ cup daily of aloe vera juice or gel in tea, or up to 10 capsules of dandelion. If you tend also to have diarrhea, add 10 drops daily of liquid gentian extract. If you have a pale tongue and fatigue, indicating adrenal weakness, add ¼ teaspoon of powdered cloves to the aloe juice daily. As a chocolate substitute, try some **Chawanprash,** a blend of clarified butter and sweet digestive spices, available in East Indian groceries. It lacks chocolate's irritating caffeine.

"WEEPY" AND "ANGRY" PMS

What can we do if PMS is extreme? A bad mood can seem paralyzing. One easy-to-use remedy cuts excess *phlegm* that underlies attacks of sadness and hopelessness that might occur during PMS. It is homeopathic pulsatilla, 30c potency. Put 10 pills in a liter of springwater and sip it during the day. Avoid use near meals. Wait twenty minutes after drinking coffee.

Pulsatilla is a tiny flower used to prevent intestinal parasites, because its *drying* effect reduces phlegm. In its homeopathic form, the remedy treats that heavy, moody feeling common in weepy PMS. It makes for deeper breathing and less fixation on negative thoughts. With increased oxygen, we can see the rainbow on the horizon more clearly.

The best remedies for angry PMS, aside from acupuncture treatments, are *cooling* liver cleansers such as aloe vera and dandelion taken in large doses, i.e., a dozen or more capsules per day. If you tend to have diarrhea, add 10 drops extract of gentian to a little water three times daily.

Lung Tan Xie Gan Wan, the Chinese patent remedy, is useful for clearing liver and gallbladder toxins, curing bilious headaches, herpes outbreaks, and constipation. Taken in doses of 10 pills or more after meals, it reduces anger (even rage) and chest pain resulting from liver congestion.

"CRAZY" PMS

PMS is sometimes a temporary madness that whacks you out of control. This extreme form may be related to hormonal, thyroid, or blood-sugar problems stemming from exhaustion, long-term addictions, or emotional trauma.

The energetic imbalance that underlies this form of PMS is related to weepy and angry PMS, although it is far more extreme. It entails a double dose of rising "fire" (inflammation affecting Wood and Earth acupuncture meridians) that is not experienced as pain but as disorientation resulting from a disruption of thyroid function and the involvement of certain brain chemicals. The result is that you feel unconnected to your body and alienated from those around you. Based on a traditional Chinese medical perspective, these are the kinds of complaints my health clients have experienced during "crazy PMS":

PHLEGM *OBSCURING THE SENSES,*
AND "RISING FIRE" OF THE LIVER

Around my period time:

- I lose my appetite.
- I smoke lots of cigarettes and drink pots of coffee.
- I take tranquilizers, antidepressants, or street drugs.
- I could stay awake for days. Or I could sleep for days.
- I hear ringing or humming in my ears.
- People on the radio are talking about me.
- I argue with members of my family or those closest to me.
- I yell myself hoarse.
- People gang up on me.
- I feel that I am in other people's bodies.
- I can become other people or animals.
- Others are controlling me.
- I can't stay inside my skin.
- I want to have sex all the time.
- People tell me things in subtle, symbolic ways.
- I know dangerous information I have to keep locked inside.
- I've got to get out of here—change my job, home, life.
- I sing at the top of my lungs, dance until I drop.
- I can't stop hearing a song or sound in my head.
- I experience this every month before my period.

Given a poor diet and a hostile or uncaring environment, this kind of disorientation can make you feel vulnerable, contentious, or lead to panic. The clinical outcome could become paranoia, mania, clinical depression, catatonia, or violent behavior. You know it is PMS because it happens like clockwork before your period—or it happens instead of your period.

Crazy PMS can be ameliorated by herbal remedies normally used to curb schizophrenia (see chapter 35). An energetic herbal approach aims to quell melancholy, rage, hallucinations, and wildly exhibitionistic or violent behavior by dissipating *phlegm,* poor circulation, and inflammation affecting brain centers controlled by the Earth and Wood elements. In that way, PMS herbs can influence hormones and brain chemicals and clear toxins.

Digestion symptoms

Digestion is a major issue with crazy PMS, although indigestion is not the problem. The imbalance is far more subtle and serious than that, because hormonal irregularities can occur along with blood-sugar problems and mood swings. When you are weak, undernourished, or disturbed by fear, rage, anxiety, or drugs, *chi,* our component of *wind* in the body, can unground you. But good nutrition helps give you the strength and clarity needed to fight off crazy PMS.

START HERE

The best way to start to heal your PMS is to use some natural method to stop smoking and taking poisons such as harsh stimulants, drugs, medicines, or anything that impedes your circulation. Try chewing cinnamon sticks and drinking oolong tea.

SUPPLEMENTS

Often recommended to prevent disorientation are mixed trace minerals that support endocrine functions, as well as zinc and chromium, which help maintain normal blood sugar. Trace minerals are called that because we need only small amounts of them, although they are very important. For example, manganese and copper help liver function and thus aid in calcium and iron absorption. Gold helps the adrenal glands work. Health-food store B vitamins usually come in fairly good proportion with each other. But for PMS, we need more of several of them. B_{12} is essential for the nervous system, and B_3 (niacinamide) is needed for the synthesis of sex hormones (estrogen, progesterone, and testosterone) as well as cortisone, throxine, and insulin. It is necessary for healthy nervous system and brain function. B_3 prevents pellagra, a disease characterized by gastrointestinal symptoms including abdominal discomfort, nausea, diarrhea, and psychosis with disorientation, confusion, manic-depressive behavior, and delirium or paranoia.

CHINESE HERBAL PATENT REMEDIES

Chinese herbs recommended to stabilize digestion while cooling inflammation include **Xiao Yao Wan** along with **Lung Tan Xie Gan Wan,** the liver cleanser. Taken together at mealtime (8 to 10 pills each), they can normalize a hyperactive thyroid mania in order to heal that spacey, out-of-your-body feeling combined with hostile or fearful thoughts.

Xiao Yao Wan, taken in high doses of 30 or more pills a day, prevents and treats hypoglycemia and depression. It is best suited for someone with a pale tongue and low *chi.* Take it anytime for as long as you need it. It will bring you into your center.

Lung Tan Xie Gan Wan is recommended for angry or violent behavior, headaches, dizziness, herpes, and constipation. If your tongue is red with a yellow coating, and you experience these inflammatory symptoms along with ear-ringing, rage, and hyper energy, take 20 to 30 pills daily (10 at a time), until your tongue becomes normal and your mood improves.

An Mien Pian are pills that improve sleep. The remedy contains blood-builders and digestive herbs that cool and regulate liver and calm the spirit. It is used for insomnia resulting from liver overactivity or congestion, agitation in heart and mind, anxiety, and mental exhaustion, along with red, irritated eyes, restless dreams, and poor memory.

The following example describes these remedies in context, and also illustrates how we may become sick with reason and purpose.

TEMPORARY MADNESS WITH A PURPOSE

I've known a number of people who have used their illness as a means to maturity. One woman changed her whole life because of her PMS. It wasn't only from personal insight; her illness forced her to leave a situation that had become untenable. We met under unusual circumstances.

It was morning in Chelsea—a pale orange-tinted sky made sticky by approaching rain—time for my breakfast green tea, trace minerals, and dandelion capsules, but I needed springwater.

Near the A&P, I stopped in my tracks in front of a girl. We each stared for a moment. There was something troubling about her. Lightly dressed, with a half-buttoned shirt, her henna red hair tangled, she wasn't dirty, just unkempt. She lacked the swagger of someone used to living on the street, but instead looked as though she'd left her bed in the middle of a nightmare.

She was thin and extremely pale. I observed her disconnected, nervous movements. Her eyes searched an unreachable horizon. I thought, "She looks anemic; maybe on drugs." She stood blankly, not begging, so I quickly went into the store. She was still there when I came out with my springwater.

It's upsetting. Living in the city, you step over people living in the street, people who say "God bless you" when you give them a dollar. I've never gotten used to it. I searched her face for a sign of recognition, and spoke to her. It was useless, so I brought her home.

She rushed to the piano, banged discordant sounds, then echoed my birds' singing. Finally she stopped short in front of Kuan Yin, striking the same pose as the statue. Her movements were fast and jerky, as though she'd leave her body behind. She wasn't on drugs—no needle marks on her arms—but her movements were frenetic so that I imagined she hadn't slept in days.

I later learned that her name was Imogene. She was tall and willowy, like a dancer. I tried to quiet her with food, but she would have none. I guessed something had scared her within an inch of her life. She couldn't put a sentence together. Later she told me in a blur of French that she had to leave. She had a little money and an address in her pocket.

I gave her a bottle of gentian extract, a bitter digestive herb. Gentian cleanses the liver, strengthens the spleen to treat hypoglycemia, and grounds rising *chi* in the center. I hoped it could bring her into her center and back to my reality. I knew it would at least help balance her blood sugar. But she needed home, food, and friends. A moment before she left, she looked me in the eyes. "She'll be all right," I repeated to myself like a prayer. Then she grasped me with a desperate hug that made me want to cry.

With diet and herbs, Imogene regained her balance in a few months. During the time we worked together, I learned that madness is not by nature different from sanity, but is, instead, an exaggerated form of suffering.

At the time we first met, Imogene's manic episode had lasted four days and included auditory and visual hallucinations. She had consumed nothing but coffee, cigarettes, and pastry during that time.

Once, weeks later, her husband brought her back to consult with me. She looked ghostly in a white lace blouse. A classical musician, she spoke softly in halting English with a thick accent. Whenever she spoke, the husband mumbled to himself, shaking his head, and picked his nose or eyed her coldly, puffed on his pipe, and corrected her grammar.

Students, they were trying to eke out a living while he attended university. They stayed in a cheap hotel and ate poorly. After describing his dissertation to me at some length—on cottage industries in the Middle Ages—he broke off abruptly and said, "She's crazy, that's all, she's crazy," implying that he was not involved.

STAGNANT LIVER CHI, DEPRESSION, AND PMS

Imogene's pulses and tongue showed *chi* tied in knots. The pulses were slow and bumped abruptly, irregularly. Her pale tongue was slightly purple and had some dark spots in the heart area, indicating poor circulation and possibly pain.

Her digestion was so weak from chronic diarrhea that it was hard to imagine she gained nourishment from their meager meals. I gave her an acupuncture treatment for depression that I had learned working in a Chinese hospital, which was intended to reduce *phlegm*, improve digestion, ground rising *chi*, and clear the senses. (See chapter 35 for herbal information on clinical depression.)

What is called madness is an energetic imbalance involving both physical and emotional components. It can be a mixture of fear, anger, anxiety, and grief all at once. When enough of the Five Elements are upset, the heart can't work smoothly. That affects mental stability. The energetic effects of these emotions can be balanced rather quickly, using acupuncture and herbs. But to maintain that balance it is necessary to understand its roots. It's important to realize that crazy PMS is not an altered state with no connection to everyday life. It arises with extreme stress from the kinds of problems we all face.

Imogene's emotional freakout was linked with PMS because the same disorientation, paranoia, and auditory hallucinations had returned for 3 months, ever since they moved to New York. Her problems were due as much to their lifestyle as to her energetic imbalance. This was not hard to imagine, considering the husband's obvious coldness and the fact that for the first time in her life she was suddenly reduced to the depths of poverty. The husband said her symptoms had improved after staying with friends who fed her well.

Herbal remedies

I gave her **Xiao Yao Wan** because it frees circulation in the solar plexus, where emotions are trapped by stuck liver *chi*. It helped Imogene regain her centering, thus improving her depression. Since she had a pale tongue, she took 30 pills daily, 10 after each meal, for three months. Her appetite and emotions improved significantly, but she needed to focus her hyper energy enough to concentrate clearly and sleep well.

Cerebral Tonic Pills balanced Imogene's manic bouts of energy. Recommended for balancing the heart energy and for reducing plaque causing hardened arteries, they improve concentration and memory and also reduce manic episodes and seizures. When the senses are cleared of *phlegm,* both sleep and attention span are improved. The recommended dose is 10 pills three times daily. They are not digestive, and consequently must be taken between meals. Neither of these remedies is a sedative that dulls the mind. They help you regain your balance.

I saw Imogene a year later, happily divorced and pursuing a successful theatrical career. What would have happened if she'd consulted a Western doctor during her PMS crisis? It's likely she would have been prescribed psychiatric drugs that would have maintained her energetic imbalance and trapped her in a situation that was killing her spirit. Imogene looks back at her PMS experience without regret. If not for that, she says, she might never have changed her life.

HERBAL PREVENTION OF PMS

If you have a red tongue and tend to be nervous or easily excitable or angry during the month, or if you have headaches and constipation, take 8 pills three times daily of **Lung Tan Xie Gan Wan** until you feel calm and well. If you have a pale tongue, hypoglycemia, depression, mood swings, irregular menstruation, or anemia, take 8 pills daily of **Xiao Yao Wan.**

As much as possible, give up coffee, cigarettes, drugs, and medicines. If you have headaches, acid stomach, bad breath, or blemishes, add $\frac{1}{4}$ cup of aloe vera juice to tea or apple juice daily.

For nervous stress, taking 8 capsules of gotu kola daily will give you smooth, steady energy.

For nervous insomnia, add 10 drops of **Wuchaseng** (extract of Siberian ginseng) to a cup of warm water before bed.

If you still have problems with PMS, add one of the following herbal combinations.

HERBAL HELP

Did you buy this book because your periods are driving you nuts? Do you feel you suffer all the symptoms of menstrual discomfort at once? There are herbal formulas that do it all—provide herbs for blood deficiency, PMS, and pain. What's more, such pills and extracts are for sale in pharmacies, herb shops, and supermarkets. Many of these are as easy to find as aspirin, but much more effective.

Several important California herbal manufacturing companies are headed by young Americans well trained in world herbal medicine. One of these is McZand Herbal, Incorporated, in Santa Monica, owned by Janet Zand, a doctor of Oriental medicine.

Herbal remedies for PMS available in health-food stores include Zand's **PMS Herbal** (capsules), which contain vitamin B₆, choline, inositol, methionine, and magnesium in a base of bupleurum, atractylodes, white peony, poria, tang kuei, ginger, moutan, gardenia, and licorice. Also helpful from Zand are **Valerian Herbal** "for support during times of stress," with nerve sedative herbs, valerian and passionflower, along with skullcap, chamomile, oatstraw, bupleurum, schizandra, and licorice. Skullcap and bupleurum cool and decongest stuck liver *chi,* while chamomile and licorice soothe digestion. This is useful for agitation, irritability, and insomnia.

I recommend additional calcium to calm nerves during PMS times. Zand makes **Women's Calcium Combination,** intended for "women over thirty-five to support optimal calcium metabolism," but since many of us did not get enough calcium in childhood and absorption is reduced in times of stress, I recommend plant sources of calcium for all women.

Another company is Crystal Star, owned by Dr. Linda Rector-Page, an author and herbalist. From among their many herbal formulas designed for women's problems, perhaps the most delicious is called **Female Harmony Tea.** It is recommended to help "balance, tone, and regulate the female system." It combines red raspberry leaf, licorice, nettle, spearmint leaf and oil, rose hips, lemongrass, strawberry leaf and oil, sarsaparilla root, burdock root, and rosebuds. In this tea, antispasmodic herbs are combined with cleansers and digestive herbs to soothe the female reproductive tract. Nettle and rose hips are included to supplement nutrition, while sarsaparilla supplies female hormones.

Health Concerns, located in Oakland, manufactures its own line of herbs by that name as well as distributing Seven Forests, Zand, Turtle Mountain, and others for herbal practitioners. (See Herbal Access.)

Health Concerns' premenstrual herbal formulas include **Women's Harmony,** which combines herbs traditionally used to help balance hormones "by working hand in hand with your liver, where hormone balancing begins." It treats PMS with abdominal bloating and breast swelling, menstrual irregularity, and menopausal distress, including mild cramps. It relieves mild depression and is especially useful for women who get headaches around period time.

Women's Harmony contains bupleurum, tang kuei, white peony, salvia, fu ling, atractylodes, cyperus, citrus peel, moutan, gardenia, ginger, and licorice to invigorate circulation, build blood, and aid energy and digestion. It should be taken for ten days before the period begins. After the period, Health Concerns recommends taking its **Restore** for a complete program of balancing.

Restore treats fatigue, pale complexion, reduced appetite, spots that float in front of the eyes, and light-headedness or vertigo. The combination is based on a formula from the Yuan Dynasty (A.D. 1279–1368) that "enriches the blood by supplying the physical and chemical components of blood as well as ensuring the proper functioning of the blood system," which includes those organs involved in making blood, the spleen and stomach. Such a formula can increase overall energy of the body.

I was surprised to discover Organic

Planet, an herbal company located a couple of blocks from me on West Twenty-fourth Street in Manhattan. A couple of traditional Chinese herbalists, Drs. Wong and Ma, have put together about twenty formulas, using loose herbs you cook at home just like in a Chinese medical clinic. What fun! These are sold in health-food stores in New York and Long Island, and can also be ordered from them by mail.

They recommend **PMS Retreat,** which contains pepper root, eclipta, astragalus, chuan xiong (Ligustrum wallichi), tang kuei, bupleurum, white peony, safflower, and licorice. Here we have blood-builders (ligustrum, tang kuei, peony) along with herbs to support and cleanse the liver (bupleurum and safflower). This combination goes further than **Xiao Yao Wan** to free stuck liver *chi,* because it uses eclipta to reverse liver damage and astragalus to lift energy and immune defenses. This approach acknowledges the view that menstrual problems come from weakness and imbalance.

Considering the large selection of herbal products readily available for treating PMS, that problem should become a "disease" of the past. Perhaps one day we'll speak of it like the times when witches were burned at the stake or angry women were locked in their attics.

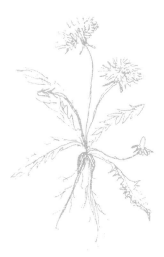

Dandelion

PREMENSTRUAL SYNDROME

What makes it worse?

Extreme hot, spicy or cold, raw diet, caffeine, chocolate, fried oils, fats, dairy; colds, emotional upsets, low progesterone-to-estrogen ratio, alcohol, drugs.

Weepy PMS: dairy, fatigue, cold, raw and sour foods (e.g., grapefruit, pickles), cold, damp weather, cold showers, colds/flu.

Angry and Crazy PMS: fasting, sugar, hot spices, alcohol, coffee, cigarettes, lack of sleep, sexual frustration, stimulants, thyroid and hormone imbalances.

What makes it better?

Cleansing and diuretic herbs that stimulate circulation: dandelion, parsley, sarsaparilla, cornsilk, nettle; iodine, trace minerals, evening primrose oil.

	HEAT SYMPTOMS	*COLD* SYMPTOMS	*PHLEGM*
TONGUE	reddish, spotted	pale, spotted	coated
SYMPTOMS	angry PMS	weepy PMS	weepy PMS
	mania	depression	
	cramps, spasm pain	weakness	bloating
	headaches, fever	fatigue	yeast infection
	blemishes	spacey feelings	
	irritability	depression	
	insomnia, restlessness		
MENSTRUATION	heavy early period	late or spotting	irregular

REMEDIES

Angry PMS: evening primrose oil, aloe, dandelion
Chinese patent: **Lung Tan Xie Gan Wan** (anger)
Crystal Star: **Flow Ease Tea** (pain, nervousness)
Health Concerns: **Nuphar 14** pills (congestion pain)

Weepy PMS: homeopathic pulsatilla (30c potency)
Crystal Star: **Female Harmony Caps** and **Vitex**
Health Concerns: **Tang Kuei 18** with **Lindera 15**

Crazy PMS: **Xiao Yao Wan** and **Lung Tan Xie Gan Win** (digestion)
Health Concerns: **Ardisia 16** with **Fu-Shen 16** (mania) or **Ardisia 16** with **Nuphar 14** (menstrual pain)

Complications cross-reference:
> *Candida,* see chapter 34
> *Headaches,* see **Anshen Bunao Tablets**
> *Depression,* see chapter 35

腎主生殖 腎主生殖 腎主生殖　　腎爲先天之本 腎爲先天之本 腎爲先天之本

[shèn zhǔ shēngzhí] The kidney is in charge of reproduction.

[shèn wéi xiāntiān zhī běn] The kidney is the foundation of the native (inborn) constitution.

28
The Miracle of Birth

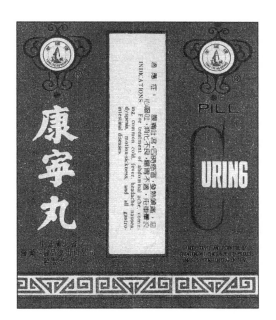

The hospital room was cold and dimly lit. In the hall, nuns in long black robes glided back and forth, rattling trays of little bottles, whispering midnight greetings. A woman pulled her chair closer to an oxygen tent to watch the child underneath. For a moment she remembered her husband's face when she had given him the news.

He'd come in from the ruined potato crop with mud on his hands. Home from war in the Pacific, he walked like a sailor. His farm clothes hung too large on his slender frame, his sensitive hands unused to dirt. When she told him she *was pregnant, he held her in his arms and smiled while crying. Her mother scolded in Hungarian, "We have nothing to eat, only eggs and mushrooms. You must not be pregnant!"*

The woman watched silently. There was no stir from the infant, hardly a breath. Two months earlier the baby had been born premature and jaundiced. All oxygen tents were commandeered by the baby boom, so the doctor had put the screaming newborn into a paper bag and attached an oxygen hose. Now the infant had pneumonia with high fever, and lay in a coma.

The nuns told the mother to go home, but she sat next to the bed, rocking gently, sending her life force into her baby with loving thoughts. When the infant finally smiled in her sleep, the woman said, "My baby is listening to angels singing."

That was Mother. She's the same now as ever: Her children always come first. It was also my first experience with complementary medicine. To this day, I believe that love heals best.

Today I shall help my friend Jane in the labor room. Unfortunately, I was unable to be with my dear sister, Michelle, at the births of her sons Nick and Henry. I think women in tribal villages get it right. We should gather our friends, stamp our feet, and all grunt together throughout a delivery to ease the new mother's fears.

Jane got acupuncture in her ear to calm her and start the contractions. The baby was taking his time, had gone past full term. Acupuncture has long been used to speed delivery by directing the mother's energy down-ward. My grandmother used to speak of women in Hungary who'd leave for harvest in the morning and return from the fields with their babies in the evening. She said the women would just squat. We forget sometimes how easy it can be.

My involvement with this baby actually began before he was conceived. Jane had come to me for advice on fertility herbs.

The Way of Fertility

We need both *yin* and *yang* to be fertile. What are the *yin* and *yang* of reproduction? Imagine a pot of water boiling on the stove. Water in the pot will not evaporate without adequate heat. The water is *yin* and the energy of heat is *yang*. We need adequate water so the pot won't scorch. We need fire so the water will boil.

YIN SUPPLIES BODY FLUIDS

We need enough body fluids—blood, phlegm, semen—to maintain healthy internal organs. Without moisture we feel hot and dry. The tongue is red and cracked. We are too thirsty or hungry; body fluids become sparse and concentrated. This leads to endocrine imbalances, blood deficiency, excess acid conditions, emotional upsets, and eventually infertility. For example, if a woman is too nervous and acidic, she has less chance to conceive because the acidic environment in her vagina kills sperm. (*Yin* deficiency, excess *yang*.)

YANG SUPPLIES ENERGY TO FUEL METABOLISM

If you lack *yang* energy, normal body processes cannot continue. Then the result is fatigue, low endocrine function, and infertility. Your eggs become weak and unable to become settled in the uterus or menstruation becomes irregular or stops (amenorrhea). Also, the monthly period of fertility becomes shorter. In January 1991, *The Journal of Medicine* from the Nanjing College of Traditional Chinese Medicine published an article on the important relationship of Chinese herbs that tonify kidney *yang* (adrenal deficiency) and luteal-phase-deficiency infertility. In their study of sixty women, pregnancy rates improved after herbal treatment to improve adrenal strength.

Both *yin* and *yang* are necessary to support life. *Yin* provides healthy hormones, sperm, and eggs, while *yang* provides the drive and energy to make and keep you pregnant.

WHAT FERTILITY HERBS CAN DO

Fertility pills dispensed by Western doctors increase your chances of pregnancy by stepping up your production of eggs. They are extremely costly and have been known to result in surprise multiple pregnancies.

An energetic approach is different from taking fertility pills because Asian herbal combining is more specific. The herbs address *your* particular problems, giving you help where it is needed most. Fertility herbs can be used to stimulate necessary hormones and maintain adequate blood, body fluids, and strength and, at times, free trapped blood circulation. They might also help with emotional balance. Here is an example showing the advantage of taking herbs that affect particular problems in appropriate places.

My friend Jane's doctor told her she could not conceive because she lacked adequate mucus. Her vaginal environment was too acidic, which killed the sperm. He prescribed a cough remedy in order to make more mucus. I laughed and told her, "You don't need phlegm in your lungs, honey. That's the wrong place!"

The cough remedy had given her a chest cold and made her put on many extra pounds because it slowed digestion. A better remedy for lubrication in the right place is an East Indian herb I recommended. The Sanskrit name is *shatavari,* but one common name is "wife with a thousand husbands." I'm sure those wives don't get chest colds from it. The herb increases *yin* where it should be, in the vagina. Shatavari, Asian wild asparagus, is full of female hormones and is a moistening tonic to the female organs.

Jane cooked the dried herb with rice, but didn't like the sticky consistency. I recommended she simmer it for an hour and drink the tea between meals. She also ate lots of asparagus from the supermarket, since it has many of the same properties and is diuretic. (See chapter 29 for other herbs in this category.)

Yin is what the doctor called mucus (or phlegm), but it is not the only *humor* sometimes needed to become pregnant. *Yang* energy is important also, when adrenal exhaustion makes it difficult to conceive.

Weak adrenal energy, exhaustion, and infertility

When I checked Jane the way an Asian doctor does, she showed signs of weakness in the Water element and possibly blood deficiency. This is typical for a lot of women who become temporarily infertile because of exhaustion. Usually kidney/adrenal gland deficiency comes first, followed by exhaustion, depression, and finally global weakness symptoms such as edema and asthma. Like many women, Jane had pursued a demanding career for a number of years before she conceived. Her job had kept Jane working long hours with no vacations.

Jane, at times, suffered from lumbago (pain in the lower back), frequent urination, or diarrhea. Her tongue was pale, with a white coating. Her pulse was deep and weak. Her voice had a soft, breathy quality, with pauses to catch her breath. She complained of late-afternoon fatigue and low sexual drive. All this showed she needed adrenal strength from herbs that increase kidney *chi* and *yang* energy. Jane needed more kidney *yang* than *yin*.

Weakness and spontaneous miscarriage

Even if she could have conceived, Jane would need added vitality and strong mus-cles to maintain the pregnancy. Otherwise, with stress and fatigue, she could miscarry.

WHAT TO AVOID IF YOU ARE WEAK

- Long, hot baths or sauna
- Cold showers
- Inadequate clothes in cold weather
- Inadequate sleep
- Deep massage with downward motions
- Laxatives, including coffee
- Sour foods (pickles, vinegar, grapefruit)
- Cold, raw foods (excess salad, ice water, ice cream)
- Anti-inflammatory herbs and drugs that may be laxative
- Acne medicines, skin peelers, or drugs that are irritating
- Arguments and anxiety

Pregnancy and laxatives

My mother got tired of waiting for my sister to be born. Her time was due the night before Halloween, and by that time Mother had waited enough.

During Mother's pregnancy with me, she had listened to classical music, which is the ancient Chinese custom. Chinese doctors felt the unborn child would be able to learn patience and wisdom and acquire increased artistic sensitivity, if the mother introduced the arts to her child during pregnancy. It worked with me, because I grew to love music.

With my sister, she must have looked at a lot of beautiful paintings, because

Michelle has a natural aptitude for art. My sister also acquired a very forbearing nature and good patience, although I don't know how that's possible, because Mother took castor oil when she became tired of waiting. Mother delivered Michelle with the help of my father in the ambulance.

If you are weak, or tend to have a pale tongue or early contractions, avoid all laxative foods, including coffee, salad, lemonade, apricots, or prunes. Laxative herbs include rhubarb, senna, cascara sagrada, and dandelion.

Baths and showers

Some Western doctors who are sensitive to the body's energy levels warn weak pregnant women not to take long, hot baths. I also recommend avoiding cold showers. Both are weakening. A hot bath relaxes muscles in the lower back and can therefore move the baby lower, weakening the pregnancy. A mother is more likely to miscarry if her muscles and *chi* are weak.

Herbal tonics

An herb is called a *tonic* because it tonifies or stimulates the body. It is more than a stimulant because it provides needed nutrition and supports the functioning of weak organs. Tonic herbs make the body stronger and more resistant to illness and weakness. They are useful in building vitality before pregnancy and for preventing miscarriage.

Blood and *yin* tonics build blood and body fluids in order to treat anemia, calm nerves, strengthen resilience, and refresh dryness and thirst. *Chi* and *yang* tonics build energy and vitality to strengthen muscles and lift energy. Moistening and soothing blood tonics make it more possible to relax and flourish during pregnancy. They protect your hair, skin, and fingernails. Energy-building *chi* tonics prevent fatigue, depression, and miscarriage.

Signs of energy deficiency include pale complexion, poor appetite, fatigue, lower-back ache, depression, shortness of breath, frequent urination, and diarrhea. When you feel achy in the lower abdomen, or chilled or spacey, you may need to do more than sit down for a rest. A *chi* tonic taken during the weaker months of pregnancy can prevent miscarriage. (For most women, that is during the third, sixth, and eighth months.)

Signs of blood deficiency include fatigue, weakness, sallow complexion, pale lips, skin discolorations, dizziness, and blurred vision. This is increased when the kidneys and adrenal glands have been exhausted by work, fatigue, too many jet flights, stimulants like coffee, and excessive sexual activity. A tonic that builds both blood and energy, taken during pregnancy, would have beneficial effects on hormone balance and would actually help prevent miscarriage.

Herbal tonics are either *cooling* or *warming*. You need a *warming* tonic if you have symptoms of *internal cold* such as a pale tongue or a deep, weak pulse. (The normal pulse changes during pregnancy; it becomes large and bounding, as though jumping over hurdles, as a result of extra hormone activity.)

You need a moistening tonic if you have symptoms of dryness such as feverishness and thirst. If you have weakness combined with headache and dizziness, you may need to take a remedy that cools those signs of inflammation as well as strengthening your pregnancy. (See the section on **An Tai Wan,** page 339.) The following Indian and Chinese patent remedies are warming and strengthening.

An Indian herbal tonic that strengthens muscles

The herb I recommended for my friend Jane was an Indian herb, famous as a rejuvenating tonic that tones muscles: ashwagandha, also called Winter Cherry (in Latin, *Withania somnifera*). The common name in Sanskrit is "that which has the smell of a horse." It is reputed to give the vitality and sexual energy of a horse. It may change the odor of the urine.

An herbal tonic, such as ashwagandha, that strengthens muscles is useful for pregnancy because it counters fatigue, lower-back ache, and it prevents miscarriage due to weakness. It also speeds delivery because, during contractions, having stronger muscles helps you push harder. She added one half teaspoon of the powdered herb to a cup of tea twice a day during her entire pregnancy. It is a *heating* tonic, so that people with red tongue can use less.

Ashwagandha is calming for people who cannot sleep from nervous exhaustion. It treats many problems of convalescence and advanced age, such as rheumatism, tissue deficiency, and loss of memory. It is useful for anemia related to weakness and deficiency, as well as for infertility. It helped Jane both with weakness and blood deficiency.

Jane bought powdered ashwagandha at a local Indian grocery in her Lexington Avenue neighborhood in New York City, but there are large Indian communities in most major cities. Also, I have seen the herb in health-food store capsules, including one called **Herbal Male Vite,** one of the Power Herbs combinations made by Nature's Herbs. Its ingredients, including Siberian ginseng and ashwagandha, can be taken by men or women for greater strength. One capsule per day is effective. High doses of ashwagandha may increase testosterone.

THREE POWERFUL CHINESE REMEDIES THAT PREVENT MISCARRIAGE

A famous tonic herb for chronic weak chi

Astragalus (in Chinese, *huang qi*) builds and lifts *chi*. It prevents weakness, especially in the legs and lower body. It protects your energy from cold, exhaustion, and chronic diarrhea or debilitating illness. It is easy to find capsules in Chinese markets and herbal shops. A tasty liquid extract is available, and you can always simmer a handful of the herb itself in a quart of water for forty-five minutes. Drink three cups daily.

Patent remedies for unstable fetus and prolapsed uterus

If you need stronger help in preventing threatened miscarriage, I recommend either of two Chinese patent remedies, "Peaceful Fetus Pill," **An Tai Wan** ("For Embryo") and **Bu Zhong Yi Qi Wan** ("Central Tonic Pills").

An Tai Wan relaxes tight muscles, calms the fetus, cools your feverish symptoms, and stops pain, premature uterine contractions, and threatened abortion due to abdominal tension. It contains four Chinese blood-building herbs that warm the uterus with increased circulation, and one *cooling* herb (skullcap) to settle your dizziness, headache, or other *heat* symptoms. The recommended dosage is 7 pills three times daily.

Bu Zhong Yi Qi Wan treats weakness, chronic diarrhea, and prolapsed rectum, uterus, or colon, as well as hemorrhoids, varicose veins, and hernia resulting from weak *chi*. It is recommended also for habitual miscarriage. Its entirely vegetarian formula contains astragalus, tang kuei, codonopsis, atractylodes, cimicifuga, bupleurum, jujube, ginger, citrus, and licorice. Dosage is 8 to 10 pills three times daily. If this makes you constipated and irritable, it is too *heating* for you; so you can either reduce the dosage or take **An Tai Wan** instead.

Sources of calcium

Other herbs that strengthen muscles are sources of calcium. These are fine to take every day as a mildly strengthening remedy for chronic weakness. For example, red raspberry leaves and nettle leaves strengthen the kidneys and adrenal glands. In *Wise Woman Herbal Childbearing Year*, Susan Weed recommends "alternate weeks of nettle and raspberry brews or drink raspberry until the last month and then switch to nettles to ensure large amounts of vitamin K in the blood for the birth." These recommendations may be useful for everyone, since we all need lots of calcium to strengthen muscles, but it is even better to be more specific about the temperature of herbs.

Pregnancy and internal heat

I knew Jane needed a *warming* stimulant capable of supporting hormone function because she had a pale tongue and a slow, deep pulse, indicating *internal cold*. But I have seen plenty of young women unable to conceive because of *internal heat* symptoms.

One such girl was Joy. Her tongue was red and her pulse fast. She was healthy, worked out in the gym regularly, and ate carefully, but was very nervous about having a baby. She wanted one, but her husband was unsure. This anxiety led to an overly acid condition of her body fluids, including those in the vagina and uterus, which killed the sperm. A Western-trained herbalist might recommend red clover flowers to balance the acid/alkaline level in favor of conception, but that is not enough.

Blood deficiency

Joy's overheated condition lasted long enough to damage her body fluids. She was often thirsty, and her urine was dark (concentrated). She felt flushed or nervous in the evening. All these *heat* symptoms became a bit worse after her period, because of blood deficiency. Other symptoms of blood deficiency might be pale, sallow skin, pale, dry lips, blurred vision, or pain after menstruation.

There are many *cooling* blood tonics. **Rehmannia Glutinosa Compound Pills** are said to "warm the uterus" and cool the liver. "Cold uterus" can result from eating too many cold or raw foods, causing lower abdominal pain that's relieved by warmth. Usually the menstrual discharge is scanty and mixed with clots. This imbalance can lead to amenorrhea. Warming the uterus stimulates blood circulation to relieve pain and normalize the period. Tang kuei (also spelled *dong quai*) is a *warming* blood-builder in this formula. Eucommia bark and cyperus stimulate blood circulation. *Cooling* herbs such as rehmannia root and skullcap are said to nourish liver and kidney blood deficiency to treat insomnia and headache.

Chinese medicine also uses processed human placenta, either cooked as a loose herb or in pill form. Although it is a very traditional herb and perfectly safe, most of my clients wouldn't think of boiling up a shrunken placenta. It looks a bit like a bumpy cookie. One client was so pure with her diet that she even complained, upon reading the label, that the placenta pills were sugarcoated. Placenta is extremely nourishing because it feeds the fetus. For adults it nourishes dry skin and hair and builds blood. It is not recommended for women who want to restrict their estrogen production. It is very moisturizing (it builds *yin*), and is therefore *cooling*. The pills are a little sweet, and leave a red dye on your tongue.

A blood tonic suitable for blood deficiency and infertility that is completely vegetarian is **Shou Wu Chih.** It can be used by men and women as a tonic for depletion from sexual excess, blood loss after childbirth, or illness. It helps strengthen bones and tendons in the back and helps aching joints. Main ingredients include he shou wu, tang kuei, polygonatum, rehmannia, and ligusticum. These all build blood by strengthening internal organs that make and store blood (the spleen/pancreas and liver). Citrus peel helps the absorption of these otherwise sticky sweet herbs.

Shou Wu Chih is a semisweet, herbal-tasting liquid, not the usual after-dinner liqueur. You can drink it plain or add 2 or 3 tablespoons to tea or water, or add it to enhance the flavor of soup each day until achiness improves and your tongue becomes normal pink.

Eventually all these tonics work. The stressed, overheated woman relaxes as she acquires adequate blood to quiet her nerves. The weaker, kidney-deficient woman becomes strong enough to conceive and maintain the pregnancy. Energy becomes more stabilized as hormone imbalances caused by both *internal heat* and *internal cold* are addressed.

Fatigue and backache during pregnancy

Backache can become an enervating problem during the last few months of pregnancy. Lower-back muscles can become weak or tight from fatigue and weight gain. The best way to counter backache during pregnancy is to take herbs that alleviate both pain and weakness. In that way the pain remedy can strengthen pregnancy.

Two kitchen spices work particularly well for this problem. Clove buds and fenugreek are pungent, hot spices that can immediately lift energy and refresh the senses. You can use either one if you have a pale tongue. They work well for adrenal weakness.

When Jane felt tired and had a backache, I recommended she add a ¼ teaspoon of powdered clove to one cup of boiling water. That tonifying spice strengthens muscles, lifts energy to protect the pregnancy, and deepens breath. You can use the same dosage for fenugreek. They are especially good to use during cold weather to build immunity and vitality. Avoid them if you have dark-colored urine from *internal heat.*

Morning sickness

Do you crave pickles or ice cream when you are pregnant? Both increase *phlegm,* which increases nausea. Congestion that collects during the night, while you've been lying in bed, turns into morning sickness. Your pickle-and-ice-cream diet makes it worse. Don't treat morning sickness by buying a bigger pillow or eating soda crackers; take **Curing Pills** from Chinatown.

Curing Pills strengthen the digestive center with bitter and *warming* herbs that stop morning sickness as well as motion sickness. The remedy comes packaged in a square red box that contains a dozen smaller plastic tubes that in turn contain many red pills. Dosage is the entire contents of one tube swallowed with warm water as needed.

A possible substitute is a cup of fresh ginger tea. Put a couple of slices of raw ginger into a cup and add hot water. Such *warming* digestive tonics do not endanger pregnancy the way anti-inflammatory or laxative herbs might.

Breech birth

In about the sixth month of her pregnancy, the doctors noticed that Jane's baby was not positioned well. He would have to be moved or he might come out as a breech birth, feet first. I remembered having met Dr. Dao, a venerable Vietnamese doctor, at a conference in Montreal. He had been head of gynecology at a hospital in Saigon before the war. He had told me how acupuncture doctors change the position of a baby *in utero* without touching the mother's abdomen. It's amazing. Chinese medicine works with a force field, invisible to the naked eye, strong enough to turn a fetus in the mother's body by setting up a torque of movement in the mother's acupuncture meridians. Her *chi* is stimulated, starting from her small toe up through her body, so that the baby moves from the force of that energetic shift.

I gave Jane the treatment, touching her right small toe at the outside upper corner of the nail with a moxa stick, a cigar of burning mugwort (Artemisia vulgaris), and the baby changed position that same night. Midwives trained in energetic medicine now use the same treatment. The National Commission for the Certification of Acupuncturists in Washington, D.C., can refer acupuncturists in your area.

Delivery herbs

When Jane's pregnancy went past full term by a day or two, she asked for herbs to speed delivery. A safe-delivery remedy is one that speeds normal contractions without endangering either mother or baby. Don't use anything until your cervix is dilated and the baby has come down sufficiently.

Then I recommend homeopathic caulophyllum (200× potency). It's especially good when you can't cook herbs or take capsules. You can take the pills along with you to the hospital, and repeat the recommended dosage every 15 minutes when contractions are occurring at regular intervals. You can continue for two or three hours under the supervision of your midwife.

Don't use abortive herbs

I never recommend abortive herbs, because they are dangerous. They weaken the body and can result in infection, blood poisoning, or other problems.

Emmenagogues

Herbs known as *emmenagogues* should also be avoided during pregnancy. They are traditionally used to regulate periods, treat PMS, stop pain from poor circulation, or clear infection, afterbirth, or uterine tumors. On page 343, I offer a traditional Chinese combination of these herbs to help clear afterbirth, but here is some general information.

Often pungent or bitter-tasting herbs, emmenagogues relieve blood congestion, clear clots in the uterus, and promote menstruation. They can be either *cooling* or *warming.*

Cooling emmenagogues help calm nerves and soothe feverish headaches and irritability. Some are also useful for uterine infection or excessive bleeding after delivery. Others are antispasmodic for uterine cramping and pain. Since they are *cooling* herbs, they stimulate the downward movement of energy within the mother's body. Many emmenagogues are laxative or affect hormones, which is why they are contraindicated during pregnancy. Some typical *cooling* emmenagogues are squaw vine, yarrow, and motherwort.

Warming emmenagogues are useful for fearful or depressed mothers with pale tongues, exhaustion, and weak muscles. *Warming* tonics build strength and courage after delivery. They also increase circulation to clear away clots. They are often combined with other herbs to help ease abdominal discomfort and heal wounds. Although they are not strong enough to promote menstruation, their daily use should be avoided, especially if you have a reddish tongue. Some typical *heating* emmenagogues are angelica, cinnamon, ginger, myrrh, and tang kuei.

Other herbs, such as tansy and pennyroyal, have unpleasant side effects and should be avoided altogether because they can be toxic.

Herbs to relax contractions and slow labor

For Jane I recommended two capsules of valerian, which is used primarily as a nervine or sedative to the nervous system. It relaxed her anxiety, sedated the nerves in the uterus to help reduce pain, and temporarily slowed contractions. That helped get her to the hospital on time. Once there, Jane, a New Age mother, lit incense, played a meditation tape, did breathing exercises, and pushed like a trouper. We watched on a monitor to see the baby move each time I stimulated acupuncture points to speed delivery. I wished we could have gotten the nurses on the floor all together to grunt and stamp their feet. No matter, Jane had a beautiful baby boy.

Afterbirth

In China, emmenagogues are used to clear the afterbirth, clean the uterus, and prevent infection. The day after delivery, make a soup with a handful each of tang kuei, persica, hong hwa (safflower), motherwort, and blackened ginger. Simmer the herbs in water for forty-five minutes, and drink three cups a day for two or three days. The ingredients stimulate circulation very strongly to treat pain and exhaustion after the delivery. They heal and tone the entire painful area of the lower abdomen and help the mother regain strength and calm.

Then, in a day or so, after those herbs have cleared the afterbirth, use herbal pills to tonify internal organs and lift fallen energy. This Chinese patent remedy improves postdelivery fatigue and depression, while it stops spotting and treats pain due to prolapse. Take 10 to 15 **Shih Chuan Ta Bu Wan** ("Ten Major Tonic Herb Pills") three times a day until strength is regained.

You will feel wonderfully improved, stronger, and more confident and relaxed when you use these tonic herbs to recover after delivery. But don't overexert yourself, even though you feel fully recovered. It still takes time to heal.

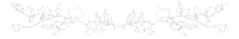

INFERTILITY

What makes it worse?

Hormone irregularities, fatigue, adrenal weakness, nervousness; spontaneous miscarriage due to exhaustion; malnutrition, coffee, cigarettes, cold, raw diet, laxatives.

What makes it better?

Chi, yin, and *yang* tonic herbs, acupuncture.

	INTERNAL HEAT	*INTERNAL COLD*	*PHLEGM*
TONGUE	red, dotted yellow coating	very pale, scalloped white or watery coating	coated
SYMPTOMS	fever, night sweats early, painful periods sharp cramps angry PMS nervousness, anxiety stuck liver *chi*	weakness, fatigue late or long periods dull cramps weepy PMS depression deficient *chi*	edema irregular heavy legs spaceyness

FERTILITY HERBAL REMEDIES

	cooling, moistening nettle, **Shou Wu Chih,** **Rehmannia Glutinosa** **Compound Pills**	*warming* tonic ashwagandha, clove tea	

MORNING SICKNESS

Curing Pills

PREVENTION OF MISCARRIAGE

	An Tai Wan	**Bu Zhong Yi Qi Wan**	

POSTDELIVERY FATIGUE AND DEPRESSION

Shih Chuan Ta Bu Wan

For skin discolorations from pregnancy, see **Patch Removing Pills** on page 299.

29
Menopause

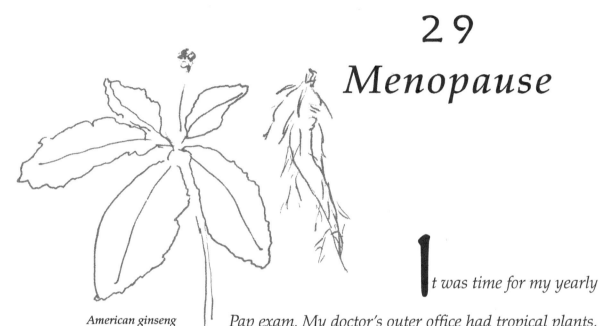

American ginseng

It was time for my yearly Pap exam. My doctor's outer office had tropical plants, beautiful furnishings, and a big brown cat lazing in a chair. In a private room I did breathing exercises, trying to visualize myself on a beach, while dreading a cold speculum. My doctor's hands have wisdom and gentleness that allow me to breathe deeper. We've been friends for years, and have exchanged Asian travel stories. When I glanced at her, she smiled, her face glowing. She was having a hot flash while asking me about herbal remedies for menopause. I was moved. Professional differences had melted.

We are in the midst of a giant "meno-boom" as more women begin menopause than ever before. Recent popular books on the subject quote scientific info-bites, "expert opinions," and dramatic testimonials of women suffering from our culture's anti-age prejudice. Authors advise improved diet, meditation, or discussion groups aimed at easing emotional distress. Although this approach may offer moral support, it does not always eliminate symptoms.

The main issue addressed is whether or not to take synthetic estrogen. The prevalent attitude seems to be, "Follow your doctor's advice, but give 'em a hard time," or simply ignore the problem: "Menopause will eventually go away." Western physicians have been known to use pressure tactics to push estrogen and progesterone replacement for hot flashes, arthritis, or hardening of the arteries. One expert on menopause left her doctor's office when he jeered, "You *must* take estrogen—don't call me in the middle of the night when you're having a heart attack!"

One dilemma is that while increasing estrogen to reduce hot flashes, ensure youthful appearance, supple joints, and adequate sexual fluids, we may protect ourselves from heart attack and osteoporosis, but risk breast or uterine cancer. If we do without added estrogen, plaque might build up, increasing risk of heart disease. Somebody said, "It's like trying to decide whether you'd rather be hit by a truck or a bus."

Another thing that makes it harder to decide what to do is that the scientific data tends to be biased. Studies on heart disease are more frequently done on men. Also, studies of estrogen replacement most often do not consider diet or smoking habits. Fat, phlegmy foods, and smoking increase the risk of both heart trouble and cancer because they impede digestion and circulation.

Theories about hormone replacement have varied greatly in past years. According to the 1977 *Merck Manual*, a standard medical text, "In a patient who is ten or more years postmenopausal and has recurrent breast cancer, estrogens should be tried first, working up to 20 mg a day." The current prevailing opinion, however, is to *eliminate* estrogen to prevent recurrent cancer. Women have been used as guinea pigs while Western medicine has done a flip-flop on hormone replacement procedures. In 1970 a standard menopausal dose of estrogen was so high it actually caused endometrial cancer! Furthermore, although both estrogen and progesterone are now given in smaller doses, they must pass through the liver. This can result in gallbladder disease, blood clotting, asthma, epilepsy, or other such disadvantages.

Traditional Asian medicine offers a different, more successful approach, which includes freeing circulation while balancing energy, blood, *yin* (body fluids), and hormones with herbs. Individual remedies are required because of differences in lifestyle, but certain factors are basic. Treatment often includes anti-inflammatory herbs that remove blood deficiency and dehydration symptoms. How do we recognize deficiency? First we must ascertain what is normal. More precisely, what is the normal age for menopause? Why has that changed recently? Ancient Greek and Chinese medical traditions described cycles of women's aging in terms of a series of seven years. According to the *Nei Ching*:

The development of the woman: at the age of seven her teeth and hair grow longer; at fourteen she begins to menstruate and can bear children; at twenty-one she is fully grown and her physical condition is at its best; at twenty-eight her muscles are firm, her body is flourishing; at thirty-five her face begins to wrinkle and her hair begins to fall; at forty-five her arteries begin to harden and her hair turns white; at forty-nine she ceases to menstruate and she is no longer able to bear children.

Although this view is sensitive neither to individual differences nor to improved diet and beauty routines, it still presents an accurate description of what was considered normal. But recently more women are beginning menopause younger than forty-nine. They're showing premature signs of aging, and also having more heart attacks, strokes, cancers, and depression than ever before.

This is because menopausal symptoms tend to be signs of *internal heat* made worse by dehydration from a variety of factors. They include not only hot flashes but night sweats, dry skin, irritability, insomnia, nervousness, brittle bones, and loss of bone mass. Nowadays younger women are smoking, drinking, working tough jobs, and raising children alone. Life has become fast, demanding, polluted, and stressful. The cost is paid in blood, energy, and *yin.*

To reverse signs of menopause and aging, it is important to take herbs that extend blood production time, and enhance beauty and vitality without increasing the risk of illness. Many menopause herbs do not directly affect hormones, but increase blood and *yin* because they are nourishing and moisturizing.

Our Fountain of Youth

Yin is a Chinese name for body fluids that moisturize the skin and prevent dry, painful vagina, prematurely gray hair, and hair loss. *Yin* keeps bones strong and joints supple. Certain herbs increase bone marrow and rebuild damaged livers by promoting the *yin* of the liver and kidney organ systems. In other words, building *yin* increases blood retention in those organs, which in turn reduces signs of inflammation. In that way, calcium absorption is improved, which strengthens bones and settles nervous tension.

Herbs that build *yin* of the kidneys and *essence* (called *jing*) increase sexual fluids and responsiveness, while easing vaginal discomfort from chafing. Because the herbs are taken internally as teas or pills, the moisture generated replenishes tissue throughout the entire body to improve beauty and vitality. *Yin-* and blood-building herbs supply our fountain of youth.

Although foods or supplements may pass through us without having a beneficial effect when we're weak and tired, herbs enhance metabolism, rebuild damaged organs, and increase energy, moisture, and blood. Menopause herbs can make us young, strong, and juicy.

COMMONLY USED MENOPAUSAL REMEDIES

The following advice is useful for anyone approaching menopause; it aims to reduce aging from dehydration and stress.

Cut out hot, spicy, and excessively fat foods, as well as caffeine and alcohol. Stop smoking! Try to get enough rest, and exercise regularly. Studies done in 1994 show that vigorous exercise of an hour or more a day reduces risk of breast cancer. Whether exercise changes hormone levels, increases endorphins to improve mood, tones muscles, or helps metabolism is not clear from the study. But for all those reasons and many more, I recommend gym workouts, dancing, swimming, or any pleasurable activity, including sex. Start an anti-aging campaign. (See the chapters on weight loss [15 and 16] and blood-building herbs for beautiful skin and hair [25].)

A DAILY HERBAL ROUTINE TO ENSURE BALANCE

Choose from among the following herbal treatments whichever ones seem appropriate, knowing they may vary from time to time, depending upon changes in symptoms. You may need to take the higher recommended dose for two or more months to ensure a smooth transition away from your symptoms, then reduce the dosage as needed. By the time your digestion has been regulated, many of your menopausal problems will be solved. Then you can use these herbs for occasional dietary abuses. The following combinations do not directly increase estrogen production, but enhance circulation and absorption and reduce nervous tension.

BEGIN WITH A HEALTHY, HAPPY DIGESTIVE CENTER

Xiao Yao Wan and **Lung Tan Xie Gan Wan** are baseline remedies that ensure good digestion and circulation. A good way to start any herbal regimen is to treat complaints located in your physical and emotional center. **Xiao Yao Wan** treats depression, hypoglycemia, irregular periods, and chest pain. It improves hormonal irregularity, irritability, anxiety, and indigestion. Take it at mealtime if you have a pale tongue and nervous indigestion, possible results of weakness or of eating too many cold, raw, creamy, or rich meals.

The recommended dose is 6 pills each time, but vary this according to your needs. The higher dose is 10 to 12 pills per dose. If you have a reddish tongue and excess *heat* symptoms such as irritability, insomnia, feverish feeling, or night sweats, this remedy is too *heating* for you. Take only **Lung Tan Xie Gan Wan** until those problems stop.

Lung Tan Xie Gan Wan, a *cooling* remedy, treats liver and gallbladder inflammation resulting in headaches; red, burning eyes; ringing in the ears; sore throat; oral fever blisters; constipation; urinary tract infections; thick or yellowish vaginal discharge; anger, rage, or violent behavior; insomnia; and oral or genital herpes. It is especially helpful for recovering alcoholics or persons with hyperthyroid or mania symptoms. It is also recommended for people who become nervous or upset after eating hot spices, oils, and sugar, or who suffer from heat and humidity.

Take 6 to 10 pills after meals until signs of inflammation, including red, dry tongue, become normal. Check regularly with an herbalist listed in the Herbal Access appendix for continued use. This remedy and **Xiao Yao Wan** are often taken together. Both are very safe and effective.

DIGESTIVE HERBS AND YOUR EMOTIONAL CENTER

Take **Xiao Yao Wan** if:
- you are weak from illness
- you have lost your appetite for life
- you are depressed or vulnerable
- you can't decide how to solve your problems
- you obsess about past or present griefs
- you are stuck in a bad personal situation that drains you

Take **Lung Tan Xie Gan Wan** if:
- you are beside yourself with anger
- you want to hit someone or say something mean, but can't
- you are very nervous and jumpy
- you can't slow your excess energy
- you think and speak so fast, you can't relax
- any little noise makes you jump
- you lie awake at night plotting revenge

QUIET YOUR NERVES FOR IMPROVED SLEEP

Siberian ginseng (**Wuchaseng**) is a highly recommended nerve tonic for menopausal and ordinary nervous tension. The liquid extract can be taken one teaspoon at a time before bed for a sweet, dreamless sleep. The powdered herb can be taken, one-half teaspoon per dose, once or twice daily between meals. This ginseng is not a sedative, but rebuilds damaged nerves. It soothes anxiety and helps concentration and depression. After your nervousness improves, you can stop using this herb regularly. If you take it for too long a period (perhaps several months), it begins to act as a nerve stimulant and can provoke insomnia. Your mind and body will tell you when you have used enough.

REDUCE PAIN NATURALLY

Evening primrose oil (in capsules) reduces cholesterol and excess weight, improves circulation, and decreases the pain of arthritis and migraines. It has been recommended as a preventive treatment for heart trouble. Nutritionists have recommended it for everything from PMS and painful periods to menopausal heat symptoms.

Healing teas

The best teas to drink at this time are those that provide taste satisfaction without injuring your nerves or aggravating thirst or appetite. Adding 10 drops or ¼ teaspoon of powdered **Wuchaseng** to a cup of caffeine tea will counter its enervating effects. Better yet, drink a non-caffeine tea. Green tea drains toxins while strengthening blood vessels. It's a better stimulant than coffee because it stirs digestion, not the nervous system.

American ginseng tea replenishes *yin* fluids, especially in the digestive tract, where it increases saliva. It is a *cooling* tonic, useful for dry skin, dry cough, and chronic thirst. It is especially good for smokers. (Look for a reddish, dry tongue with cracks down the center and near the tip.) Drinking American ginseng tea eventually replenishes moisture of skin and hair. For *internal heat* conditions such as hot flashes, night sweats, drink American ginseng tea made from the cooked root (also edible in soup), the powdered root, or the instant granules daily, until the tongue turns from red and cracked to normal pink. Do not use American ginseng during a cold or flu because it increases phlegm.

Chinese medicine aims primarily to cure illness, not correct beauty problems. A traditional Chinese doctor may never tell you this, but I will: American ginseng increases water retention (*yin*) in the digestive tract, which means, for some people, that it can increase cellulite (horrors!), which is made up of water and toxins. Persons with slow metabolism should combine American ginseng with stimulant and weight-loss herbs. Do not use American ginseng alone if you have bloating, slow digestion, water retention, or digestive phlegm. (Look for a large, puffy, pale, and phlegm-coated tongue, or lots of saliva.) Persons with chronic thirst and dry, red tongue can safely take American ginseng between meals, until moisture is regained.

Herbs that build yin

The herbs and combinations discussed below also rebuild damaged *yin* of the liver resulting from stress, hormone imbalances, or dehydration from poor diet or alcohol. They treat a variety of *internal heat* problems such as hair loss and premature graying, and also skin blemishes and fragile fingernails. These can be symptoms of blood deficiency for men and women. (See the Blood Questionnaire in chapter 24.)

Han lian cao (in Latin, *Eclipta alba* or *herba ecliptae*) replenishes the liver *yin* and blood. It's useful for liver and bone marrow damage from alcohol, chemotherapy, or inflammatory disease. It treats cirrhosis and chronic hepatitis. It helps replenish thinning hair and damaged bone marrow, and also reduces enlarged liver and spleen and eases nervous insomnia and anemia.

Han lian cao is a major *cooling* rejuvenator herb used to reverse aging. It builds *yin* for luxuriant hair, improved skin texture and tone, and stronger nails. Take powdered han lian cao internally if the tongue is dry and red and you feel heated, dry, or feverish during the afternoon or night. Start by mixing ½ teaspoon powder in just enough water to swallow it, once a day between meals. Then increase the dosage to twice a day. Stop taking the remedy if it makes you feel chilled. Remember, refurbishing the liver will make you doubly sensitive to hot, oily foods and alcohol.

He shou wu (also called shou wu and fo ti) comes as a loose herb, in pills (**Shou Wu Pian**) or liquid (**Shou Wu Chih**). It is used mainly to treat prematurely gray hair, but has other moistening benefits. It's said to increase *jing* (vital essence), which means that in men the herb increases semen, while in women it produces vaginal fluid for sexual comfort. It will not increase estrogen.

Simmer a handful of he shou wu for at least one half hour and drink one cup as tea or soup stock daily. You can also take **Shou Wu Pian**, 5 pills three times daily. This is a very moistening herb. If your digestion is slow (look for a pale, puffy tongue), avoid the herb at mealtime and take it along with at least 6 pills of **Xiao Yao Wan.** You may have to avoid taking any form of he shou wu during a spell of humid weather, because it can dampen your energy with excess *phlegm.* I have also combined he shou wu with cinnamon, one handful of the loose herb to ¼ teaspoon of cinnamon powder. Drink this between meals. The diaphoretic cinnamon spreads the moistening herb to refresh the skin.

Herbal combinations that increase estrogen

The following herbal combinations do increase estrogen. They might be taken to revitalize moisture and energy by women not already taking medications that reduce estrogen. Natural estrogen-increasing herbs are safer to take than synthetic hormones because they are absorbed better, and also because they encourage your body to perform a natural process. But if you are at high risk of developing breast cancer, take the following herbs with the supervision of your herbalist. Most women take one of them for three to six months in order to rebalance hormones and reverse menopausal complaints. If you have chronic arthritic or headache pain, also add evening primrose oil capsules daily.

Placenta Compound Restorative Pills is a *warming* Chinese patent remedy containing blood-building herbs and processed human placenta. Available in Chinese herb shops, they are traditionally used to restore vitality after illness, and to improve fertility. Many people object to using human or animal products, so I recommend several modern vegetarian combinations available in health-food stores.

Change-O-Life and **Fem-Mend** are made by Nature's Way. Herbs found in these formulas that can affect hormone production are false unicorn, squaw vine, blessed thistle, black cohosh, and sarsaparilla. Of the two, **Change-O-Life** is more *cooling.* **Fem-Mend** contains cayenne and ginger, but is cooled somewhat by goldenseal (an antibiotic, not meant for long-term use) and red raspberry leaf.

Health Concerns manufactures **Menaplex,** available in stores and by mail. Health Concerns is said to be the first American manufacturer of Chinese herbal formulas to bring together biochemists, herbalists, clinicians, Asian medical doctors, and translators to introduce centuries-old formulas adapted to modern needs. **Menaplex** is based on a formula developed at the Shuguang Hospital of the Shanghai College of Traditional Chinese Medicine. To the original formula were added the Western herb black cohosh, because of its estrogenic properties, and the metabolite vitamin E.

Menaplex treats menopausal symptoms including amenorrhea, hypertension, hot flashes, excessive sweating, nervousness, fatigue, lassitude, insomnia, palpitations, irritability, tinnitus (ringing in the ears), depression, urinary frequency, low-back pain, and graying of hair. In terms of traditional Chinese medicine, it addresses "kidney *yin* and kidney *yang* deficiency and spleen *chi* deficiency." The combination contains black cohosh, epimedium, circuligo, morinda, tang kuei, anemarrhena, phellodendron, and vitamin E. Feverish symptoms are removed by the anti-inflammatory herbs anemarrhena and phellodendron, while "kidney *yang*" (adrenal and immune strength) is increased by *warming* herbs such as morinda and epimedium.

Crystal Star makes herbal teas and capsules available in pharmacies and health shops. For prevention of menopausal complaints, Crystal Star offers **Est Aid Tea.** It combines rosemary, anise oil, and sage (strong *heating* stimulants); motherwort, blessed thistle, wild yam, and damiana (for hormones); and tang kuei (for circulation and blood-building). Most of these herbs are stimulants, so that the remedy puts into effect the principle "Strengthen what is

weak," in order to prevent excess stress to the heart. Such a combination could be helpful for fatigue, anxiety, and palpitations for persons with *internal cold* symptoms (look for a large, pale tongue).

Est Aid Capsules contain black cohosh, wild yam, squaw vine, sarsaparilla, blessed thistle, tang kuei, damiana, and false unicorn. All the herbs except tang kuei are a source of female hormones. **Easy Change Caps,** from Crystal Star, contain Western, Chinese, and Indian herbs, including black cohosh, tang kuei, cramp bark, damiana, skullcap, false unicorn, squaw vine, red raspberry, sarsaparilla, bayberry bark, blessed thistle, trifala fruits, pennyroyal, and carrot. This creative formula combines estrogenic herbs with anti-inflammatory cleansing herbs for the liver and intestines along with emmenagogues (herbs that increase menstruation).

Zand makes **Changes for Women** "for the changing needs of women over thirty-five." Zand's combinations contain plenty of Chinese tonic herbs; this particular one has tang kuei, vitex, peony, and polyporus for support of blood production and circulation; bupleurum, gardenia, nettle, and skullcap for *cooling* and cleansing; and oatstraw, astragalus, and others for strength. I've already mentioned their **Women's Calcium Combination** (see page 330).

When in doubt about herbal hormone replacement, I recommend starting with nourishing formulas that do not affect hormone production. Then check with one of the herbal practitioners I've recommended for more specific advice.

Heart disease

You can prevent a great many heart-related problems by changing your diet. Circulation will improve after reducing caffeine, alcohol, and cigarettes. Cholesterol will become more normal from eating fewer unhealthy fats and sweets.

A favorite remedy for prevention of heart trouble and stroke is hawthorn berries, a stimulant antiphlegm herb. The herb is bitter and sour in flavor, though *warming* in effect. Overuse of the single herb can cause excess stomach acid, bad breath, or skin rash. Combinations that include hawthorn are usually safer for long-term use. Hawthorn works for menopausal women or overstressed persons of any age by strengthening the heart and reducing cholesterol over a period of time.

Hawthorn capsules and combinations containing it, such as **Heartsease C.H.F.** made by Crystal Star, are widely available in supermarkets and health-food stores. (See Slimming Teas in chapter 5.) You can take a hawthorn capsule after meals, especially if your tongue is pale and gray-coated and your chest occasionally feels heavy or tight. Persons with a reddish tongue and hypertension should take herbs to reduce blood pressure (see chapter 21).

THE CLASSIC ANXIETY ATTACK

Sometimes during peri-menopause (the year or so before the period completely stops) or after the onset of menopause, women will awaken during the night with heart palpitations, feeling feverish, sweaty, and terribly anxious. I have also seen this happen to men and women who are exhausted or overweight, and to women as a result of taking birth control pills. It is a *heat* condition that must be treated with calming herbs that reestablish a smooth heart rhythm.

For example, **Fu-Shen 16,** a Seven Forests formula, is recommended for mental agitation, insomnia, heart palpitations, convulsions, and inflammation or sores in the mouth. It contains several natural forms of calcium found in oyster shell and bones, along with blood-builders for mental agitation and nutritive herbs appropriate for persons easily frightened—also for hallucinations, hysteria, or convulsions.

One dose of 3 to 5 pills can calm an agitated heart so you can get a good night's sleep, but that is not the final answer to your anxiety problem.

People with chronic inflammatory illness, or *heating* and *drying* addictions like smoking, or hormone imbalances, sometimes have to choose between taking *cooling* antibiotic, moistening, or sedative herbs, depending upon which they need the most. Heart-relaxing herbs such as passionflower tea, or combinations like **Fu-Shen 16,** can release you from temporary crippling fear and sharp chest discomfort. But after their period of effective use, you should stop taking heart sedatives or switch to other appropriate herbs.

For example, if your chronic chest discomfort is related to high cholesterol, use anticholesterol herbs such as Chinese slimming teas. If it's due to hypertension, see chapter 21. If acute chest pains or palpitations come from poor circulation and heartburn or indigestion, use digestive herbs such as **Xiao Yao Wan.** If chest discomfort, anxiety, and insomnia correspond to exhaustion and stress, **Wuchaseng** extract will help you. Also, chapter 33 will offer useful herbal combinations that can promote tranquil sleep without harmful side effects. The point is that taking a sedative herbal combination to settle anxiety may not be enough to eliminate the core of the problem.

A FINAL WORD ON HORMONES AND HEALTH

Although we don't have a complete picture of the causes of postmenopausal heart disease, arthritis, or cancer, they are clearly more complicated than a matter of hormone balance. Hormones are one thing Western medicine chooses to study when regarding women's problems, but we are much more than our hormones. Diet, exercise, physical stress, and our thoughts and emotions are all underlying factors because they affect our vitality, circulation, and internal cleansing.

For example, when I studied breast cancer in a Shanghai medical school, I was told that it is very complicated, involving internal and environmental toxins, weakness, poor immune strength and circulation, hormone imbalances, and emotions.

More specifically, I was told, "Breast cancer is a disease of melancholy."

It may be argued that chronic depression can be provoked by hormone imbalances, but our life can also induce depression. Taking natural or synthetic hormones cannot change your life. But when you choose to live purely, sanely, and simply, your immune health improves because your body and emotions stop fighting stress. You must choose to change your life now, or else lose a precious gift: health gained from insight.

Menopause is your chance for a second coming, a new adulthood. The first time arrived during the blazing heat of puberty. Now, from a distance, at menopause, you have a chance to reflect upon your life plans and hopes, seeing which have been accomplished and which have failed. You can now learn from experience, then act. Now is the time to claim all you need and want for maturity. Freed from youth's awkwardness, ignorance, and timidity, you can finally fulfill your desires. You might end a bad marriage or begin a good one. You might start a new life enriched by artistic endeavor, study, or travel. I have met women who, after retirement, have sold their homes, said goodbye to their adult children, and traveled the world; and others who gave birth for the first time at the threshold of menopause. They had a glow of fulfillment in their eyes and serenity in their voices. The herbs in this chapter can keep you cool, calm, and strong as you grow, knowing that the best is yet to come.

MENOPAUSAL COMPLAINTS

What makes it worse?

Hot flashes, irritability, insomnia, inflammatory arthritis, headaches, muscle cramps, heart trouble, and breast cancer:
Coffee, cigarettes, alcohol, hot spices, rich or fat diet, fatigue, weakness, drugs, environmental toxins, aggravation.

Depression, fatigue, indigestion, cholesterol, dull joint pain, and swollen joints:
Rich, creamy, sweet, or oily foods, also cold, raw, and sour foods, lack of exercise, excess *phlegm,* stalemate, frustrating relationships.

What makes it better?

Cleansing, blood-building, and moisturizing herbs, tonic or nervine herbs as needed, simple wholesome diet, rest, exercise, fulfilling personal and professional life.

	HEAT SYMPTOMS	*COLD* SYMPTOMS	*PHLEGM*
TONGUE	red or quivering	pale, scalloped	coated
SYMPTOMS	headache, fever	pallor	sinus, congestion
	irritability	depression	cloudiness,
	insomnia	hypertension	spaceyness
	hot flashes	(kidney weakness)	weight gain
	hypertension	rheumatoid arthritis	swollen joint pain
	inflammatory arthritis		

BASELINE NONHORMONAL REMEDIES

Hot flashes: 1 teaspoon skullcap powder or 20 drops extract, 3 times daily
Pain and inflammation: evening primrose oil, aloe vera
Indigestion: **Xiao Yao Wan, Lung Tan Xie Gan Wan**
Irritability, anger: **Lung Tan Xie Gan Wan**
Anxiety insomnia: **Wuchaseng, Fu-Shen 16**
Cancer prevention: green tea, astragalus, beta-carotene, mixed trace minerals
Prevention of heart disease: vegetables, grains, fruits, green tea, hawthorn (capsules or slimming teas)
To increase vaginal moisture and comfort, reduce premature gray hair and dry skin: **Shou Wu Pian** (between meals)

HORMONAL SUPPORT FORMULAS

Crystal Star: **Est Aid, Female Harmony**
Nature's Way: **Fem-Mend, Change-O-Life**
Nature's Herbs: **Blessed Thistle Combination**
Health Concerns: **Restorative Tablets, Women's Harmony, Menaplex**

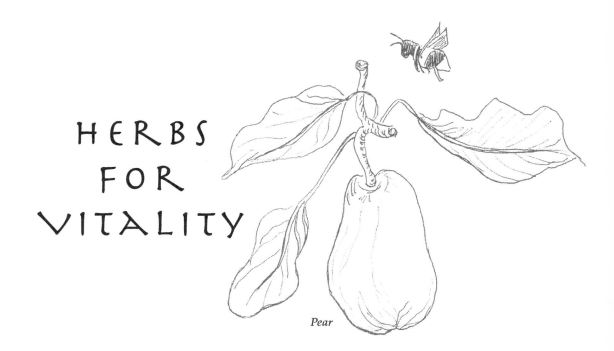

HERBS
FOR
VITALITY

Pear

Vitality is the ripe fruit of springtime's budding. It is the bloom of beauty and the solace of peaceful sleep gained from blood-building herbs. It is the fire that burns in the heart of the lover, the steel that hardens the bones and muscles of the warrior. It is the mature wisdom that comes from taking the herbs of each season.

For spring, we cleanse with bitter, sour dandelion. For summer, we cool and purify our bodies with chrysanthemum flower tea. In autumn, we lift our spirit and breath with astragalus. In winter, we secure our mind's clarity and memory and increase our sexual and creative energy with lycium and epimedium. Every season has its herbs. The way to vitality is to know how to use them even before they are needed.

This section concerns the prevention of problems that devitalize you, such as colds, flu, and also insomnia. In addition, it contains two chapters on energy-building herbs, including several kinds of ginseng and others to suit your specific needs. Finally, it contains a chapter on sexual tonics to help you put your increased energy to good use.

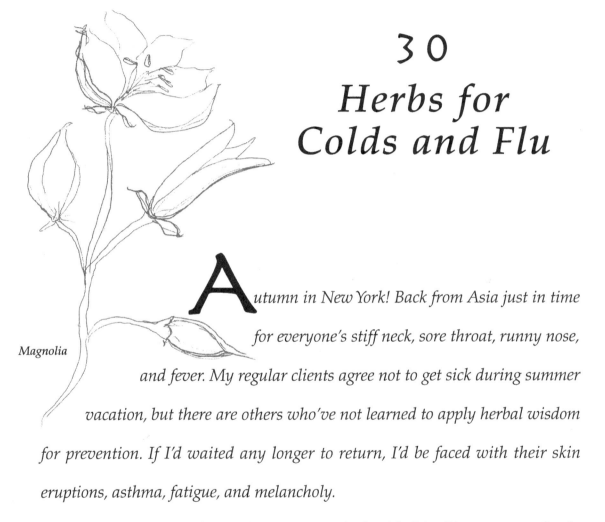

Magnolia

3 0
Herbs for
Colds and Flu

Autumn in New York! Back from Asia just in time for everyone's stiff neck, sore throat, runny nose, and fever. My regular clients agree not to get sick during summer vacation, but there are others who've not learned to apply herbal wisdom for prevention. If I'd waited any longer to return, I'd be faced with their skin eruptions, asthma, fatigue, and melancholy.

After two months in the tropics, I deal with Big City reentry, slowly unpack clothes from Thai jungles, paintings of Krishna from Delhi, or suitcases of books and herbs from China. When I finally listen to my phone messages,

most New Yorkers have hung up upon not find-
ing me there. Some said, "Could you see me
this afternoon?" or "Call me collect from any-
where in the world!" Most people are impatient
with cold remedies too, demanding fast-acting
pain relief. I sweat out a cold before it develops
with **Gan Mao Ling** *or ginger tea. It's the*
same every year: The autumn air may be gray
and dense, but October, like a gift from the
gods, lifts its veil. The weather clears and
everyone stays out late, enjoying iced drinks,
wearing light clothes. They play ball in the park
or get caught in the rain. They catch colds and
my work continues.

Seasonal Colds and Flu

In this chapter we'll discuss a natural approach to cold and flu prevention and
treatment, using diet and herbs. You will
discover remedies to keep in your medicine cabinet and briefcase this autumn and
winter so that you won't have to call your
herbalist until spring cleansing time.

In general, for prevention of colds and
flu, the best approach includes wearing adequate clothing in cool, damp weather and
eating a good diet that is low in fats and
phlegm-producing foods. For cold treatments, you should use fast-acting, powerful herbal remedies such as those discussed
in this chapter. They include diaphoretic
herbs that make you perspire, clear your
sinus congestion, and keep the cold from
penetrating beyond your immune defenses.
The herbal formulas also contain anti-
inflammatory herbs that reduce fever, muscle aches, and headaches, and antibiotic

herbs that stop infections. It is best to use
the recommended herbal cold remedies
only while symptoms persist. The kinds of
herbs used for prevention and treatment of
colds and flu will vary somewhat according
to the season.

SPRING PHLEGM AND ALLERGIES

Spring and summer colds are characterized by thick phlegm. This is because, after
winter's lethargy and rich food, you can
develop coldlike symptoms more easily
because your body's detoxification has
slowed. Often a one-day cleansing fast
early in spring will prevent colds. If sneezing, coughing, and tearing continue after a
day or two of cleansing teas or cold remedies, you may have a seasonal allergy that
requires additional cleansing. You know
it's an allergy if it happens like clockwork
every spring (see chapter 23).

AUTUMN FATIGUE AND DEPRESSION

Autumn is a time when most people frequently catch head colds that can turn into
upper-respiratory infections and pneumonia. Autumn is associated with the Metal
element, according to Chinese medicine,
which presents problems related to the
lungs, the large intestine, and the skin. For
that reason, many persons suffer shortness
of breath, poor elimination, or blemishes at
that time. It is not uncommon for a Chinese

herbal antibiotic to treat simultaneously infection from influenza, mumps, dysentery, and furuncles (nasty blemishes).

Fall is the season of colds and flu because the lungs, our most superficial organs, are also our most vulnerable. And to make things worse, with chronic weakness and mucus, a late-summer cold may turn sooner or later into asthma. Smokers are subject to bronchitis because of inflammation.

WINTER BLAHS AND ASTHMA

All the coughing and sneezing of spring or summer colds are kid stuff compared to the problems we face in winter. In cold weather the Water element (the kidneys and adrenal glands), governing our vital energy, is compromised. If you become sick in winter, you can easily get depressed, exhausted, and demoralized. Because of adrenal weakness, you may lack courage and stamina. Pale, breathless, and crabby, you have the "winter blahs," lacking adequate strength and oxygen to cope. The deeper problem of blahs actually starts earlier, on a superficial level. The trick is to know how to avoid a cold in the first place, so it can't turn into asthma or bronchitis.

PREVENTION

Prevention is better than the best cold and flu drug, because it makes your body stronger. How does an herbal cold-prevention remedy work? It's not always simple and fast-acting. To be most effective, it should vary somewhat with the season. A springtime cold preventer should clear the body of excess acid and phlegm, while an autumn cold-prevention plan should build a strong defense against weakness and cold weather. This is a general rule, although there may be digestive problems, internal imbalances, troubling emotions, fatigue, or addictions that can complicate things at any time.

Also, because a cold or flu weakens you in stages, herbs used for prevention are different from those used for treatment. In brief, cold-prevention plans aim to alleviate chronic weakness, while cold remedies treat acute problems, not weakness but inflammation.

SPRING COLDS

Because ridding your body of excess acid and mucus can eliminate underlying toxins that aggravate colds, the best prevention plan for persons who tend to have *internal heat* is one that is cleansing. Many inflammation problems increase in spring and summer, so this method is especially well suited to those seasons. (Look for a reddish tongue with a yellow coating, thirst, and nervous insomnia.)

To reverse chronic *internal heat*, I sometimes drink a tea made from one quarter teaspoon each of cumin, coriander, and fennel powder, added to a cup of boiling water. It's best taken after breakfast. This mild tea helps prevent fevers, rashes, stomachache, and nervousness from chronic illness, hot climate, and spicy foods. It is also useful for preventing spring's headaches and inflamed joints. But a tea for chronic inflammation such as this will not treat a cold. It only clears impurities that make a cold and fever worse.

AUTUMN COLDS

In autumn or whenever you tend to be tired and stretched beyond your limits from overwork, addictions, or emotional stress, it pays to take some special precautions in order to avoid becoming sick. (Look for a pale, scalloped tongue, shortness of breath, anemia, chronic diarrhea, and fatigue.) Cleansing teas such as the one above can reduce inflammation when it is necessary, but you may also need to build resistance.

Your daily herbs for chronic weakness might include Chinese ginseng, garlic, daily vitamins, minerals (especially zinc), antioxidants, or spirulina.

I also recommend a daily dose of astragalus, a potent immune builder. It is convenient to take one teaspoon of the powder per day, added to tea, water, or juice. This lifts energy, prevents fatigue, and keeps the cold, damp weather out. None of these will reverse the onset of a cold, although they may prevent one by building resistance.

CHRONIC FEVER CONDITIONS AND IMMUNE WEAKNESS

Persons who are chronically ill or have low immune strength, HIV, or diabetes are at risk of developing asthma or TB. They often suffer fevers, night sweats, excess thirst, rashes, and exhaustion. A good daily soup for them would help reverse weakness and fever in order to improve vitality. This is especially recommended for long-time drug and alcohol users, for persons with fevers from HIV or AIDS, or for others damaged by toxic chemicals and cancer drug therapies. It is not a cold or flu remedy, but can be used to protect immunity throughout the year, because it improves breathing and promotes calm and balance.

A soup stock for chronic fever and weakness

Simmer one handful each of anemarrhena (zhi mu) and epimedium (yin yang huo) in a quart of springwater for forty-five minutes, and drink 3 cups per day.

Anemarrhena reduces fever, and epimedium builds adrenal strength. Together they reverse inflammation and weakness. The soup is easy to prepare and mild-tasting. Persons with chronic diarrhea along with fever and weakness can take a dose of **Curing Pills** after meals (see page 341).

PILLS FOR RESISTING ILLNESS AND ENHANCING STRENGTH

There are several increasingly popular, modern, American-made Chinese herbal remedies that rebuild damaged immune weakness to protect and stimulate good health. Originally used by the AIDS community because of their effective, fast-acting results, they have now become widely recommended to reverse damage done by modern medical intervention. They greatly strengthen natural immunity in order to treat anemia, exhaustion, chronic inflammatory symptoms, and poor circulation. They are used for cancer chemotherapies, chronic fevers and infections, herpes, colitis, and liver damage from drugs, toxic chemicals, and radiation. They can protect you against contagious diseases by building your natural strength and vitality.

Enhance, made by Health Concerns, contains ganoderma mushroom and Chinese blood and moisturizing tonics including American ginseng, kidney tonic herbs including epimedium, several herbs used to help circulation, and a relatively high number of anti-inflammatory antibiotic herbs including andrographis, isatis, lonicera, oldenlandia, and viola. It would be well used by persons with a dry, reddish tongue indicative of *internal heat,* and also thirst, dry cough, and chronic infections. During fever, more than the recommended dose could be used until symptoms are reversed.

Composition A, made by I.T.M. and available from Health Concerns, contains a slightly higher dose of *chi*-building herbs, moistening herbs for the lungs, and blood tonics. It adds deer antler as a kidney tonic, along with epimedium. Like **Enhance,** it contains many of the major *cooling* antibiotic herbs used in Chinese medicine: andrographis, hu zhang, isatis, lonicera, oldenlandia, phellodendron, and sophora.

These combat *damp heat,* characterized by feverish conditions with excess phlegm affecting the lungs, or other sticky, yellowish pus discharges anywhere in the body. The two formulas are rather similar; both are balanced and improve resistance to infection because they cleanse the body and build health at the same time.

Resist, made by Pacific Biologics in California, is another herbal combination widely used to fight chronic infection and stave off acute attacks. It comes in two parts: **Resist** is to be taken daily and **Resist II** is for acute outbreaks of fever, colds, flu, herpes, or other *damp heat* conditions. **Resist** contains mainly *chi*-building herbs, and the sister combination contains more anti-inflammatory herbs to be used in a dose high enough to stop the outbreak.

Monthly costs for these herbal combinations are comparable and quite reasonable, considering the high costs of getting sick. I recommend any of the formulas to be taken during times of stress resulting in inflammatory symptoms, and as extra protection if your work exposes you to many sick people. If you find the formulas too *cooling,* you can alternate them with Chinese ginseng. It makes much more sense to take strengthening herbs than to wait for a problem to happen or to get the flu from a flu shot.

These herbal pills are available through APP in New York City, Georgia, and Florida, Health Concerns in California, and local herb shops. I recently found them in the Action Care Nutrition Center in my Chelsea neighborhood. It's a regular pharmacy that also sells herbs and has an acupuncturist on staff. This East/West approach may become the new wave in local health care. When I walked in to take a better look, I found a pleasant German man who said, "If it were up to me, I'd sell only Asian herbs. They are very popular where I come from."

Cold and Flu Treatments
COLD TREATMENTS ARE ACUTE REMEDIES

A cold is an acute problem, not a chronic one. It must be treated immediately and carefully, or else it will linger. The best method for cold and flu treatment is to stimulate a natural immune response by sweating out the cold. People develop serious colds because they do not recognize the early symptoms. Once your stiff neck, chills, or stuffed sinus begins, you have to reverse the problem within an hour so the illness does not penetrate defenses deeper to weaken you.

For this purpose, a diaphoretic cold remedy such as ginger or cinnamon tea encourages sweating. It also builds defensive *chi.* Therefore the cold is eliminated from the inside out, thus strengthening defenses. This means that during cold and flu season you may have to carry along with you an herbal cold remedy like the ones we'll study.

Asian medical theory is lost to modern people. They wait for a full-fledged cold to hit, then they want fast relief, feeling that the stronger the cure, the better. But strong *drying* drugs can scorch sinus passages, lungs, or skin. Certain cold medicines may drive or depress the nervous system in an attempt to suppress symptoms. Quick-fix cures risk not only damage to immune strength, but can cause addiction to over-the-counter narcotics as well as producing other long-term side effects.

WHERE COLDS BEGIN: AN ASIAN PERSPECTIVE

Not all Asian doctors agree on the origins of colds, but most recommend similar cures that build immune strength. Ayurveda believes colds and chronic illnesses such as rheumatism are caused by excess toxins (*ama*) of an internal origin. Thus, cold remedies clear the body of undigested food and other wastes. Chinese doctors believe that when resistance is low, we catch colds and flu from outside influences brought on by "evil winds." In other words, cold symptoms are *excess* symptoms such as fever and chills coming from the outside. The appropriate remedy, according to that healing tradition, eliminates excess *cold, dampness,* and *wind* from the body.

Cold remedies shared by most herbal traditions clear toxins and excess conditions by increasing sweating, killing germs, and reducing fever, pains, stiffness, and congestion. Since natural cleansing is increased, immune strength is augmented. The idea of "evil wind," "evil dampness," and "evil wetness" is more than an amusing footnote. This belief is shared by American Indian healers, who also thought illness came from external malevolent forces. Scratch the surface of an herb used for "evil" influences, and oftentimes you'll find an antibiotic. "Evil" was perhaps an early description of infection.

CARDINAL RULES FOR COLD PREVENTION AND TREATMENT

1. The first step in cold prevention and treatment is to "sweat it out" with a diaphoretic herbal tea and rest.
2. *Never* take tonic or *heating* herbs like ginseng and garlic for a cold; they only drive the cold deeper. Instead, take herbal cold pills to sweat it out and kill germs.
3. Avoid cold, raw foods, extreme fatigue, long baths, or deep massage during a cold, because they weaken your defenses.

HOW COLDS ORIGINATE

Here is an example of how colds often originate from both internal and external causes.

Chuck and Marion are having a fight. They can't decide on a vacation spot. He wants to see the Caribbean, while she prefers Paris. He wants the beach. She wants to shop, practice her French, go to plays, and eat crêpes. They've each collected brochures, contacted travel agents, lost sleep over the matter, and still can't decide. Finally, one morning after a long debate, Chuck bolts down his coffee and leaves to walk the dog. He's wearing only a shirt. It's raining and cold. He's tired and exasperated. He catches a chill.

By the time he gets back, he's soaked to the skin and has a stiff neck. But he's remembered the French words for "I love you." She, meanwhile, has been admiring her bikini, thinking how nice a cozy small island could be. They kiss and make up. The next day he has a cold with a stiff neck, a sore throat, chills, and fatigue. He doesn't sweat out his cold with cinnamon tea or herbs, so that the following day he starts sneezing, feels stuffed up, loses his voice, and gets a fever.

THE COMMON COLD

Stage one

At the first sign of a cold, which usually includes chills, stiffness, and fatigue, take a diaphoretic herbal tea or pill remedy (cinnamon tea or **Gan Mao Ling**); wrap up in warm sleepwear, go to bed, and take a sweat-bath vacation for about an hour. Then eat warm barley soup during the rest of the day to clear phlegm. You will tend to have more congestion symptoms if your diet is rich, creamy, sweet, and fatty, because those foods slow digestion and create phlegm.

Stage two

If you have ignored your cold, your symptoms will become inflammatory, with headache, fever, sore throat, and cough. This is because your immune system is battling with your cold. At this stage, take antibiotic herbal combinations to ease your symptoms and kill infection (**Gan Mao Ching** or **Tablets Kang Yan**; add other herbs as needed to soften thick phlegm and move congestion or treat cough).

FIRST-STAGE COLD REMEDIES: SWEAT IT OUT

Natural doctors may debate whether you catch a cold because of depression or excess phlegm (perhaps from your daily bagel and cream cheese), or from some "evil wind" smacking you in the face as you walk the dog; but their remedies would clear congestion and pain by increasing sweating. Sweating both clears toxins and lifts excess conditions away. This is very easily accomplished with home remedies.

How do you know if you have gotten rid of the problem? If the diaphoretic herbs give you chills for a few minutes, then make you feel much stronger, you probably have "sweated out" the cold. You needn't literally perspire. Rest and liquids will also help colds, but if you take the right herbs at the first sign of discomfort, you should not have a long, difficult cold. The following remedies are listed in the order you will most likely need them: herbs for stiffness, chills, sinus congestion, cough, and sore throat, and a number of strong-acting cold pills that treat a cold's pains and infection.

REMEDIES FOR STIFFNESS AND CHILLS

The cinnamon-scallion cure and other teas

Here is a Vietnamese home cure: Finely chop one scallion; put it into a teacup and add two slices of raw ginger and a dash of powdered cinnamon. Fill the cup with hot water, let the herbs steep, and drink the tea. Cinnamon and ginger induce sweating, while scallion clears the sinus.

Yogi Tea Company makes a tasty herbal brew that works just as well and is available in tea bags from health-food stores. **Yogi Tea** is said to treat the whole person, including the Five Elements and the seven chakras. That is in keeping with Yogi Bhajan's philosophy, "Doctors diagnose and God cures." The tea, which contains ginger, eucalyptus, licorice, basil, black pepper, cardamom, orange peel, celery seed, valerian root, lemongrass, peppermint, clove, oregano, and yarrow flowers, increases sweating, dries phlegm, and builds energy.

These herbs are said to increase *agni* (heat or fire energy), which encourages the body to fight off a cold. A pinch of basil leaves or cinnamon powder (diaphoretic herbs) is also easily made into a cup of tea.

A SIMPLE REMEDY FOR SIMPLE PHLEGM

Sometimes the only discomfort you may notice with a cold is thick, phlegmy congestion. This is especially the case with a spring or summer cold, because you may not be aware of muscle stiffness or chills. In that case you might as well take a remedy that stops phlegm. Homeopathic pulsatilla (30c potency) works well for congestion, shortness of breath, and lethargy that accompanies phlegm. You know you need it if you feel you must go outside to breathe, if your chest feels tight and your head stuffed. You can add 10 pills to a quart of water or a pot of tea and drink it all day.

THE BEST HERBAL APPROACH FOR SINUS PROBLEMS

I have met a number of people who have taken decongestant pills regularly for as long as fifteen years. After that length of time, they had scarred their lung tissue and caused nearly irreversible damage. They would develop weepy, itchy eczema when they felt better, or asthma when they felt worse. All their symptoms were those of *internal heat*. The dehydration had spread from the lungs to almost everywhere else in the body. Some of them even became blood-deficient.

There are more sensible ways to dry excess phlegm in the sinuses. Herbs are more gentle. Also, it is understood that they should be taken for a limited period of time, while the symptoms persist. If a person took *drying* herbs (for example, those that increase sweating) for a long time, they could provoke dry cough, thirst, or dehydration symptoms. The following herbs should be used no longer than a few days, or combined with *cooling,* moistening herbs.

Bayberry (in Latin, *myrica*) is a diaphoretic herb that cleanses sinus passages and lymph glands. It works on the respiratory, circulatory, and lymphatic systems as an expectorant. It clears excess phlegm from the throat because it is astringent and diaphoretic. And it relaxes nervous cough because it is antispasmodic.

Bayberry capsules can be used for colds, flu, laryngitis, sinus and nasal congestion, sore throat, asthma, bronchitis, adenoids, fever, chronic sores in nasal passages, and bleeding gums. Some sources say it improves the voice and opens the mind and senses. It is one of the best herbs for the initial stage of a cold because it mobilizes the body's defensive energy. About the only precaution advised for bayberry is that it should be used sparingly by people with hyperacidity or hypertension.

Echinacea is a powerful *heating, drying,* astringent/diaphoretic herb. It kills germs and dries phlegm. But this herb comes with a warning: It is so strongly *heating* and diaphoretic that it can cause dizziness and bronchitis. Do not take it at all if you have a fever, night sweats, or dry cough. I do not recommend its daily use. Some herb doctors have had good results combining it with *cooling* herbs such as goldenseal and honeysuckle flowers and isatis. Even so, long-term use can dry the lungs and impair blood production.

AN HERBAL SNUFF FOR CONGESTION AND PHLEGM HEADACHE

I remember one lady with a thick nasal voice, who complained of adenoids, nasal polyps, and stuffed-up headaches from excess phlegm. No wonder: Her favorite food was a sticky bun she bought in Chinatown, made from white flour and pork. She was exhausted because her breathing was difficult.

I recommended diet changes along with bayberry capsules between meals, and gotu kola capsules used as snuff. Its *drying* effects open the sinuses and stimulate the brain.

A SIMPLE SORE THROAT REMEDY AND A GRAND OPERA CURE

If you need to speak or sing and have a cold, it can really hurt. The best and fastest remedy is homeopathic calcara sulphate (30c potency). When you take a dose, usually 5 pills, once or twice before your performance, your throat will be relaxed and moist. It also helps fight weakness and improves the cold.

SINGER'S COUGH

I usually recommend easy-to-take pill remedies for colds, but have been known to concoct special herbal soups for friends. One friend's symptoms were complicated because she smoked a few cigarettes daily and used her voice a lot. She was experiencing hot flashes, so she couldn't tell whether she had the usual feverish, achy flu symptoms. She was fatigued from work and travel and had received a sedating massage that left her depressed. She needed a more complicated remedy than **Gan Mao Ling.**

The soup I made had to accomplish several things at once: ease sore throat, clear congestion, and eliminate dizziness or headache. This requires anti-inflammatory, expectorant, and diaphoretic herbs. The best approach is often aromatic and antibiotic herbs, and those that move phlegm outward. To loosen thick phlegm, it must first be softened, then cleared with expectorant herbs. The baseline recipe contains moistening and antibiotic herbs, but you can add others for fever and sore throat as needed. Here is an example:

A GRAND OPERA COLD CURE

Simmer all the ingredients listed below together for 10 minutes in 1 liter of springwater.

A handful each of forsythia, pinellia, and ophiopogonis (in Chinese, *mai men dong*). These *cooling,* moistening herbs soften phlegm in the upper respiratory tract.

Add a handful of cracked magnolia buds. The camphorlike aroma clears the sinuses.

Add two main ingredients always included in patent formulas for colds: honey-

COLD AND FLU REMEDIES

FIRST STAGE

SWEAT OUT THE COLD WITH CINNAMON, GINGER, SCALLION, OR GAN MAO LING

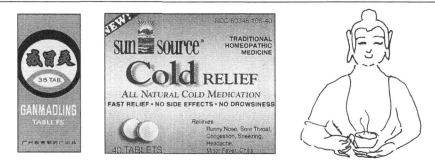

FEVER STAGE

USE ANTI-INFLAMMATORY COLD REMEDIES THAT REDUCE FEVER AND ACHES

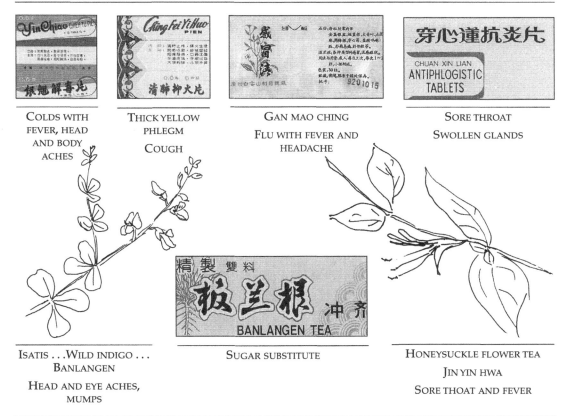

COLDS WITH FEVER, HEAD AND BODY ACHES

THICK YELLOW PHLEGM

COUGH

GAN MAO CHING

FLU WITH FEVER AND HEADACHE

SORE THROAT

SWOLLEN GLANDS

ISATIS . . . WILD INDIGO . . . BANLANGEN

HEAD AND EYE ACHES, MUMPS

SUGAR SUBSTITUTE

HONEYSUCKLE FLOWER TEA

JIN YIN HWA

SORE THOAT AND FEVER

suckle flowers (an anti-inflammatory antibiotic) and chrysanthemum flowers (a *cooling* diaphoretic used to eliminate fever and headache). Chrysanthemum flowers and magnolia buds are traditionally used together to clear sinus congestion.

To overcome unpleasant spacey feelings from diaphoretic herbs, add two that strengthen digestion: one piece each of dried orange peel and atractylodes.

Optional: If necessary, add a pinch of coptis for headache and fever. Or for singer's sore throat from fatigue and overuse, add several fructus scaphigerae.

This brew is slightly sweet, bitter, and pungent, yet *cooling*. It worked wonders for my friend. In a short time she felt less congested and stronger. Tension and pain left her eyes and throat. She could breathe and sing. With this remedy, much of our work to get rid of her cold was done. **Gan Mao Ling** pills would be strong enough to take for the rest of the day.

CHINESE PATENT COLD REMEDIES

These are for stage two of a cold, when it is often too late to sweat it out. Symptoms include fever, chills, aches, congestion, cough, thick phlegm, and weakness from infection. Chinese patent cold remedies contain antibiotic and anti-inflammatory plants.

I have listed them in the order I recommend, using the first one for milder cold symptoms and the others for deeper, more serious colds with fever, chills, and

infection, including complications associated with AIDS. You can take the first one anytime to prevent and treat a cold. But the stronger ones work best if your phlegm is thick, yellow, or green, or if you have a dry cough or fever.

Gan Mao Ling pills can usually turn my colds around in an hour or less. Three pills four times a day is recommended for prevention and treatment of colds and flu. It contains ilex, vitex, chrysanthemum, evodia, lonicera, isatis, and menthol.

It works for chills and fever, swollen lymph nodes, sore throat, and stiff neck from colds. Ilex (holly) increases energy circulation in the chest. Chrysanthemum is an anti-inflammatory diaphoretic. Isatis (wild indigo) and lonicera (honeysuckle flowers) are natural antibiotics.

Other popular remedies include **Yinchiao Chieh Tu Pien,** a pill containing honeysuckle flower, forsythia, mint, other anti-inflammatory ingredients, and also antelope horn, designed to relieve stiff neck, swollen lymph nodes, sore throat, fever, and headache. Some manufacturers in Hong Kong add caffeine, so read the label to avoid those brands.

Gan Mao Ching, a strongly detoxifying herbal capsule, contains, among other ingredients, andrographis paniculat (chuanxinlian), which, according to *Chinese Herbal Medicine Materia Medica* compiled by Bensky and Gamble, "clears heat and detoxifies fire poison" (in this case flu), and also treats a variety of *heat* patterns in the lungs, throat, and urinary tract, and on the skin, such as sores and carbuncles.

For serious colds: How can I be sure which cold remedy to use?

If you have ignored a cold, if you smoke or are weak from fatigue or stress, symptoms will become more like bronchitis or pneumonia. Phlegm will be thick and yellow or green. You may cough and feel short of breath. Stronger antimicrobial, anti-inflammatory, and expectorant herbs are necessary.

What color is it?

With herbal antibiotics, the question is "What color is the phlegm?" Thick yellow or dark phlegm requires a *cooling* antibiotic such as **Specific Chi Kuan Yen Wan,** recommended for cough, bronchitis, and asthma accompanied by *internal heat* symptoms. These include thirst, shortness of breath, panting, excessive thick sputum, restlessness, painful chest, and bronchial asthma. The remedy contains pummelo peel and tangerine peel to dry phlegm; fritillary, an expectorant; coltsfoot to cool *heat* and *dryness;* and ginger to build *chi.*

If the phlegm is watery and white and the cold is accompanied by chills, weakness, nausea, or watery diarrhea, a *warming* remedy is more appropriate. One popular remedy that is strengthening and balancing is called **Curing Pills.** Normally recommended for nausea and diarrhea, it also treats early stages of a cold with diaphoretic herbs.

A THREE-PART CURE

In severe cases of infection, such as colds of long duration, pneumonia, or AIDS, several remedies are often combined: one for cough along with one for fever, and an antibiotic. You might take all three of these several times daily. The dosage will vary according to your symptoms. Do not be afraid to take more than the dosage recommended on the bottle. You know the herbs have done their job when your phlegm turns from green or yellow to thin white. Then continue taking the herbs for another couple of days to knock out any remaining infection.

Powerful Linche Anti-inflammation Pills is an herbal antibiotic for upper respiratory infections. The pills contain chuen-sun-lin-noi-gee (herba andrographis) and san-gee-machum-ko (wild sesame seed).

Ma Hsing Chih Ke Pian is a lung demulcent and expectorant for colds and coughs that contains ephedra, pericarpium citri, radix glycyerrhizae, semen armeniacae amarae, radix platycodi, gypsum, talcum, and honey.

If the expectoration is thick, yellow, or greenish, add **Ching Fei Yi Huo Pien.** These pills treat fever, cough, excess phlegm, swollen sore throat, oral and nasal boils, bleeding gums, toothache, constipation, and dark urine. They contain skullcap, rhubarb, sophora, platycodon, gardenia, peucedaunum decursiv., trichosanthes, and anemarrhena.

WHEN TO TAKE COLD AND SINUS HERBS

It is best to take herbs that affect sinuses or breathing after meals or between meals, because they do not directly affect digestion. They may be overpowered by phlegm-producing foods such as pasta, milk, cheese, tofu, rice, and wheat. You may wonder why. According to Chinese medical anatomy, the acupuncture meridians that pertain to the large intestine pass through the sinus area to the brain.

Celebrate the season

One way to prevent a cold is to celebrate the cold season with a healing meal with friends. You may wish to prepare barley, radish, or other antiphlegm foods, guided by the recipes from section I of chapter 13, but you ought to top off the meal with the following:

LETHA'S BREATHE-BETTER VODKA

I've been known to make some potent potions. These home brews are an enjoyable way to have an inexpensive tincture. Here is my recipe for a vodka or brandy that clears your head. I add osha root, gathered from the mountains in New Mexico (but you can buy the dried root in herb shops).

Add about three 3-inch osha roots to a bottle of vodka and let it steep in a cool, dark place for at least three weeks.

Alcohol is by nature *heating*, so don't use this drink if you have a fever or dry cough. It does not treat a cold, but prevents excess phlegm because it is mildly diaphoretic, and dries wet mucus from lungs and sinuses. (Good for chronic asthma and weakness with pale tongue and wheezing.)

Enjoyed in front of a cheery fire with friends, it offers a delicious way to prevent winter's colds and blahs.

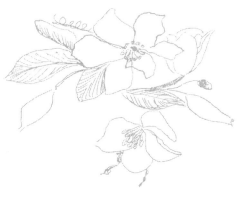

Magnolias

COLDS AND FLU

What makes it worse?

Cold, raw, and sour foods; unwise dress in cold, damp weather, fatigue, depression, drugs, cigarettes, phlegm-producing diet, low immunity from illness.

What makes it better?

Stage One:

For chills, stiffness, and fatigue, use diaphoretic herbs (cinnamon, ginger, scallion tea) to sweat out the cold.

Stage Two:

For fever, cough, congestion with yellow phlegm, use anti-inflammatory antibiotic herbs.

	INTERNAL HEAT	*INTERNAL COLD*	*PHLEGM*
TONGUE	reddish coated yellow, brown	pale	coated
SYMPTOMS	flushed appearance fever stiffness yellow phlegm dry cough night sweats thirst insomnia rash	pallor chills white or gray phlegm loose cough, wheezing	nausea nasal congestion wet cough thick phlegm

Prevention: For chills and stiffness, cinnamon, scallion, ginger

Stage One (no fever): **Gan Mao Ling,** bayberry, echinacea

Stage Two (fever): **Yinchiao Chieh Tu Pien, Gan Mao Ching**

Serious or chronic lung infection, asthma, or bronchitis: **Powerful Linche Anti-inflammation Pills** and **Ma Hsing Chih Ke Pien**

For thick yellow mucus, add: **Ching Fei Yi Huo Pien**

For recovery of strength after the cold is completely finished (no yellow or green phlegm): **Ping Chuan Wan**

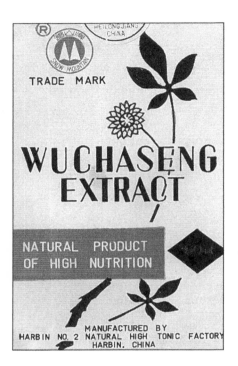

31
Energy Herbs: Why Are You Tired?

M y exhaustion is intense, physical and emotional. I feel it collapse my spine toward

the chair. In bed, my muscles jump and my ears ring. Sleep and Siberian ginseng

(Wuchaseng), a nerve rejuvenator, could revive me, but I'm leaving for Tibet in

two days and have left no time to pack. Listening to a blur of phone messages, I

list people to call: One telephoned at midnight for advice on an herbal "something

or other with a long name." Another wants to know how to cook barley. Others

ask where to buy herbs. And can I suggest an herb for someone's sick aunt in

Washington, and can't I make an exception to see one client before I *leave? Several have sent me postcards for years. Others have simply wanted to move in.*

My health clients and I share a most intimate relationship: We explore their pain together. Hardened from rich diet and neglect, emotional pain turns to physical illness. Melting these with herbs, we open Pandora's box of childhood fantasies. Adults taking transformative herbs for the first time become suddenly vulnerable. It turns a mirror on their hidden desires and old agendas. They need to be loved again, better than their mother and father ever could. That is the work of an alternative health professional.

Why are *you* tired? The answer is not always simple. Good health requires adequate blood, energy, nourishing food, and adequate rest, as well as mental and emotional balance. Most people experience fatigue as weak or aching muscles or poor concentration, without realizing that their digestion, breathing, and emotions are also affected. They need an herbal tonic that will address many of these factors at the same time.

Most people take some sort of stimulant when tired, which often does them more harm than good. The origins of fatigue can be overactivity that drains the body of needed oxygen and nutrition, or slow metabolism that leads to a buildup of toxins. Fatigue is always affected by weak immune strength and illness. To be most helpful, our energy tonics must also address these individual issues. To ignore underlying weakness is to invite illness, trouble, and sorrow.

DO YOU DRINK COFFEE TO MAKE YOU NERVOUS?

Healing herbs maintain health better, because they nourish as well as stimulate normal reactions. Caffeine pushes nervous drive—sometimes to the limit. Our addictions can be long-term so that we lose sight of their damage. Some people can drink coffee before bed and still fall asleep because their baseline energy is so low there is nothing left to push.

Determine Your Baseline Energy

As an experiment, for one day, avoid your usual stimulants: caffeine, sugar, alcohol, vitamins, drugs, television, or sports. Get your usual amount of sleep. Eat and work as you usually do, but note your energy throughout the day to see under what circumstances it lags. Notice when you would like to take a nap or have a second cup of coffee. Are you addicted to stimulants? If so, what are they?

The observation on page 374 includes the hours when most people complain of fatigue, along with possible interactions from the Five Elements involved.

HOW TO USE THE OBSERVATION

This observation can illustrate the extent of your dependence on external factors such as diet, environment, and habits. After you

Determining Baseline Energy

I FEEL MOST TIRED:

When I get up in the morning (7 A.M. to 9 A.M.)

- Did you overeat before bed (Earth and Water)?
- Does excess phlegm impair your breathing (Earth and Metal)?
- Did you stay awake angry, thinking, planning (Wood)?
- Are you depressed (weak Earth and Water, *stagnant* Wood)?

At 10:00 A.M.

- Does your heart also feel slow or weak (Fire)?
- Do you get depressed then (Fire)?

When I don't drink coffee

- Do you also get a headache? Are you constipated and irritable (Wood)?
- Are you addicted to coffee to help you think (Metal, Fire)?

After meals

- Do you experience bloating or stomachache (Earth)?
- Do rich or fat foods disagree with you (Wood)?

From noon to 2:00 P.M.

- Do you lose mental focus (Fire)?
- Would you like to take a nap then (weak Fire)?

Midafternoon, 3:00 P.M. to 5:00 P.M.

- Do you feel tired, sleepy, inattentive (Water)?
- Is that your favorite nap hour (Water)?

From 5:00 P.M. to 7:00 P.M.

- Does your energy and enthusiasm lag (Water)?
- Is your sexual energy low, or do you feel vulnerable (Water)?

Mid-evening, 8:00 P.M. to 10:00 P.M.

- Do you feel tired when you don't have friends or television to distract you? (Nervous energy requires stimulus.)

During unpleasant weather conditions

- Humidity or rainy weather (*phlegm,* Earth)
- Windy, cold weather (Wood, Water)
- Hot weather (*stagnant chi* or *heat* affecting Wood, Earth, or Fire)

During emotional turmoil

- Do you feel anger (Wood)?
- Do you feel grief (Metal)?
- Are you depressed (Water, Earth, Fire, Metal, Wood)?
- Are you paralyzed by fear (Water, Wood, Fire)?

determine what makes you sleepy and what keeps you awake, you will be able to determine the quality of your vitality when unaffected by stimulants. Notice, during your day of stimulation privation, how much energy you have, compared with other days. That is your baseline energy, your actual vitality without props.

ANALYSIS OF YOUR FINDINGS

If your daily fatigue is predictable—if it happens at about the same time, under the same circumstances—it is most likely part of an energy and behavior pattern you have had for some time. This debility will be reflected in the health of your Five Elements.

You may need to take steps to bolster immune strength or *chi* affecting one or more organ systems. This will determine, in part, how well they work together. For example, if you have fatigue related to the Earth element, you may have to pay attention to the chapters on digestion and weight loss (14–16). You should be aware, however, that if your energy is low after eating, it may reflect either problems with digestion or heart weakness.

If your energy is low in mid to late afternoon, your sexual energy may also be affected. This is because the organ systems involved (kidney, adrenal glands, and other components of the Water element) are taking from your baseline energy the energy they need to maintain their functions. You may need a global energy tonic like the ones I'll discuss, and extra rest, and you may also want to refer to the chapter on sexual problems (34) or see the section on blood pressure in chapter 21. When taking an herbal combination tonic, your vitality and mental clarity will improve as your *chi* and blood production improve.

Chi *and Sleep*

Have you ever felt so tired you could not sleep or could not work? With low vitality and blood, we can neither work nor rest. Asian energy tonics treat both exhaustion and insomnia. A stimulant alone is rarely the best measure, because it causes more fatigue. Also, the causes of fatigue are individual.

Although there are times when adequate rest or a change of pace is all that is required, you may be prone to fatigue states related to your element. For example, an Earth-type person experiencing digestive weakness will feel fatigued after eating rich meals. The weaker the digestion (and eventually the heart), the deeper the fatigue.

The chart on page 376 illustrates each of the Five Elements, their associated internal organs, and some causes for fatigue. In each case, underlying causes for fatigue include *chi* and blood deficiency. There may be more cause for your fatigue than you think.

The Deeper Causes of Fatigue

Clearly it's not enough to take ginseng or pep pills when you are tired. Such stimu-

The Five Elements and Your Fatigue

Fire (heart, pericardium, small intestine, Triple Heater)
- irregular heartbeat from physical or emotional stress
- rich diet, high in fats and sweets (Earth-related)
- chronic heart weakness (Wood- or Water-related)

Earth (stomach, spleen, pancreas)
- hunger
- poor eating habits (fasting then feasting)
- blood-sugar irregularities
- chronic diarrhea from "weak spleen" or parasites
- slow metabolism, chronic indigestion, phlegm
- sweets and alcohol addictions

Metal (lungs, large intestine)
- shortness of breath (Water- or Earth-related)
- emphysema, bronchitis, asthma, lung damage (smoking, TB, or other)

- excess phlegm (Earth-related)
- blood deficiency (Earth-related)

Water (kidneys, adrenal glands, hormones, sexual energy)
- exhaustion (overwork, sexual excess)
- stimulants (sweets, salt, coffee, cigarettes, drugs)
- poor diet (cold, raw foods, undernourishment)
- jet lag
- depression
- hormone imbalances
- low immunity
- environmental poisons

Wood (liver, gallbladder)
- fat diet, alcohol, or drugs
- conflicting emotions (poor *chi* circulation)
- infection, chronic inflammation
- environmental and drug poisons (chemotherapy, radiation)
- insomnia (blood deficiency, worry, stress, indigestion)

---

lants are too *heating* for someone already weakened from *internal heat*. Also, increasing stress in that manner lowers immune strength. Instead, it is better to rest when required, and take the right remedy at the right time.

Many home remedies and Chinese patent combinations are of great value for increasing stamina. Recently, for this purpose, a large number of herbal pills and teas using Chinese herbs have become readily available. The following selection is not entirely representative, because new products are appearing all the time in supermarkets, pharmacies, and health-food stores. Monitor the use of these with a health specialist such as one of those listed in the Herbal Access appendix. Also pay particular attention to your tongue diagnosis, realizing that an energy tonic is only part of the bigger picture of health.

Herbs to Create Energy in the Five Elements

FIRE, WOOD, AND EARTH ELEMENTS

To increase energy in these elements, it is important to eliminate excess protein, fats, sweets, and alcohol. Poor digestion leads to weakness, poor circulation, and eventually heart trouble. For that reason, energy remedies for the Fire, Wood, and Earth elements include herbs that process fats, move stuck circulation, and remove water retention.

Indigestion and fatigue

- Do you suffer from bloating, indigestion?
- Do you have irregular eating habits?
- Are you addicted to junk food?
- Do you have food allergies?

If you feel tired after eating richly, you may lack adequate digestive *chi*, or circulation may be stuck. I suggest starting with a few days of **Xiao Yao Wan** if you tend toward hypoglycemia (look for a pale tongue with scallops and possibly dark-colored spots). If you have water retention in the middle (a large waistline, and gastric discomfort after eating), it pays to increase your circulation in the area by taking **Shu Gan Wan.** (Look for a bloated, darker reddish, or purplish tongue and a coating.) Then, after your digestion and circulation improve, you can notice how much your energy recovers.

Heart irregularities and stress-related weakness

- Does your heart feel weak and irregular?
- Do you have anxiety attacks and fatigue?
- Does your energy lag at about 10:00 A.M.?
- Are you pale and listless? Lack enthusiasm?
- Do your hands occasionally feel numb?

For heart irregularity and weakness from stress (pale or purplish tongue), take a hawthorn berry capsule after meals once or twice daily. It tends to gradually lower cholesterol by increasing heart action. Be aware, however, that hawthorn can cause stomach irritation with long-term use. Some prefer to take it every second day. You may require an additional blood pressure remedy. Also see chapter 5 for anticholesterol slimming teas.

For tachycardia resulting from poor diet, stress, or depression, accompanied by pain in the chest (with pale tongue), **Xiao Yao Wan** works wonders. The usual dose is 6 pills after meals, but you can take them anytime for tachycardia. For digestive disturbance leading to bloat, pressure in ribs,

PREVENT FATIGUE!
HERBS FOR MAKING SOUP STOCKS

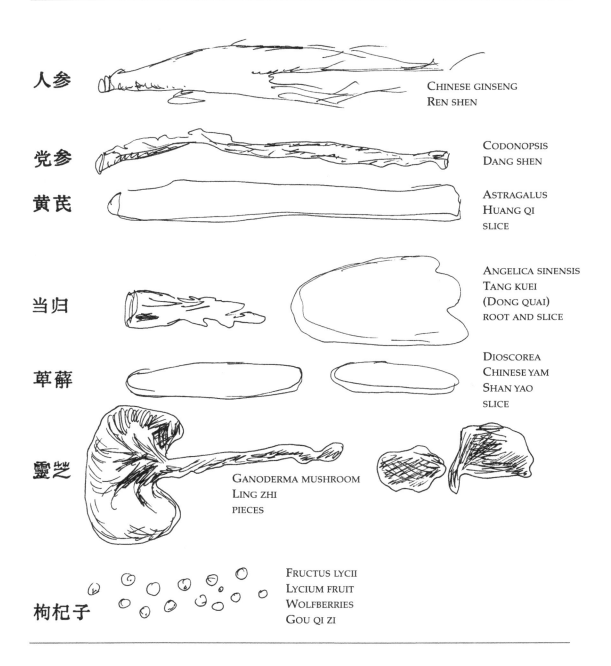

人参   CHINESE GINSENG
REN SHEN

党参   CODONOPSIS
DANG SHEN

黄芪   ASTRAGALUS
HUANG QI
SLICE

当归   ANGELICA SINENSIS
TANG KUEI
(DONG QUAI)
ROOT AND SLICE

草薢   DIOSCOREA
CHINESE YAM
SHAN YAO
SLICE

靈芝   GANODERMA MUSHROOM
LING ZHI
PIECES

枸杞子   FRUCTUS LYCII
LYCIUM FRUIT
WOLFBERRIES
GOU QI ZI

excess fat, and water retention in the abdomen, take **Shu Gan Wan,** 8 pills three times daily, or more if you have serious water retention in the abdomen (ascites).

Overweight

🌿 Do you often eat sweet, creamy, or rich foods?

🌿 Do you frequently suffer from heartburn?

🌿 Do you feel bloated and suffer indigestion more when fatigued?

🌿 Is your cholesterol count too high?

Losing excess fat and water retention is an important factor in heart health. Having a strong, even heartbeat and a low cholesterol count improves not only vitality but also longevity. Given a rich diet and little exercise, it is wise to add lecithin, vinegar, and vitamin B_6 (for water retention) to your diet. This combination of fat-fighters sometimes appears in bodybuilding supplements such as **Razor Cuts,** made by National Health Products.

With a gym-lingo name like **Razor Cuts,** you know it's meant for those who want to lose water weight and turn fat into muscle. It combines lecithin, vinegar, vitamin B_6, and diuretics such as cornsilk, juniper berries, buchu, and parsley, with chromium picolinate, spirulina, and digestive herbs. Follow directions on the bottle.

Even if you don't need a diuretic combination such as this, take at least 1,000 mg daily of lecithin to normalize brain function. Persons who drink coffee or tea require double that dose.

Low energy, indigestion, and low appetite

For chronic indigestion from inadequate acid and enzymes, drink **Yogi Tea** (see page 364), or use digestive remedies from Chinatown or purchased by mail order, such as **Digestive Harmony, Bupleurum S,** or **Bupleurum 12** by Seven Forests, distributed by Health Concerns. **Bupleurum S** treats stomach pain and abdominal bloating, while **Bupleurum 12** treats digestive tension, depression, irritability, nervousness, and cold limbs. Both improve digestion. They can be taken over long periods to help normalize blood sugar, appetite, blood production, and energy.

Blood deficiency fatigue

🌿 Are you pale, or do you have pale lips?

🌿 Are your fingernails brittle or pale, or do they have white spots?

🌿 Do you have a chronic feverish condition or menopause?

🌿 Do you smoke or take drugs?

🌿 Have you recently given birth or had surgery?

🌿 Are you tired after your menstrual period is over?

Fatigue related to blood deficiency is worse after menstruation or blood loss. It is best to build back your health every month by taking a blood tonic. You will need to know if you require a *warming* or *cooling* tonic. The questionnaire in chapter 24 will help in your selection of blood-builders.

For example, for fatigue related to

heart, spleen, and kidney weakness associated with aging, insomnia, palpitations, poor memory, and fatigue, take **Ren Shen Yang Ying Wan** or one of the other blood and energy tonics listed in chapter 25. General tonics such as this can be taken over a long period. Be sure to monitor changes in your energy and tongue.

METAL AND WATER ELEMENTS

Lung inflammation or dryness will in time reduce oxygen intake and energy. It gives you a dry cough and panting shortness of breath. Take measures to stop smoking now. Reduce hot, *drying* foods or those that cause sweating (especially echinacea, ginger, or ma huang) if you have dry cough and thirst.

Cooling *remedies*

- ℘ Do you smoke?
- ℘ Is your throat dry? Do you have dry cough and thirst?
- ℘ Is your skin dry and ashen?
- ℘ Do you pant or breathe very rapidly?
- ℘ Do you have halitosis?

If your tongue is dry and red in the lung area, near the tip (see chapter 11), you may need a *cooling* remedy to ease inflammation, cough, or shortness of breath. Such a remedy will help to ensure healthy tissue, adequate oxygen intake, and calmness.

For example, sweetening recipes and drinks with cubes of **Lo Han Kuo Instant Beverage** cools lung inflammation (for a

dry, reddish tongue). See chapters 29 and 30 for individual problems, including fatigue with fever and sweating.

Exhaustion and cloudy thinking

When you are exhausted, it is hard to take a breath, hard to talk or be social. Then you need to address your intake of oxygen. If you are strong enough, you can take in adequate breath, but exhausted *chi* can lead to chronic imbalance.

Heating *remedies*

- ℘ Do you struggle to inhale?
- ℘ Are you so short of breath, it's hard to sleep when you're lying down?
- ℘ Do you wheeze and cough every morning?
- ℘ Is the mucus watery and white?

For profound fatigue and shortness of breath from lung and adrenal weakness or exhaustion (very pale tongue), TB, asthma with chills and wheezing, or emphysema, you need a remedy that improves your breathing. **Sexoton** (called by a variety of names, including "Ba Wei Di Huang Wan," "Eight Flavor Rehmannia Pill," and "Golden Book Tea") treats spleen and adrenal weakness with abdominal distension, weak digestion with watery stools or urinary incontinence, shortness of breath, cold, clammy hands and feet, sore back, and sexual weakness. It is known as a high-class tonic that fortifies both the *yin* and *yang* of the kidney.

This vegetarian formula contains

rehmannia, dioscorea, evodia, moutan, fu ling, alisma, cinnamon, and prepared aconite. Rehmannia, a blood-builder, is the *di huang* in the name. Other ingredients such as cinnamon and dioscorea, the Chinese yam, warm digestion and ensure absorption. "Leading" herbs such as fu ling and alisma take the *yin*-building herbs (rehmannia) and *yang*-building herbs (cinnamon) to affect the kidneys and adrenal glands.

Ping Chuan Wan, a Chinese patent remedy, deepens your breath and builds *chi.* It contains plant herbs to resolve phlegm and other, more exotic ones to strengthen lungs and kidney energy, such as the fungus cordyceps, and gecko lizard.

A simple home remedy that works well for asthma-related fatigue and shortness of breath is one pinch of clove powder (the kitchen spice) as hot tea. One pinch in a cup of hot water will revive your breath and energy and clear your chest and sinuses with its hot, sweet, pungent flavor. You might keep a bottle of the spice in your pocket during cold weather. A shake of the powder onto your tongue will revive your energy and refresh your breath.

High nutrition in a capsule

Blood-building herbs require *chi*-building herbs to ensure their digestion and absorption. For this purpose I recommend a particularly good combination, **Liquid Ginseng Extract with Royal Jelly,** a nutritious stimulant. Do not use such a stimulant instead of sleep. Rather, cook a piece of ginseng along with soup ingredients and blood-building herbs to improve the general health of the entire family.

I also strongly recommend two excellent capsules that are not complicated formulas, though they are very effective as energy, vitality, and beauty enhancers.

Sherong Sow Woo Wan contains sika deer antler, North Korean ginseng, and polygoni multiflori (shou wu), a major rejuvenating, moistening, blood-building herb. It is recommended for nervous exhaustion, poor circulation, and premature or abnormal whitening of hair due to stress. Dosage is 2 pills twice daily. Even though it contains ginseng, you can take it if your tongue indicates *internal heat* because the herbs are nutritious and neutral in temperature.

Pollen, Ginseng, Ling Zhi Capsules is a favorite of mine because it builds solid nutrition and helps prevent illness, while curbing fatigue. Bee pollen is one of the richest sources of amino acids known, a high-energy food that is very easily absorbed. Ling zhi is a famous health food known in China. Regular use is said to build heart strength and help prevent cancer.

After illness, surgery, or childbirth

A useful Chinese remedy that treats exhaustion following illness, surgery, or childbirth is **Jen Shen Lu Jung Wan.** These pills are recommended for poor appetite, anemia, weak legs and back, mental restlessness, insomnia, spermatorrhea (loss of sperm), heart palpitations, lumbago, sciatica, and poor memory. They come either as a large, gummy pill you can chew twice daily, or in a condensed form (5 pills three times daily is the recommended dosage).

Both forms contain a mixture of plant and animal ingredients, including deer horn in the large pill and deer horn, "tiger bone," and seahorse in the condensed pills. Real tiger bone is, of course, prohibited, and the substituted herb likely comes from a domestic source.

A complex warming *blood and energy builder*

For long-term weakness, chills, sallow complexion, blood deficiency, and poor appetite from mental and physical exhaustion and sexual weakness, you may need to add an additional *heating* tonic from chapter 25 or 34, on sexual remedies. They do more than increase sexual capacity. Often they improve appetite, mental powers, and longevity. I would take them also to improve stamina and well-being after a course of chemotherapy or following surgery or childbirth.

For example, **Tsepao Sanpien Wan** invigorates lungs, spleen, and kidney/ adrenal glands. Expect to use the remedy a long time (perhaps several months) until the exhaustion is reversed, but watch your tongue. You know you have taken enough when your energy is revived and backache is eliminated. You should definitely stop taking it if it makes you nervous, angry, or insomniac.

Brainpower herbs

Our ancestors may have gotten tired from chopping trees or building pyramids, but we get tired from thinking. Brain tonics do more than improve memory; they can prevent serious mental and physical burnout.

A cooling *remedy for "burnt brain" syndrome*

- Are you tired, but jumpy and nervous?
- Do your ears ring (tinnitus)?
- Do you have chronic nerve-related skin rash?
- Do you feel forgetful when you are fatigued?
- Do you have to work late hours with few vacations?

Gotu kola, available as tea or capsules, is well suited to modern stressful living. It cools and nourishes the brain and nervous system without delivering a big jolt of energy. It builds steady vitality, cooling inflammation without increasing phlegm. It works fine all day, and can be used before bed to balance both sides of the brain. For nervous insomnia, it combines well with **Wuchaseng** extract.

I often recommend 6 capsules daily, taken between meals, for students, artists, and businesspeople, or for those who drain themselves daily with thinking.

Ma huang: A warning

You can find Chinese ephedra, or ma huang, in several sorts of health-food store herbal products these days—decongestants, diet aids, and pep pills. I must issue a strong word of warning concerning the general use of ma huang in stimulant formulas: Traditionally it was never intended as an energy tonic or a weight-loss remedy, but instead as a powerful diaphoretic herb. Ma huang increases sweating, speeds metabolism, and can raise blood pressure. It can result in hyperactive thyroid, headaches, dizziness, or tachycardia.

Avoid ma huang if you tend to have *internal heat* conditions, including heart conditions and hypertensions, or feel spacey and out of balance. Never use the herb alone, because combination formulas are safer.

From health-food stores or mail order

A growing number of American health manufacturers have combined traditional Chinese herbs in formulas for popular use. Since they can be used by many people to build a solid foundation of health, they are for long-term vitality. Such energy and blood tonics combine herbs that help restore overstressed organs to ensure stamina and improve immunity to disease. In other words, they are not quick-fix energy boosters.

The herbal formulas listed below are nourishing and support chronic weakness. I list them here even though they are more expensive than traditional patent remedies, because they are widely available and some people prefer their packaging.

Several can be used to reverse chronic illnesses that result in weak muscle strength and poor coordination. Many of the tonic herbs used have adaptogenic qualities. That means the herbs have a homeostatic effect on immune problems, i.e., they can strengthen deficient immune systems or calm overactive ones.

HEALTH CONCERNS

Astra 8, available to the general public from Health Concerns, increases immune strength and energy. It treats fatigue, excess weight loss, chronic lymph swelling, nervousness, diarrhea, night sweats, weakness, chills, lethargy, poor digestion, aching muscles, and adrenal weakness leading to a variety of complaints, including poor concentration. A combination such as **Astra 8** can be used in support of Eastern and Western cancer therapies. It's often recommended for athletes and students to boost performance.

Astra 8 contains astragalus, ligustrum, ganoderma, eleuthero ginseng, codonopsis, schisandra, oryza, Chinese malt, and licorice. All the herbs are *chi* tonics that support the work of astragalus, an herb that has been the subject of much research because of its immune-enhancing ability. For digestive disorders and weakness, **Astra 8** can be combined with **Digestive Harmony,** also from Health Concerns.

NUTRITIONAL LIFE SUPPORT SYSTEMS

This company, located in San Diego, makes **Emperors Restoration** for deficient energy and blood due to stress and anxiety. The formula combines traditional tonic herbs that support nutrition and circulation.

Ginseng Root Compound contains Chinese ginseng and *yin* tonics such as lychii fruit and the *chi* tonics astragalus and schisandra.

Oxygen Acquisition builds lung *chi* for fatigue related to shortness or loss of breath on minor exertion, and weak voice. Possible causes are weak constitution, chronic degenerative lung disease, and stress. **Oxygen Acquisition** contains poligonati, schisandra, platycodum, ophiopogonis, panax ginseng, pseudostellaria, ligusticum wallichi, lily bulb, and licorice.

Nourish treats general weakness from poor digestion, illness, overwork, emotional stress, and advanced age. It builds *chi* and blood.

Two Tigers "helps prevent short- and long-term burnout." A *chi-* and blood-builder, it strengthens internal organs and slows premature aging. It is appropriate for persons weakened by long illness, congenital factors, or damaging lifestyle.

CRYSTAL STAR

Crystal Star, in Sonoma, makes several energy remedies, including **Ginsengs of the World, Ginseng 6 Restorative Caps,** and **High Energy Tea.** This last contains gotu kola, red clover, damiana, American ginseng, kava kava, red raspberry, peppermint, and cloves. It's *heating.*

Other energy combinations from Crystal Star include **Hi Performance,** used for stamina. Similar to other combinations for bodybuilders, it contains Siberian ginseng, which in high doses is a source of testosterone. The formula has herbs for nutrition—bee pollen, sarsaparilla, gotu kola, licorice, dandelion, wild yam, yarrow, al-falfa, yeast, spirulina, barley grass, and ginger—as well as the *heating* energy stimulants ma huang and capsicum. Ornithine and arginine are amino acids that speed metabolism. In this formula, high nutrition, found in pollen, alfalfa, and spirulina, combine with herbal *heat* and *speed* (pepper and ma huang).

Be sure to drink adequate fluids and avoid the use of *heating* stimulants if you have a red, dry tongue indicating dehydration, fever, or night sweats.

Finally, from Crystal Star, **Rainforest Energy Caps** help shorten healing time from injury, fight fatigue, and prevent depression. This eclectic combination adds stimulant and digestive herbs to nutritional sources that could be helpful for recovery from addictions and stress.

This formula blends guarna seed, kola nut, suma, bee pollen, ginger, capsicum, astragalus, and 30 mg of L. glutamine. The recommended daily dose of L. glutamine is 1 to 4 grams (1,000 to 4,000 mg). It's the natural source of glutamine and glutamic acid, a brain fuel for improved intelligence. Avoid this *warming* tonic if you tend to have headaches or rashes.

Quick-energy herbs

Ampoules of bee pollen, royal jelly, or ginseng are now ubiquitous in food and herb markets, and present an up-to-date health substitute for fattening snacks.

Also highly recommended for quick energy is **Vrrooom Power Tabs.** With a name like that, you know it comes from California! Health Concerns, in Oakland, makes and distributes it. It offers quick relief for acute fatigue without sacrificing balance. I like the company's approach, described in an accompanying brochure: "This formula can neutralize the burnout induced by overuse of ma huang and caffeine-containing stimulants. The herbs and nutrient companions [used] are the perfect antidote for the diet and lifestyles of most Americans."

Some of the herbs in **Vrrooom Power** help decrease water retention, while moistening tissues dried by consumption of sweet or fried foods and alcohol. Other ingredients settle nerves and boost energy. The combination contains wild yam (dioscorea); L. phenylalanine; isosine; pyridoxal alpha ketoglutarate (which helps convert blood sugar into energy, calm the nerves, and increase oxygen in the tissues); prince ginseng (pseudostellaria) and white yam (which help promote fluid balance); and a couple of others, including malt and oryza, which help the ingredients to affect digestion. Such a balanced formula provides help for people who are fried from too much work, worry, or good times.

THE LONG VIEW

There is an important link to understand between this chapter and chapter 33, on insomnia. I have already mentioned that many energy tonics treat insomnia because increasing *chi* and blood improves both. What underlies this phenomenon is an important concept: Health is a gradual process. We are easily misled by words. Fatigue and insomnia are real events that took time to develop. Not coincidentally, they also take time to reverse, because the body needs time to heal.

To be more specific, an energy tonic will sometimes cause sleepiness for a while because the body needs rest and nourishment before it can be stimulated. As we have seen, what we mean by adequate rest and nourishment is in part individually determined.

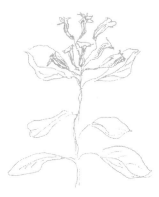

Clove

FATIGUE

What makes it worse?

Illness, overwork, stimulants, pollution, stress, emotional upheaval, and diet leading to indigestion and circulation problems.

Causes of fatigue according to the Five Elements

Fire: stimulants, thyroid or hormonal problems (mania), anxiety, fat/sweet diet, age

Earth: sweet/fat diet, thyroid imbalance, worry, lack of exercise, coffee

Metal: phlegm-producing diet, cold weather, grief

Water: overwork, too much sex, hormone imbalances, caffeine, fear, age, jet lag, weak immune strength

HEAT SYMPTOMS	*COLD* SYMPTOMS	*PHLEGM*
mania, insomnia	depression, insomnia	indigestion
palpitations	pallor, weakness	shortness of breath
anxiety, anger	obsession, fear	cloudy thinking
rashes, headache	rheumatism	

REMEDIES

Herbal stimulants that are

Cooling or neutral	*warming*	digestive
gotu kola	Chinese ginseng	**Xiao Yao Wan**
Vrrooom Power	**Tzepao Sanpien Wan**	
	Ren Shen Yang Ying Wan	

For adrenal weakness (aching back, sexual fatigue, poor concentration, lethargy, pale tongue and face), *warming* remedies: **Tzepao Sanpien Wan, Astra 8**

For blood deficiency or anemia associated with menstruation or childbirth, diabetes, hypoglycemia (pallor, weakness, depression):
Warming or *cooling* blood tonics (see chapter 25)
Warming: **Sexoton**
Cooling: **Liu Wei Di Huang Wan**

For asthmatic weakness and phlegm congestion:
Ping Chuan Wan, clove tea

西洋參 西洋參 西洋參 西洋參 西洋參 西洋參 西洋參 西洋參 西洋參

[xīyángshēn] American ginseng; radix panacis quinquefolii; radix ginseng americana.
The drug consists of the root of Panax quinquefolium L. (family Araliaceae).

32
The Ginsengs: A Root for All Seasons

Ginseng, long praised by Asians as a panacea, has become as familiar as vitamins. The North American ginseng story began during the eighteenth century, when Iroquois Indians near the Great Lakes trapped for fur and gathered the man-shaped root for trade with both the French and English in exchange for guns and liquor. A few medicine men complained that braves would forget their hunting skills because they spent so much time gathering roots. In the nineteenth century, ginseng was sent to China from a port in my New York neighborhood, Chelsea. Today ginseng is grown in Wisconsin and Vermont,

FIVE GINSENGS

LISTED BELOW ARE COMMON NAMES, FORMS FOUND, AND FUNCTIONS

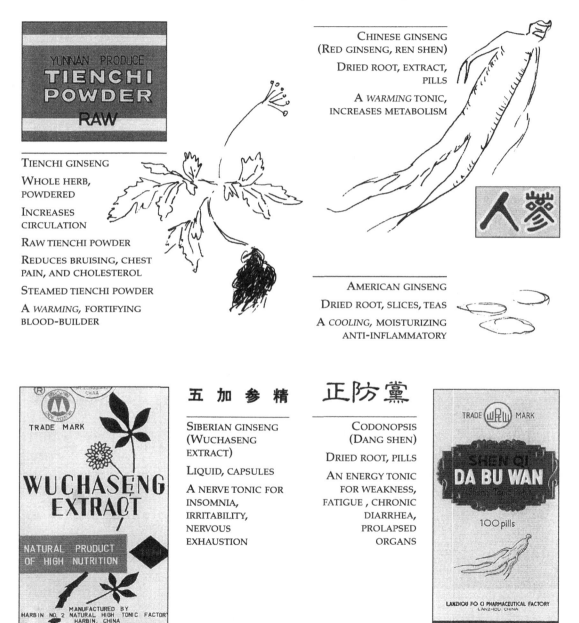

YUNNAN PRODUCE
TIENCHI POWDER
RAW

TIENCHI GINSENG

WHOLE HERB, POWDERED

INCREASES CIRCULATION

RAW TIENCHI POWDER

REDUCES BRUISING, CHEST PAIN, AND CHOLESTEROL

STEAMED TIENCHI POWDER

A *WARMING*, FORTIFYING BLOOD-BUILDER

CHINESE GINSENG
(RED GINSENG, REN SHEN)

DRIED ROOT, EXTRACT, PILLS

A *WARMING* TONIC, INCREASES METABOLISM

AMERICAN GINSENG

DRIED ROOT, SLICES, TEAS

A *COOLING*, MOISTURIZING ANTI-INFLAMMATORY

TRADE MARK

WUCHASENG EXTRACT

NATURAL PRODUCT OF HIGH NUTRITION

MANUFACTURED BY
HARBIN NO. 2 NATURAL HIGH TONIC FACTORY
HARBIN, CHINA

五 加 参 精

SIBERIAN GINSENG
(WUCHASENG EXTRACT)

LIQUID, CAPSULES

A NERVE TONIC FOR INSOMNIA, IRRITABILITY, NERVOUS EXHAUSTION

正防黨

CODONOPSIS
(DANG SHEN)

DRIED ROOT, PILLS

AN ENERGY TONIC FOR WEAKNESS, FATIGUE , CHRONIC DIARRHEA, PROLAPSED ORGANS

TRADE MARK

SHEN QI
DA BU WAN
(Shen Qi Tonic Pills)

100 pills

LANZHOU FO CI PHARMACEUTICAL FACTORY
LANZHOU CHINA

but the root derives its name not from its origin, but from its type. Ginseng refers to several different plants variously called Chinese ginseng (panax ginseng); American ginseng (panax quinquefolium); Siberian ginseng (eleuthero); dang shen (codonopsis); and tienchi (pseudoginseng). All the ginsengs have unique qualities and are not interchangeable. In fact, the types and temperatures of plants in the ginseng family vary enough to provide a root for all seasons.

The five kinds of ginseng sold by Asian merchants fall into these categories: *warming* (speeds metabolism), *cooling* and moistening, neutral (neither *warming* nor *cooling*), those that affect the nervous system, and others that increase circulation. Some forms of ginseng are referred to as "red" or "white." In general, red ginseng is a stimulant, while white is moistening and anti-inflammatory. Usually the root is tonic (builds energy), and the leaves and flowers are moistening (increase saliva).

The country of origin has nothing to do with ginseng's quality or properties. Whether it's Chinese, American, Siberian, or Korean is not as important as its energetic effects, its "temperature," and its color.

You can use the ginsengs as seasonal remedies if you have no overpowering energetic imbalances (such as *internal heat*) that might prohibit their use.

Chinese ginseng: During cold weather, use a *warming* or neutral form of ginseng to increase energy and vitality.
American ginseng: In summer or for hot, dry conditions such as radiator steam heat, use this *cooling,* moistening form of ginseng.
Tienchi ginseng: In spring, use tienchi to stir circulation, reduce blood lipids, and ease muscle soreness.
Siberian ginseng: In autumn, Siberian ginseng helps you adapt to stress, to relax and sleep better.

The correct use of these ginsengs will vary depending upon the local weather conditions as well as your individual energetic needs.

Ren Shen: Stimulant/ **Warming/*Red***

- Are you chronically weak?
- Do you have slow metabolism?
- Do you have low blood pressure?
- Are you overweight, with global water retention?
- Is your tongue large, pale, puffy, scalloped?
- Are you frequently short of breath?
- Do you feel low enthusiasm or experience sexual fatigue?

Chinese ginseng (in Latin, panax ginseng; in Chinese, ren shen) is the best-known Oriental herb. It's considered a panacea for fatigue and aging because it stimulates energy and metabolism as a *warming* tonic. Chinese ginseng (ren shen) is best used by those with a pale, puffy tongue indicating slow metabolism. It helps reduce global water retention by stimulating energy.

Runners, bodybuilders, and martial-arts students use Chinese ginseng for endurance and strength. According to traditional Chinese medicine, ren shen also increases blood volume, promotes life and appetite, quiets the spirit, and gives wisdom. It treats anemia, shortness of breath, spontaneous perspiration, nervous anxiety, forgetfulness, and impotence stemming from weakness.

It contains saponins, carbohydrates, sugars, organic acids, nitrogenous substances, amino acids, vitamins, and minerals. A lot of research has been done here and abroad to prove ginseng's effectiveness as a strengthener, anticonvulsant, antipsychotic, digestive, and energy and brain rejuvenator. It contains antioxidants that decrease liver and eye diseases, atherosclerosis, and nerve aging. Research is being done on its use in treating diabetes and geriatric illnesses.

Ren shen should not be used by anyone with high blood pressure, headache, fever, or flu symptoms. Because panax stimulates all aspects of metabolism and endocrine function, it speeds the heartbeat and encourages hunger, faster breathing, and insomnia. Ren shen is believed to promote longevity because it improves weakness resulting from aging. But not everyone

ages in the same way: If you have a dry red tongue or one with a thick yellow coating, chronic fever, hot flashes, or night sweats, avoid Chinese ginseng altogether; it is too strong a stimulant.

DAILY USE OF CHINESE GINSENG

Most westerners use Chinese ginseng like jet fuel, to drive themselves beyond their capacity. But that's a mistake. Chinese ginseng should not be used to replace rest. It's a nutritive tonic that has, for generations, been added to stew pots in China with vegetables and meats. In soup stock, a ginseng root helps digest starch and protein. One quarter teaspoon of ginseng powder or liquid extract can be added to tea.

In traditional patent remedies, ren shen is often combined with hard-to-digest herbs in order to ease their absorption. It treats chronic problems such as lethargy and low blood pressure, not acute fatigue symptoms. Therefore, if you are weak, anemic, or undernourished and have *internal cold* symptoms (but not the common cold!), I advise you to include Chinese ginseng as an ingredient in your *warming*, fortifying soups.

Si Yang Seng: *Moistening*/**Cooling**/*White*

🌿 Do you need more saliva? Are you often thirsty?

🍃 Is your skin dry and parched?

🍃 Do you have chronic fever, menopausal hot flashes?

🍃 Do you smoke, or take drying acne medications?

🍃 Have you recently had a fever and now need moisturizing?

American ginseng, once abundant on rocky, shaded slopes from Quebec to Appalachia and Florida, is now endangered. It is cultivated by the Tenren company in Wisconsin. American ginseng is a white ginseng (in Latin, panax quinquefolium), sweeter tasting than Chinese ginseng, with anti-inflammatory properties.

The person who needs American ginseng the most has a dry, red tongue (possibly with a thick yellow or dark coating), thirst, dry mouth, ruddy complexion, or chronic fever. Since we can get drier as we get older, it pays to replenish natural juices with American ginseng. In the long run it is calming and beautifying, because it renews internal organs while refreshing the body fluids.

It was highly prized in the nineteenth century by a number of American Indian tribes. The Penobscots steeped the root to make an infusion to increase fertility in women. (Modern research has shown that ginseng increases the weight of seminal vesicles and prostate glands, and enhances sperm counts and fertility.) The Menominees used the root as an energy tonic and to strengthen mental powers. The root is stimulant and stomachic. It gently energizes the central nervous system, has anti-fatigue action, and can increase motor activity. It stimulates DNA and RNA production and protein synthesis. Several species of ginseng help us to adapt visually to darkness, to tolerate high and low temperatures, and to increase work efficiency.

Traditional Chinese doctors recommend American ginseng tea made from either the root or leaves, after fever, in order to cool the body by increasing fluids, especially saliva. If you're often thirsty, have a dry cough, or smoke, this should be your choice among ginsengs. American ginseng is appropriate for anyone who is weak and tends to have systemic inflammatory symptoms such as hot flashes and night sweats. It cools and refreshes while strengthening the body. This makes it an important remedy for menopause and chronic fever illness such as AIDS or diabetes. It has been recommended for excess uterine bleeding, nosebleeds, and blood in the urine and stools from *internal heat*.

Older Asians drink American ginseng tea daily as a beautifying rejuvenator that refines the skin and diminishes dryness, patchy areas, wrinkles, and fragile capillaries. In China it is also a popular remedy for excess drinking.

HOW TO PREPARE AMERICAN GINSENG

Make a tea from sliced American ginseng root, or enjoy a cup or two of the instant granules (sold in health-food stores) after drinking alcohol, in order to detoxify the body.

American ginseng is sold in many forms: The whole root can be cooked in soup stock or steeped as tea, one half teaspoon of powder to a cup of boiling water. For variety, you might add the powder to juices. The dried root is often sold on the street by Chinese vendors, and is also found in herb shops, sold as thick roots, as long, thin "tails," or powdered. If you don't enjoy the taste of the tea, put the powdered root or instant granules into empty capsules bought at the health-food store, and take several a day.

You can even find American ginseng chewing gum sold at Asian fruit and vegetable stands. Named **Haitai,** it's actually made with Korean white ginseng, named after the country that grows and sells it, not for its type. There is nothing better to chew while flying in an airplane: It refreshes and cools you, increases saliva, and unplugs your ears.

Dang Shen: Chi Tonic/ Neutral/White

🌿 Do you have chronic diarrhea?

🌿 Do your legs feel weak or frail?

🌿 Do you have vaginal bleeding related to fatigue?

🌿 Do you have prolapsed uterus or rectum after surgery or illness?

🌿 Do you have frequent colds or allergies?

A neutral ginseng called dang shen (in Latin, *codonopsis*) strengthens energy without increasing inflammation. It is said to tonify and lift *chi* and therefore is used for prolapsed organs and chronic diarrhea from weakness. It has also been recommended for lack of appetite, fatigue, tired limbs, chronic cough, and shortness of breath. It "nourishes fluids" and so has been used for diabetes.

Dang shen is included in several weight-loss herbal formulas such as **Keep Fit Remove Fat Pills.** It turns fat into muscle by strengthening digestion and speeding metabolism. Western research has found that dang shen improves performance and increases red blood count and hemoglobin. In general, its functions are analogous to those of Chinese ginseng, though it is not as strong or *warming.*

HOW TO USE DANG SHEN

If you suffer from colds, flu, allergies, or general weakness, with shortness of breath and chronic diarrhea, prepare a fortifying soup using dang shen and astragalus, before cold season strikes. It will prevent fatigue and weakness (but not treat frequent colds and allergies). This remedy for chronic weakness is easy to make. Add a handful of each herb to a ceramic-coated pot along with 1 quart of springwater, and simmer the ingredients for forty-five minutes. You can drink 3 cups per day between meals.

Wu Cha Seng: Nerve Tonic/Warming/Red

- Are you nervous and insomniac?
- Are you very anxious?
- Are you under tremendous stress?
- Do you get tired and cranky from very hot or cold weather?
- Do you have menopausal irritability?
- Do you get tired from exercise or work, and become unable to rest?

Siberian ginseng, Eleutherococcus senticosus, has been known as "touch-me-not," "devil's shrub," "wild pepper," and "eleuthero." Chinese forms of wu cha seng first became available in America in the 1970s, but the plant was mentioned in Chinese herbal literature as early as two thousand years ago. I recommend the liquid extract from China, **Wuchaseng,** available in herb shops and by mail order.

Traditional Chinese medicine considers Siberian ginseng a nerve tonic—i.e., it treats nervous disorders. It is recommended for stress, anxiety, and insomnia, and is an important adjunct remedy during menopause or chronic debilitating illness such as AIDS and cancer.

It grows wild in northeastern Asia, including the former Soviet Union, China, Korea, and Japan, with the major producing region being the northern Chinese province of Heilongjiang (formerly part of Manchuria). But seedlings have been introduced as far west as Montana and Oregon.

Soviet clinical studies done in the 1960s, involving more than 2,100 normal and stressed persons, established Siberian ginseng as an adaptogen, a medicinal substance that increases resistance to adverse influences. Since then, Siberian ginseng has been widely used by Soviet deep-sea divers, mine and mountain rescue teams, explorers, soldiers, factory workers, cosmonauts, athletes, and anyone else who wished to reduce stress from damaging heat, noise, motion, excess work, or exercise. Significant improvement was noted in auditory functions, in mental alertness, and in both the quality and quantity of work accomplished and performance achieved under stressful conditions.

Another Russian study, done with more than 2,200 people, showed improvements and, in some cases, total normalization of symptoms with few side effects for a wide variety of ailments, including neuroses, atherosclerosis, several forms of diabetes, hypertension, hypotension, chronic bronchitis, cancers, acute head trauma, and rheumatic heart disease.

HOW TO USE SIBERIAN GINSENG

The dosage affects the herb's action—a smaller dose being sedative, and a larger one stimulating. This may be true of other adaptogens as well. For example, one teaspoon of **Wuchaseng** liquid extract is recommended before bed for nervous insomnia and anxiety. This should be taken as needed during times of stress. When anxiety and insomnia are reversed, the herb can be stopped. I've noted with several of my clients that continuing the herb after its period of effectiveness has produced excess energy, even restlessness and irritability.

Cautions

Athletes take a higher-dose energy booster found in Siberian ginseng capsules for sale in health-food stores. Some bodybuilding formulas made with an unusually high concentration of Siberian ginseng are so strong they may eventually affect hormone function, producing extra testosterone. It's wiser for women to take **Wuchaseng** (the liquid extract—not the capsules) or a balanced herbal formula, because extra male hormone could possibly effect secondary sex changes or create problems in menstrual cycles. Individual dosage is always required. Start with a low or minimum dose, pay attention to the results, and watch changes in the tongue.

Tienchi: Circulation Stimulant/Warming and Cooling/Black

- Do you have bruises, swelling, or pain from injury?
- Do you have chronic chest pains from poor circulation?
- Is your cholesterol count high?
- Are you anemic, with *internal cold* symptoms?
- Do you have colitis? Bleeding gums?

Pseudoginseng (tienchi) is another one of those Chinese miracle herbs that seem to do everything. It was valued more than gold by ancient doctors. Long-term use reduces stress as an adaptogen does, but it is known primarily for its ability to increase blood circulation. Both raw and steamed forms are used internally for treating wounds, pain, and bruises.

Raw Tienchi Powder is *cooling*, reduces cholesterol buildup around the heart, and contains a natural corticosteroid that reduces inflammation and pain. It also stirs circulation to reduce bruising quite effectively, although it requires several days' use. I have found it to be a near-miracle remedy for persons with colitis or bleeding gums.

HOW TO USE *COOLING* RAW TIENCHI POWDER

Persons with a dry, reddish tongue are advised to add one half teaspoon to a cup of *cool* water daily. Hot water cooks it and changes its effects. I've found the raw herb to have good results among clients with chronic bleeding gums and tooth infections, and in higher doses for colitis (usually 1 to 2 teaspoons per day for acute colitis). It speeds healing of bruises and is often helpful for inflammatory joint pain.

For chronic fever and bleeding symptoms

Raw tienchi could be a good daily remedy during menopause, for chronic fever, or with bleeding symptoms such as excess uterine bleeding or blood in urine, sputum, or stools, and bleeding ulcers. Use it if the bleeding is accompanied by fever, or if pain feels hot and throbbing.

STEAMED TIENCHI IS WARMING

Steamed Tienchi Powder is a blood tonic that increases circulation and reduces pain due to blood stasis. Add prepared **Steamed Tienchi Powder** to hot tea if your tongue is pale and your complexion sallow, if cold makes pain worse, and if exercise or increased circulation makes it better. Try one or two cups per day, depending upon the effects. You will immediately feel warmed as your circulation improves.

Menstrual pains

Either raw or steamed, tienchi powder can be used to correct menstrual pain, depending upon the symptoms. We discuss such pain symptoms in relevant chapters. The most frequent use of tienchi is in capsule form.

A MIRACLE CURE FOR INJURY

Both raw and steamed forms of tienchi are combined with five other herbs in a formula called **Yunnan Paiyao** to stop hemorrhaging and speed healing (see chapter 18). Take **Yunnan Paiyao** capsules after surgery, injury, or a tough gym workout—anytime you are sore, stiff, injured, bruised, or severely bleeding.

Tienchi flowers

Essence of Tienchi Flowers, an instant drink, is available in food and herb shops in Chinatown. The flowers' anti-inflammatory action treats bilious liver symptoms such as headache, nausea, stiff jaw, grinding teeth during sleep, anger, insomnia, hypertension, and skin blemishes due to liver inflammation. This form of ginseng flower is sweet enough to be used as a sugar substitute.

The Root of the Problem

The ginsengs offer a full spectrum of herbal cures ranging from *heating* tonics to *cooling*, moistening rejuvenators, to cures for acute injury and chronic inflammation. They have so many benefits for improving metabolism and healing that it makes sense to take them often. The problem is to choose the right kind for you.

When you use Asian diagnosis to determine your choice, the ginsengs can be combined with foods in soup stocks for daily meals. Or they might be enjoyed as a delicious sweet treat. For example, when Chinese ginseng is combined with a rich nutritional supplement such as royal jelly, it makes a time-tested "thousand-year tonic."

33
Herbals for Insomnia

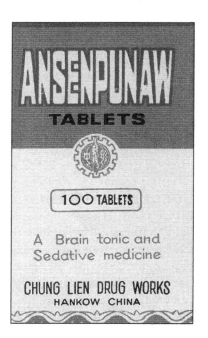

ANSENPUNAW TABLETS

100 TABLETS

A Brain tonic and Sedative medicine

CHUNG LIEN DRUG WORKS
HANKOW CHINA

"Why Can't You Sleep, Honey?"

Are you restless? Overtired? Can't stop thinking? Millions of Americans suffer from insomnia. Many take over-the-counter drugs, drink warm milk, or watch David Letterman. This can cause them to wake up groggy, out of sorts, or congested, depending upon several factors, including Letterman's opening monologue. We will approach the problem of insomnia by redefining Asian concepts concerning the *humors.* Although the ancients could not take such factors as modern illnesses, street drugs, environmental pollution, or jet lag into consideration, they did describe insomnia in terms of physical and mental imbalance. Chinese medicine holds that insomnia results from a deficiency of blood, *yin,* or *chi,* and also from disturbed *shen* (emotional problems). Given this rationale, Chinese insomnia cures endeavor to increase blood, body fluids, and digestive energy, or to repair nerve tissue or adrenal strength.

Ayurveda believes that insomnia and indeed all discomfort stems from problems concerning *wind, bile,* and *phlegm.* Understanding such imbalances helps in the choice of remedies by determining individual needs. But we can't really understand the effects of the *humors* on insomnia or anything else until we redefine them in terms of the modern world.

Wind-induced insomnia can be translated into nervous exhaustion; *bile*-provoked insomnia involves inflammation or blood deficiency; and *phlegm* insomnia can be the result of eating too much, too late at night. Each requires a different remedy, and curing one kind can make another kind worse.

Nervous Exhaustion and Wind Insomnia, or "Anyone for Tennis?"

- Do you often feel agitated or have a nervous twitch?
- Do you use coffee or other stimulants daily?
- Do you have jet lag?
- Do you frequently lie awake, unable to stop thinking?

Persons who experience too much *wind* energy overstimulate the nervous system. They use stimulants, extreme diets, high emotions, and excess physical activity to drive them. When they lie awake at night, unable to sleep, they're likely thinking of work, wooing a lover, drinking their tenth cup of coffee, or planning their entire life. Perhaps they are cleaning house, telephoning friends, or watching late-night movies. In short, they don't know when to quit because they are suffering from nervous exhaustion.

Chinese traditional doctors explain nervous insomnia as a deficiency of blood and *chi.* When the body is exhausted, we can maintain neither physical nor emotional health. When weakness results from illness, stress, or injury, both blood and energy production become impaired, and eventually hormone balance suffers. We receive nourishment and energy from food and oxygen, but require a healthy metabolism in order to have adequate *chi.* The vicious cycle of fatigue, weakness, and insomnia, prompting more fatigue, gets out of hand at some point, so that many people will take a sedative. But that doesn't correct the underlying nutritional weakness. In other words, the body must be adequately nourished and strong to be able to rest, but most often people just try to quiet their nerves.

NERVINES (*WARMING*, MOISTURIZING, AND SEDATIVE)

For insomnia resulting from excess *wind*, Ayurveda recommends nervines, which are herbal sedatives—for example, one or two capsules of valerian before bed. I like to use valerian for simple nervous insomnia as well as for nerve pain (neuralgia) during winter and to eliminate dizziness after flying. This is because, even though it is slightly *warming* in effect, it calms and settles nervous inflammation.

Many popular over-the-counter sleep remedies contain valerian. For example, Zand makes a well-rounded combination of sedative and digestive herbs called **Valerian Herbal.** Available in health-food stores, it combines valerian, passionflower, and skullcap to sedate nervous insomnia, along with chamomile and bupleurum for digestion.

Crystal Star makes a combination called **Night Caps,** capsules containing valerian, skullcap, passionflower, kava kava, hops, carrot crystals (a source of calcium), and other vitamins and minerals needed for deep sleep. Both combinations are useful for calming nervous irritation. The dosage for **Night Caps** includes these directions: "Take 2 caps before retiring. Use for two to three weeks at a time if needed, then rest for a week to allow for body rebalance between courses." This points up the fact that the body can become habituated to a nerve remedy. In fact, the necessary dosage depends upon its desired healing effects.

A little dose will do

To be more specific, you should use caution in taking nervines because their sedative effect varies with the dosage. One or two capsules of valerian work as a nerve sedative, although a higher dose becomes a nerve stimulant and can result in restlessness and nightmares. In the same way, we learned in chapter 32 that a low dose of Siberian ginseng liquid extract (**Wuchaseng**) is a sedative for anxiety and insomnia, while a concentrated dose, found in capsules and in bodybuilding formulas, stimulates energy. A nerve sedative, when overused or taken in higher doses, can become a nerve stimulant.

I once recommended **Wuchaseng** for a friend going through a crisis. It helped him sleep for a few weeks while he was particularly stressed. Believing that more would work better, he continued the teaspoon of **Wuchaseng** before bed for a couple of additional weeks, long after his nervous anxiety had healed. The result was that his energy became so high, he developed insomnia and irritability.

The rule of thumb is this: For nervousness or insomnia, use an herbal nerve sedative only as you need it. Start with one capsule of valerian powder or 10 drops of extract, and wait at least one half hour to feel the results. If you still need a nerve sedative, take another dose an hour after the first. Unlike drugs, herbs may not be physically addictive, but they do have their optimum dose and period of effectiveness. Improper use can result in imbalances.

If a nerve sedative makes you feel relaxed, but you still can't sleep, it is likely that other factors are at work. You may be feeling the enervating effects of blood deficiency or troubled emotions.

Blood-Deficiency Insomnia

🍃 Do you have insomnia after your menstrual period?

🍃 Do you stay awake because your ears ring?

🍃 Do heart palpitations keep you awake?

🍃 Do you wake up feverish or anxious?

🍃 Do you feel tense and weak?

Imagine yourself stretched out on a bed, breathing deeply and smoothly, your muscles long and relaxed. You feel refreshed and light, as though floating on water. Your eyes are heavy. You feel calm, quiet, and sleepy. That's how adequate *yin* feels. It nourishes and moisturizes body/mind/spirit. With blood and fluid deficiency, the opposite occurs: You feel tense, tight, hot, thirsty, and anxious.

Herbal formulas for this type of insomnia treat troubled emotions (agitated *shen*) by improving blood quality and moderating heart action. Often they contain mineral sources, such as oyster shell for calcium, along with blood tonics that reduce dehydration and reduce stress. They can strengthen circulation and calm anxiety by moderating the heart. We can thus improve normal waking and sleeping patterns with nourishing herbs. The following selection of formulas is useful for insomnia resulting from blood deficiency, worry, and stress.

INSOMNIA HERBS THAT BUILD BLOOD AND REDUCE STRESS

Certain blood-building remedies reduce inflammation to treat dizziness and poor memory as well as restlessness, palpitations, and nightmares. Ingredients include blood tonics, herbal mineral supplements, and sedatives.

One such insomnia remedy, available in health-food stores, is **Emperors Restoration,** made by Nutritional Life Support Systems in San Diego. It is said to support the heart and promote calm.

Chinese patent remedies recommended for restlessness and insomnia include **An Mien Pian** ("Peaceful Sleep Tablets"), **Cerebral Tonic Pills, Ding Xin Wan** ("Calm Heart Pill"), **Tian Wang Bu Xin Wan** ("Emperor's Tea"), and **Jian Nao Wan** ("Healthy Brain Pills"). In most cases, a couple of weeks' usage is necessary to support normal heart functions and calm high emotions, but there are exceptions.

"The better to bite you with, my dear"

I cannot guarantee that herbal insomnia pills will always have the same effect. Although they may not always induce sleep, they will certainly promote calm. I remember once recommending **Ding Xin Wan** to a lady insomniac. A razor-thin, hard-driving, high-strung actress, she enjoyed staying awake to read Victorian novels. She shared her apartment with her lover, a good-natured Irish carpenter. While she read *Wuthering Heights,* he drank Budweiser and watched Charlie Chaplin. She ate a macrobiotic diet, and he smoked cigars. She told me that she took **Ding Xin Wan** pills, not to help her sleep, but because they cleared her mind so she could argue with him better.

This proves that not all insomnia is caused by stress. Taking "knockout drops" that sedate the heart, muscles, or nervous system will not cure insomnia if the cause is more complicated. Another possible complication is that insomnia can stem from anger or indigestion. A liver remedy might have helped both problems.

Inflammation and Bilious Insomnia, or "You Are What You Heat"

✍ Do you get headaches, rashes, boils, or cold sores?

✍ Do your palms feel hot?

✍ Do you grind your teeth during sleep?

✍ Do you have insomnia because of anger or frustration?

✍ Do you frequently experience nausea, dizziness, or palpitations?

✍ Do you feel overheated or look flushed?

Biliousness refers to more than bile. It refers to a set of complaints that arise when bile cannot flow, aiding later stages of digestion, clearing tension, chest pain, excess acid, and irritability. Asian doctors think of bilious

conditions as energy that is "hot and stuck."

Bilious insomniacs often stay awake late, aggravating themselves over people and things, cooking hot, spicy foods, or suffering pain. For headaches, rashes, and nervousness that result from stuck bile, naturopaths recommend laxatives. For insomnia, though, a laxative may not be the cure.

Bile-type persons tend to overheat, but they need *cooling* brain and nerve tonics, not sedatives. One excellent remedy is gotu kola, which cools and clears the mind. Gotu kola (in Latin, Hydrocotyle asiatica; in Chinese, man t'ien hsing) is a rejuvenative nervine recommended for nervous disorders, including epilepsy, senility, and premature aging. As a brain tonic, it is said to aid intelligence and memory. It strengthens the adrenal glands while cleansing the blood to treat skin impurities. The herb does so many things that in India it is called *brahmi,* that which imparts knowledge of the supreme reality. It is an aid for meditation that is said to balance the two sides of the brain. It is particularly helpful for super-stressed city folk who feel as though they're juggling both sides of the brain.

Chinese patent remedies that treat insomnia resulting from fatigue and inflammation include **Eight Flavor Tea** ("Anemarrhena, Phellodendron Eight Flavor Pill" or "Zhi Bai Ba Wei Wan") and **Er Ming Zuo Ci Wan,** a variation of **Six Flavor Tea.** Ingredients include antifever herbs as well as *cooling,* blood-building herbs to treat a variety of symptoms such as night sweats, heat in the soles of the feet or in the palms, insomnia, and high blood pressure. Take these while the symptoms last. You should also reduce all stimulants such as coffee, cigarettes, hot spices, and hot debates before bed.

Indigestion and Phlegm Insomnia, or "Make Mine Mit Schlag"

- 𝒻ᴀ Do you toss and turn at night with a stomachache?
- 𝒻ᴀ Do you awaken at dawn with cramps or diarrhea?
- 𝒻ᴀ Do you suffer from chronic excess mucus or stuffed sinus?
- 𝒻ᴀ Do you feel bloated or congested after meals?
- 𝒻ᴀ Do you eat before bed or take a nap after eating?

A little phlegm can be a wonderful thing. It makes us feel heavy, dull, and sleepy. But persons with the *phlegm* body type already make too much. When they're insomniac, it's usually from slow digestion, eating the wrong thing at the wrong time. Often digestive remedies or aromatic decongestant herbs are required before sleep is possible.

Sleep remedies for indigestion insomnia can be either *warming* or *cooling*. *Warming* digestive herbs such as basil, bayberry, and eucalyptus work best for persons with weakness, chills, and sinus congestion. They may be tired and achy, with pale tongues and low pulses. It's hard for them to sleep because it's hard to breathe and their *chi* is low. Insomniacs with joint and muscle pain from cold, damp weather should take a cap-

sule of myrrh or a cup of cinnamon tea to sweat out the cold well before bedtime. A few bay leaves brewed with a pinch of cloves makes an aromatic digestive tea for persons with *internal cold*. It's especially good for insomnia from indigestion, depression, and shortness of breath. (Look for a very pale, scalloped tongue.)

Cooling digestive nervines such as catnip, chamomile, jasmine, peppermint, spearmint, and vervain work well for people with both *phlegm* and inflammation. (Look for a reddish tongue with a thick yellow coating.)

One major problem for people with poor digestion is that excess *phlegm* makes it difficult to think clearly. They may not be able to figure out which remedy to take for insomnia, although they probably won't lie awake nights worrying about it. Instead, they'll obsess about the past or about some current sticky problem. They are likely to need a sleep remedy containing both *warming* and *cooling* digestive herbs along with those used to quiet palpitations and nightmares. One such is **Jie Yu,** made by Nature's Sunshine.

Jie Yu is said to treat pain in the ribs, depression, PMS, breast lumps, general aches, irritability, and headaches. It treats heart symptoms such as palpitation and insomnia as well as digestive complaints such as bloating and slow digestion. It contains stimulants such as ginger and ginseng; anti-inflammatory herbs such as coptis, bupleurum, and ophiopogonis; and tang kuei and cyperus, herbs that free stuck circulation.

Traditional Chinese patent remedies

that work in a similar way to treat depression and *phlegm* from poor digestion are **Xiao Chia Hu Tang Wan** and **Xiao Yao Wan.** Although they are not, strictly speaking, insomnia herbs, they work to free congestion and ease discomfort. That is the source of the *phlegm* person's insomnia. If, as the story goes, a princess was kept awake from a pea under her mattress, many more suffer insomnia from a lump in the middle.

Insomnia and the **Humors:** *Treating the Correct Imbalance*

Traditional Asian doctors have attributed all sorts of things to the *humors,* not just sleep patterns. It is said, for example, that *wind* types also tend to be reckless, guided by desire; that *bile* types are ruled by anger, and *phlegm* types by greed. That may or may not be true. But it is certainly an oversimplification.

Wind people, those insomniacs with nervous exhaustion, are not necessarily lying awake craving more excitement. They may not always be sex/travel/adventure maniacs. They may just be overtired. They may have eaten too much cold, raw food or been blasted by superamplified music or jet lag. For them a warm bath, nourishing cooked food, and a quieting, grounding herb such as valerian will do the trick.

Bile types are not necessarily angry. They may not lie awake at night planning to blow up buildings or burning with fever.

They do need cooling and moistening, or else they'll get thirsty and develop premature gray hair and wrinkles. That alone may be enough to make their ears ring. A nerve sedative such as valerian would only push inflammation deeper, not cool them.

Phlegm types are not always greedy. I have known some lovely *phlegm* types— generous, devoted, sweet people, who just eat too much before bed. *Phlegm* may not refer to their tendency toward cloudy thinking as much as their difficulty in digesting rich food. For them, eating pasta and cheese, then going to bed, results in an insomnia stomachache. For them a sedative like valerian or gotu kola would not help.

The "greed" of *phlegm*-type persons can arise when their eyes are too big for their stomachs. It would be better to eat lightly, eat less, and take a walk before retiring. The best insomnia remedies for persons with difficult digestion are digestive stimulants.

Picking the right sleep remedy involves a lot more than choosing the size of the hammer to knock yourself out. The wrong choice of a sleep remedy can cause insomnia. When we take time to study ourselves, we can predict what herbs will work. Using methods of self-diagnosis such as observation of the tongue can help determine herbs. So does paying attention to diet and personal habits. It's part of the adventure of self-knowing. Referring to such cohesive traditional systems of thought as the ones we're studying in this book also helps. But we must apply their ancient logic to our times.

INSOMNIA

What makes it worse?

Nervous insomnia: Stimulants, excitement, illness, loud music, television, jet lag, cold, raw foods, iced drinks, caffeine, drugs, decongestants, acne medications, inclement weather, overwork, fear, anxiety, age.

Bilious insomnia: Blood deficiency from illness, menstruation, hormone imbalances, hot, *drying* foods and spices, stimulants, hot weather, overwork, stress, anger, frustration.

Indigestion insomnia: Rich, heavy foods, cold drinks, eating too much food or too often, late meals, inadequate exercise, humid weather, worry, aggravation, depression, grief.

What makes it better?

Nervous insomnia: Rest, herbal nervines, *warming,* nourishing foods, massage with sesame oil, quiet music, sweet fragrances.

Bilious insomnia: Lighter, *cooler* diet, digestive herbs that increase and free stuck bile, brain and nerve tonic herbs, rest, cool weather, swimming.

Indigestion insomnia: Light, antiphlegm diet, exercise, sweating, decongestant and digestive stimulant herbs, cool, dry weather.

	HEAT SYMPTOMS	*COLD* SYMPTOMS	*PHLEGM*
TONGUE	reddish, dry, shaking	pale, large, scalloped	coated
SYMPTOMS	irritability	depression	obsession
	headache, rash	chills, dull aches	sinus congestion
	bad breath, hunger		
REMEDIES			
	liver cleansers	nutritive tonics	digestives
	anti-inflammatory herbs	*chi* tonics	decongestants
	blood-builders		
	sedatives		
	Night Caps (Crystal Star)		
	gotu kola,	valerian,	bayberry
	Wuchaseng (liquid	**Ding Xin Wan,**	**Xiao Yao Wan,**
	extract), skullcap,	linden leaf, hops	chamomile, ginger
	vervain, passionflower,		
	tulia		

精 精

[jīng] (1) Essence of life: the fundamental substance that builds up the physical structure and maintains the body function; (2) semen

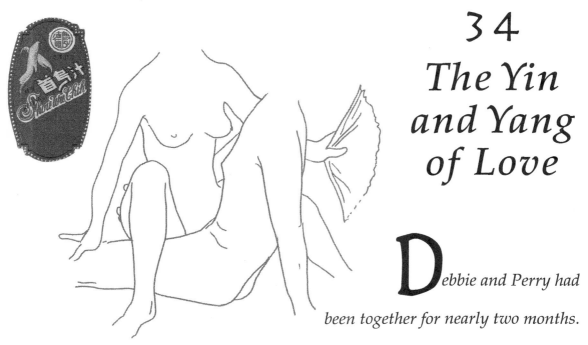

34
The Yin and Yang of Love

Debbie and Perry had been together for nearly two months.

They'd settled into a comfortable routine of having lunch on Wednesdays and spending the weekend together. Saturday night she'd cook his favorite Italian dinner and they'd have dessert in bed. Sunday they'd walk the dog in the park and go to a movie. It felt just right for both of them: He loved her cooking; she loved his lovemaking. They both loved the dog.

One Sunday morning Perry stayed in bed with his head hidden under a pillow. Nothing had happened the night before. In fact, nothing had happened for several weeks. Debbie thought that their problem, which Perry called "impotence," proved he was tired of her. She tried to entice him with his favorite cheesecake. It didn't work. He got indigestion and complained that his mother's was better. Debbie became furious and threw the chicken cacciatore on his best tie.

What's wrong with this picture? Perhaps it just needs more kindness and an herbal aphrodisiac. In this chapter we'll cover a number of herbs and kitchen spices that improve sex. But first we have to redefine the entire problem, because our mindset has become limited by vocabulary.

The "Sexual Dysfunction" Mind-set

In cases of what doctors call "sexual dysfunction," *kindness* requires greater understanding. Often that's impossible because the terminology used by health professionals to describe sexual energy imbalances is inappropriate or insensitive to the point of threatening self-esteem. Such terms as "impotence," "frigidity," and "premature ejaculation" may or may not be currently used by your health professional, but the mindset that determined their use is still in vogue. It comes from a belief that we have to be strong and "hot" to be virile or sexy, or from another fallacy, that we can *control* our sexuality entirely with the mind. This leads to misunderstanding when sexual issues are seen as "disease states," not as temporary imbalances. They can, in fact, be

improved in a variety of ways with herbs and diet. Traditional Asian doctors treat sexual imbalances by improving *chi* and blood.

CULTURE AND SEX

Western medicine may have problems with sexual terminology, but traditional Asian medicine has problems with prejudice. Its approach to sex must conform to modern needs. One case in point is female sexuality. The fourteen original Chinese medical texts on female sexuality have been lost over time. According to one source, some were literally "eaten by worms." A sexist approach has been prevalent for a long time because traditional remedies for women's sexuality deal primarily with menstruation and fertility. This leads to moral blinders: What about those of us who do not want children as much as increased sexual desire, pleasure, and stamina? What herbs address the needs of homosexual men and women, or persons who are celibate? When the main issue to address in modern sexuality is not reproduction, it becomes satisfaction, well-being, and relationship. The answer becomes an energetic one.

Asian (male) doctors used to think that women were not sexually strong because they were "shy." There is a book on Ayurvedic medicine that even claims that women have sexual problems because they are "ashamed." (Imagine!) This ignores not only all the stimulant and rejuvenating aphrodisiac herbs Ayurveda has to offer, but all the other integrated energetic medicines as well, throwing the whole problem instead into the realm of the purely psychological.

Sexual Problems and Energy

We are not shy! We've chosen lovers and husbands without the help of arranged marriages for quite some time. We're just tired and strung out from too much work, from staying up late at night, from jet lag, coffee, drugs, and too many lovers, not to mention stress from the threat of AIDS. Gentlemen! Wake up and smell the oolong tea!

Certainly psychological factors can be inhibiting, but to think that only men need aphrodisiacs is to see only half of the picture. Each of us needs vitality from adequate production of blood and *chi*, not just sexual arousal. We need strong muscles and adequate breath and *chi*, so that we don't feel tired after sex. Physical weakness makes anyone feel emotionally vulnerable. Often it's that vulnerability which limits our ability to express love, to find happiness. Both men and women need help. We're under stress the ancient Daoists could never imagine.

Many of my clients, sensitized by either a clinical or a relationship-oriented approach, are hesitant to talk about sexual issues for fear of being labeled as sick or as "failures." I've seen them for years, sitting quietly in my office, hands neatly folded on their laps as they sniff the incense and admire Guatemalan weavings and Ladakhi masks upon the wall. My birds, silent and watching, sense that they're nervous. Finally they say, "By the way, do you have any herbs for sexual strength?"

Of course I do. They didn't have to tell me. When I took their pulses at the radial artery, I could hardly feel the bottom two, the ones that correspond to the Water element, the kidney and adrenal organ function. That's what the Chinese doctors call the "*yin* and *yang* of the kidney."

Yin *Makes Love Wet,* Yang *Makes It Hot*

To be able to enjoy a full and healthy sex life, we require what Chinese doctors call "kidney *yin* and *yang*." This does not refer merely to the kidneys or the adrenal glands themselves, but also encompasses sexual fluids and hormones, and sexual drive and energy. *Yin,* as an energetic function, nourishes the sexual organs with adequate blood and moisture; while *Yang* furnishes adrenal strength and vitality. The two *humors* must be both adequate and balanced in order to function well.

Ancient Chinese medical texts say that "*yin* nourishes *yang*, while *yang* protects *yin*." This means that if *yin* is deficient, internal organs cannot retain enough fluids to prevent inflammation and dehydration. Without adequate *chi, yang* cannot be energized and all vitality stops. Here's an analogy: To make sexual steam, we need water (*yin*), heat (*yang*), and a stove (*chi*).

Sometimes I will ask a health client who has a pale tongue and a weak kidney pulse, "How is your sexual energy?" But I usually can tell without asking. It's lousy. Maybe they're too tired to date, to seek fulfillment in love. Maybe they're just not interested. To have enough sexual enthusiasm and energy, we need adequate kidney *chi*. But what are the signs of good sexual energy (kidney *chi*)?

THE EYES SAY IT ALL

During Casanova's time, there was a popular Italian folk belief to the effect that a good lover would have a large nose. This was substantiated by Casanova himself, because he had an ample Roman schnoz. But Asian traditional doctors look at the complexion and the eyes.

Chi, or vital energy, is necessary for maintaining all functions of metabolism. A weakness in kidney or adrenal functions could include dark circles under the eyes, pale, dull, or ashen complexion, low enthusiasm and vitality, shallow breathing, and depression.

THE TONGUE

Using Asian diagnosis, we see that the person with low kidney *chi* has a very pale tongue with scalloped edges, and a slow, deep pulse. Persons with *stagnation* symptoms such as purple tongue and irregular pulse might also have sexual weakness

from stuck *chi* that originates from blockage of circulation, not deficiency. In any case, when the kidney organ system is not furnished with adequate *chi*, our sexual energy suffers. We develop temporary symptoms that Western doctors might call "impotence" or "frigidity."

WHY WE USE SEXUAL HERBS

Sexual strength is only one indicator of the quality and quantity of *chi* that originates in the Water element. By improving the level of *chi* in that element, we improve urinary function, sexuality, and immune strength. There are added advantages to taking herbal formulas that support sexuality: Often they treat a variety of other complaints at the same time. (For types of *chi* and the associated Five Elements, see chapter 6.)

First we'll study some well-known herbs that rebuild exhausted sexual strength accompanied by symptoms of *internal cold*. We'll examine some Chinese patent remedies that work by building blood, *chi*, and what the Chinese doctors call *jing*, or "essence." Then we'll look at another category of sexual problems. What happens when our energy is too hyperactive from fatigue or stimulants? Sexual capacity can become limited by anxiety. How can we distinguish these two types of problems, one arising from deficiency and *internal cold*, the other from *internal heat*? Questions such as these make up our study of Asian energetic medicine.

WHAT HAPPENS IF YOU GET IT WRONG?

Many of you are unused to choosing medicinal herbs, and inexperienced in holistic diagnosis. You may wonder what would happen if, based on energetic principles, you chose an inappropriate herb for sexual problems. Would it harm your sex life? The answer is that any herb passes through the body quickly, without doing harm. There may be temporary simple discomfort or else no improvement of your problem. For you to suffer a bad side effect, you would have to misuse an herb repeatedly. Here are the most common examples.

Excess yin

If you had a pale tongue indicating *internal cold* or chronic weakness and you used a *cooling* herb, the result would be that the *cooling* herb would create unneeded phlegm. You might temporarily feel tired or get a head cold. This is not because the herb or food (such as salad) is a sedative, but because it simply is too *cooling* (anti-inflammatory or laxative) for your current needs.

Excess yang

The same holds true if you were to choose a *warming* herb and you didn't need it. For example, if you noticed that your tongue was reddish and dry, that you had thirst and insomnia, and you still chose a *warming* herb such as Chinese ginseng, the result would be that the inflammation would be in excess. You might experience insomnia or irritability, or get a headache or a moment of dizziness. Chinese ginseng itself is not harmful, but it would have been used incorrectly.

Types of Sexual Problems and Herbs to Treat Them

The following discussion of sexual problems is based upon possible imbalances of the *humors*. First we will cover sexual fatigue, timidity, and indifference resulting from nervous exhaustion (excess *wind*). The remedies in this section will be primarily *warming* stimulants useful for weak adrenal strength, including problems usually designated "impotence" and "frigidity," as well as shortness of breath and depression caused by weakness.

The second section, Hot and Fast, covers problems associated with inflammation and dehydration (*bile* problems), including nervousness, deficient semen or vaginal fluids, and premature ejaculation. The moisturizing herbal tonics will replenish needed blood and *yin* while helping ease tension, without sedating drive or capacity.

Exhaustion and Sex, or "I'd Rather Be Knitting"

℀ Does your lower back feel weak and hurt?

℀ Is your urine clear and frequent (every hour or two)?

- Do you have urinary incontinence from fatigue or illness?
- Do your legs feel heavy, bloated with water?
- Are you tired, short of breath, pale, listless?
- Are your feet often ice-cold?
- Is your menstrual period too heavy and long?

Sexual exhaustion can result from either *internal heat* (exhaustion of fluids) or *internal cold* (just plain exhaustion). In this section we will study sexual signs of *internal cold*. Did you answer "yes" to several of the above questions? They all pertain to adrenal weakness indicating *internal cold*.

People with *internal cold* symptoms will often look wan or speak with a breathy voice. This indicates that their energy is low. But their appearance doesn't always give evidence of their sexual strength. For more serious diagnosis, Asian doctors look at the tongue. You can conveniently do this just before a kiss.

TONGUE DIAGNOSIS FOR *INTERNAL COLD* SEXUAL EXHAUSTION

The appearance of the tongue that indicates *internal cold* is most often large, pale, and puffy. It can be scalloped, with lots of saliva, or coated with thin phlegm. If you or your lover has such a tongue, do not despair. There are *warming* herbs that are wonderful remedies.

LOW VOLTAGE

What kinds of sexual problems manifest themselves along with a pale tongue? The terminology used to describe the most common symptoms is very poor and inexact. So-called impotence and frigidity seem to indicate a failure of power on the one hand and an icy coldness on the other. Neither is correct. A power failure might normally be corrected by adding more electricity or more high-voltage circuits. But increasing *yang* or *chi* energy with a stimulant such as ginseng does not always work. Sometimes we need more blood or sexual fluids, not more *chi*. We need more *chi* or *yang* only when we have a very pale, scalloped tongue. Then cooked foods and warming aphrodisiac herbs will strengthen muscles, legs, lower back, and sexual energy.

Women can also experience the equivalent of low voltage. It has nothing to do with feelings of love and desire. It has nothing to do with acting "cold." It can be caused by fatigue, diet, or injury. Here is an example of the latter.

Martha was elegant, tall and attractive. She was an artist, and her paintings were bright swirls of emotion. She had come to me for herbs to treat her fatigue, but soon she spoke of her sexual problems in an agitated manner: "When I was first married, I had a wonderful girlfriend named Meg. We shared our first-year-of-marriage troubles together and learned what we could about sex from books. She told me that for a long time she had felt nothing physical during sex. Then one day she read that the sensitive nerves involved in orgasm are embedded very deeply inside the walls of the vagina. To feel something, we have to squeeze. I forgot about Meg's advice until now. I'm too tired to feel anything."

Here she broke off to cry quietly. She had suffered an injury to her waist (near the right adrenal gland) during a car accident. It had left her in severe spasm for a week. Her tongue was very pale and her pulses slow, deep, and hard to find. She experienced the sexual weakness, fatigue, lower-back pain, frequent urination, and depression that indicate *internal cold* affecting the Water element. She experienced no orgasm, and was exhausted after sex. She feared her sex life was ruined. Western doctors called her problem "frigidity," even though she assured me several times that she was *in love* with her man. Clearly something else was wrong, and Western medicine had no answer.

SOME CAUSES OF SEXUAL EXHAUSTION

Fatigue, childbirth, or injury to the kidney-adrenal area, also steroid drugs or excess use of stimulants, including caffeine, to the point of adrenal exhaustion, can all harm sexual strength for men and women alike. Muscles can become weak. Blood circulation and nerve sensitivity can become impaired. These are important factors in sexual strength. Some sexologists think of the vagina as a muscle. Their advice is to strengthen sexual muscles with squeezing movements like those we use to stop urina-

tion. Other experts say the vagina is not as important as the clitoris in orgasm.

In either case, when there is adequate *chi* and blood circulation in that area, we feel stronger surges of sensation. It's very likely that strengthening the lower back and kidney-adrenal area with tonic herbs can also help maintain a healthy hormone balance necessary for satisfying sex. Many Chinese patent remedies for sexual exhaustion also contain beneficial hormone-increasing substances.

KITCHEN SPICES FOR *INTERNAL COLD* SEXUAL EXHAUSTION

Because Martha suffered from *internal cold* affecting the kidney organ system, I recommended a hot, sweet spice: cloves. They increase the "*yang* of the kidneys." This would correct her excessive clear-colored urine and feelings of physical and emotional exhaustion. After our session, she called me to report the results of the cloves.

She was bubbling. "When I drank it the first time, I shouted 'Hooray!' Clove tea warmed my lower back and lungs. I felt it cleared my lungs and strengthened my back. Immediately I took a deeper breath and had more energy. I've started adding one eighth teaspoon of clove powder or one drop of pure essential clove oil extract to my afternoon tea. What a difference!"

Her sexual energy returned that same week, and remained high despite a back-breaking workload. Cloves work equally well as a stimulant for both men and women. *Caution:* They should be avoided by persons with *internal heat* signs such as dry, reddish tongue, fever, and flu symptoms, or dark-colored urine.

The easiest-to-use sexual tonics come from your kitchen. It is also a good excuse to give a dinner party for someone you wish to know better. If you've checked out the tongue and found it to be very pale and puffy with scalloped edges, you can add some special *warming* herbs to your delicious meals. According to Dr. Yves Requena, a French endocrinologist and doctor of traditional Chinese medicine, fennel herb and seeds, lemon, ginger, clove, rosemary, and sage all stimulate the adrenal glands (the *yang* energy of the Water element) to treat a variety of problems, including sexual weakness, exhaustion, depression, and poor memory.

In his book *Acupuncture et Phytothérapie*, he goes on to say that clove improves deafness brought on by adrenal fatigue as well as Crohn's disease. Rosemary treats heart weakness, asthma, and low blood pressure. Lemon, high in vitamin C, strengthens our immunity against illness. It is heartening to realize that if you use these cooking herbs, your friends and family will not only have more energy, but will also hear you and remember you better.

Other *warming* aphrodisiacs well known to Eastern and Western herbalists include fenugreek and damiana. Fenugreek, used as a stimulant tonic, increases sexual strength. Also an expectorant, it is recommended for asthma and bronchitis. Steeped as a tea, fenugreek is a useful food for con-

valescence and debility of the nervous, respiratory, and reproductive systems. Add one pinch of fenugreek seeds per cup of hot water. *Caution:* Fenugreek should not be used during pregnancy, because excess use can promote vaginal bleeding.

SEXUAL IRRITANTS AND SEXUAL TONICS

Some foods and herbs irritate sexual desire when eaten because they increase blood circulation or inflammation locally affecting the sexual organs. They are known as *sexual irritants.* Other herbs build adrenal strength or supplement hormones. They are called *sexual tonics.*

For example, damiana is not only a stimulant, but also provides needed sexual hormones for both men and women. It is sometimes included in formulas related to menopausal or menstrual problems because it provides hormone support.

All the above herbs enhance sexual strength. They are not considered aphrodisiacs, because they "irritate" the sexual organs to excite sexual behavior. Rather, they are healing remedies that treat weakness, whereas onion, garlic, asafoetida, and persimmon are just irritants that may build desire, not vitality. Dr. Vasant Lad, in his beautiful book *The Yoga of Herbs*, puts it this way:

Vajikaranas (substances that improve sexual vitality and functioning) reinvigorate the body by reinvigorating the sexual organs. . . . Many are tonics that actually nurture and give direct sustenance to the reproductive tissues. Others help promote the creative transformation of sexual energy for the benefit of the body-mind.

By starting in the reproductive system, these herbs invigorate the entire system, just as a tree is invigorated from the roots. They have a strong revitalizing action on the nerves and bone marrow, and increase the energy of the mind.

Ayurvedic doctors recommend a number of medicinal herbs that are available in some Indian groceries. One famous remedy used for exhaustion and sexual weakness is called *ashwagandha* in Sanskrit (in English, winter cherry; in Latin, Withania somnifera). It is a tonic rejuvenator similar to Chinese ginseng, used for weak muscles, nerve exhaustion, loss of memory, paralysis, rheumatism, anemia, overwork, and mental exhaustion. Short of a vacation on the beach, it seems to fix everything that could go wrong due to fatigue and old age. At the same time, it is safe enough for children and pregnant women. It actually strengthens pregnancy by firming muscle tone. (See chapter 28.) If you are weak, you can add one half teaspoon of the powder to hot water and drink it as tea daily. Be sure to watch your tongue as your energy improves. Stop the herb after it has done its work to strengthen you; otherwise you may develop irritability or insomnia.

SPEED OF ACTION AND DURATION OF HERB USAGE

How long should it take to improve sexual problems with herbs? This varies with the individual. Sometimes, for simple fatigue from overwork, one dose of stimulant herbs will do the trick. Your energy and enthusiasm will rise quickly. At other times you may need to give more than one dinner party. Certainly, if you use tongue diagnosis, you will know if the remedy is working well.

Here are the guidelines: With the correct use of *warming* stimulant herbs, an overly pale, scalloped tongue will eventually become pink. With *cooling*, moisture-building herbs, a reddish, dry tongue will become more moist and lighter pink. This is because you will have reversed imbalances in metabolism.

Cooking for Sexual Strength

What can you cook to cure a Romeo or a Juliet of a pale tongue and inspire their ardor? Remember, not all hot, spicy herbs tone the adrenal glands, enhancing sexuality. Some pungent herbs, such as thyme, stimulate breathing, while others, such as ginger, anise, and black or cayenne pepper, stimulate hunger. If you use those herbs instead of kidney tonics, Romeo may want a smoke or more food instead of wanting *you.*

This is a problem. People sometimes group themselves into either the type that loves oral satisfaction—eating, drinking, smoking, talking—or the type that loves to love. The eaters and drinkers might put on weight. The smokers get nervous. The lovers eat less and take dance classes. We need to find a happy middle way. For that reason it may be wise for some people to add the additional herbs provided for speeding digestion to the following basic recipes. You will also enjoy creating your own recipes using the right healing herbs. Here's one hot dish that can inspire interest.

HOT CHICKEN SOUP

1 diced Bermuda onion

2 cloves minced garlic

1 teaspoon extra-virgin olive oil

juice of ½ lemon

1 teaspoon thinly sliced lemon peel

1 quartered chicken with the skin removed

salt substitute

pepper

1 cup diced fennel herb (sometimes called anise-fennel)

¼ cup Spanish green olives

¼ cup chopped mild pimientos

½ teaspoon clove powder or ¾ teaspoon whole cloves

¼ teaspoon ginger powder or 4 slices raw ginger

1 pinch saffron

1 sprig rosemary

1 small piece Chinese ginseng (ren shen) or 1 level teaspoon ashwagandha powder

Brown the diced onion and minced garlic in a little olive oil. Strain the oil and set it aside. Add the lemon juice and peel to the onion mixture.

Brown the chicken in the oil. Add salt and pepper. Cover with water and add the onion mixture. Then add to the chicken mixture the chopped fennel herb, olives, pimientos, clove powder or clove buds,

ginger, and saffron. *Optional:* To make this soup an even more powerful (*warming*) adrenal stimulant tonic, add rosemary, Chinese ginseng, or ashwagandha powder.

Simmer 15 minutes or until nearly done. Turn off the burner and let it steam 5 more minutes. Serve hot with cooked vegetables: peas, red potatoes with parsley, or other.

If digestion is unusually slow, with bloating or indigestion, or for an overly large waistline, use ½ cup of the following soup stock:

¼ cup pinellia

3 pieces magnolia bark

1 piece chen pi (citrus peel)

1 handful dried licorice root

2 tablespoons chopped raw ginger

Make a soup stock with the above herbs by boiling them in 5 cups of water for at least 20 minutes. (This soup stock can also be precooked and added to any dish to ease digestion.)

See chapter 14 for other slimming soups.

Warming *Herbal Pills for Internal Cold Sexual Exhaustion*

We don't always have time to cook. For our convenience, many pill remedies are available. The Chinese patent remedies for sexual weakness caused by deficient *chi* or *internal cold* are complicated and sometimes include questionable ingredients such as the private parts of several animals. But here are a few that are particularly effective.

Kang Wei Ling, translated as "Excessively Limp Efficacious Remedy," is primarily for "male impotence." ("Excessively limp" refers not to the remedy but to the complaint it is meant to cure.) It is a *warming* remedy only for men with pale tongues. It contains 30 percent each of tang kuei, paeonia, and licorice, also 10 percent dried centipede, an irritant used to stimulate circulation, presumably in the "limp" area. Take it orally, following directions: 10 to 15 pills, two times a day with wine, for fifteen days. It is said to "increase sexual drive and help prevent premature ejaculation, build sperm, and invigorate the liver." It is an example of a remedy that is at once a stimulant tonic as well as an irritant.

Hai Ma Bu Shen Wan ("Seahorse Tonify Kidney Pills") is a general-purpose tonic for energy and blood-building. According to Jake Fratkin in his book *Chinese Herbal Patent Formulas,* it is recommended for persons whose "kidney deficiency has affected the heart or digestion." It is useful for those who are elderly or recovering from childbirth, or who have symptoms associated with congestive heart failure, including fatigue, lowered sexual drive, impotence, lower-back pain, and cold limbs. It contains many tonic herbs, including seahorse, deer ligament, deer horn, gecko, ginseng, and several blood-builders.

The above two remedies are pills. Another quite effective remedy is **Tzepao Sanpien Wan,** a large, chewable pill. It can be used by men or women as an acute one-time remedy for exhaustion, severe back pain, and sexual weakness caused by *internal cold,* or as a strengthening tonic for several months. It comes packaged in a lovely little red box containing the wax "egg" used to protect the herbal ball. You can't add it to your cooking. It tastes strange, but at least it's fun to use. After you break open the wax egg, you'll find the soft ball, which contains some forty-two ingredients, both animal and vegetable. I recommend that you cut it into four pieces and swallow it with water, though some people like to chew the ball. It "strengthens kidneys, spleen, and lungs, improves mind and spirit, strengthens lower back, empowers sexual function, counters fatigue, spontaneous sweating, poor memory, and chronic asthma."

You may not have a Chinatown available in your area, or the FDA may be raiding your Asian community's food and herb markets, so you will need some other reliable sources. The supermarket *warming* aphrodisiacs I mentioned above will work quite well as long as you choose the remedies according to observations of the tongue. For persons with *internal cold* and slow metabolism (a pale tongue) chapter 13, especially the sections on reducing phlegm and reducing nervous exhaustion, will be helpful.

MAIL-ORDER SOURCES FOR HERBS

You may need mail-order sources for herbs, and referrals for health professionals in your area. If so, see the Herbal Access appendix. For example, **Woman's Treasure** and **Man's Treasure** are two formulas, made by Seven Forests, that treat sexual weakness. The first of these is indicated for menstrual disorders such as irregular periods or blood deficiency caused by kidney and liver weakness; infertility, reduced sexual drive, low energy, back pain, and cervical dysplasia are also treatable with this remedy. (We studied menstrual and menopausal problems in chapters 26 and 29.)

Man's Treasure treats "impotence, male infertility, reduced sexual drive," and low energy, lumbago, and frequent urination. The ingredients include herbs such as cistanche, cynamorium, epimedium, and achyranthes, used for low sperm count or immobility of sperm. The remedy also includes the blood-builders rehmannia and lycium, and tonic herbs such as seahorse and deer antler that provide *chi* for treating sexual weakness. Other Seven Forests remedies can be added to **Man's Treasure: Gecko A,** for "impotence"; **Eucommia 18** for backache; or **Cuscuta 15** for premature ejaculation. (Available at your health-food store or from Health Concerns and other distributors.)

HEALTH-FOOD STORE HERBAL FORMULAS

There are many new herbal sexual formulas available in herb shops, pharmacies, and supermarkets. They can be recognized by names such as **Loving Mood Extract for Men, Love Male,** or **Love Female** (made by Crystal Star); or by more subtle names such as **Ginseng-Damiana Combination** (made by Nature's Herbs). They often contain hormonal herbs, including damiana, sarsaparilla, Siberian ginseng, and saw palmetto, as well as energy stimulants such as Chinese ginseng (ren shen), gotu kola, and guarana.

Some formulas contain stimulants or irritants that can cause overheating with symptoms such as headache, dizziness, thyroid imbalances, or irritability. These strongly stimulant herbs include ma huang, garlic, capsicum, and yohimbe bark, a known aphrodisiac. Avoid these if you have signs of *internal heat* such as sparse, dark-colored urine, irritability, insomnia, or prostate inflammation or pain.

Otherwise, any of the above herbs are safe to take by persons who suffer from weak *chi* with *internal cold* symptoms such as very pale tongue, slow, deep pulse, lethargy, fatigue, pallid, lusterless complexion, shortness of breath, backache, depression, and poor concentration and memory. But what if you have sexual weakness with *internal heat*?

Hot and Fast: Anxiety and Sex

What is *internal heat* as it refers to sexual strength? Here's an amusing example. One day a couple was arguing in Kam Man, the big Chinese grocery store on Canal Street. She, in tight leather pants, spike heels, and teased hair, was pushing him to buy herbs. She was loud and red-faced, with dry skin and a smoker's voice. He was withdrawn and nervous, flushed and fidgeting with the groceries. I didn't have to take their fast pulses or look at their reddish tongues to know that they both suffered from *internal heat*. Hers made her angry; his made him nervous. She snapped at the Chinese sales staff, "My boyfriend needs ginseng, a strong one." From his embarrassment, I could tell she was frustrated and driving him. He wanted to leave, but that made her insist even more loudly.

The problem is that even with the most expensive Chinese ginseng, their sexual energy would not improve. They were already too "hot." Chinese ginseng (ren shen), a *warming* stimulant, would only have made her more angry and him more nervous. Instead, traditional herb doctors would recommend *yin*-building tonics, which would be *cooling*, moistening herbs to soothe internal tissue, build sexual fluids, and restore calm. So-called impotence or frigidity can result not only from weak *chi*, but also from inflammation and dehydration, otherwise known as *internal heat*. We need both *yin* and *yang* to be healthy.

SEX, DRUGS, AND ROCK AND ROLL

Stimulants wake us up and keep us smiling, dancing, or marching toward our goal. They are so familiar that most people ignore any side effects. Some are hot, spicy foods, street drugs, or medical prescriptions without warning labels. Please heed this warning: Medical drugs as diverse as diuretics, acne medications, antidepressants, and blood pressure pills have been known to cause sexual problems. The misuse of *heating* or *drying* stimulants such as Chinese ginseng, ma huang, echinacea, and *heating* aphrodisiacs; also excessive salty food, garlic, hot spices, and especially *heating* substances, such as cigarettes, coffee, and cocaine, can affect your sexual life. I've met cocaine users who've lost their sex lives or suffered strokes. Using too many stimulants is like driving an overheated car without gas.

Do You Have Internal Heat *and Speed?*

- Are you frequently nervous, angry, anxious, or fearful?
- Is your urine dark, infrequent, urgent, or sparse?
- Do you have a stiff or tight lower back, sciatica, or headaches?
- Do you get too excited and come too fast during sex?
- Do you desire sex very frequently— never get enough?
- Are your palms or the soles of your feet hot and dry?
- Is your tongue red? Are you flushed, feverish, or dry?
- Do you have bad breath, body odor, bloodshot eyes?
- Do you feel exhausted and overwrought after sex?

Did you answer "yes" to the above questions describing *internal heat*? Many people who complain of anxiety attacks are suffering from *internal heat*. Some are fearful or jumpy, while others have palpitations or night sweats. They need to cool down. Their tongues will be red, dry, and cracked. They may have bad breath, headaches, dizziness, or insomnia. They may avoid romantic contacts with people because they are nervous or unsure of themselves. After sex, they may feel even more "wired." Their adrenal glands are so hyperactive they could just about jump out of their skins. Men may complain of "coming too soon." Women may feel physically or emotionally "dry and brittle." They are too "hot." Nurturing remedies most appropriate for them are herbs that have a *cooling, moistening* quality. Traditional Chinese doctors describe these as remedies that "increase blood and *yin*" (see chapter 24).

Internal heat problems that affect sexuality are often chronic, whereas acute inflammation and dehydration more often originate from colds, flu, or other fever illnesses that must be addressed separately. Many people who smoke, stay up late, travel frequently, eat too many hot foods, or perspire a great deal have chronic *internal heat* conditions. This is also true for people with certain illnesses, such as diabetes, that involve long-term dehydration or other blood-deficiency conditions. Because the problems tend to be chronic, they may take longer to treat, but the time is worth it.

People who are overheated need to regain a comfortable speed. Their frenetic pace may not change, but with the right herbs they will be able to breathe with ease. They will be able to make contact with their bodies again. Too often, speedy persons are so hyperactive that they hardly take time to reflect on what they are doing. With *cooling,* moistening remedies, they may even take more time to notice you.

When treating sexual problems caused by inflammation and dehydration imbalances, we must make a distinction between chronic and acute problems. *Internal heat* takes many forms. Do you want to invite dinner guests to help with their gray hair? Do you wish to be friends for a thousand years? Or do you need faster results? Many of the *yin-* and blood-building herbs qualify as true health tonics; they accomplish many good things and take a long time to work. They may not necessarily enhance sexual fluids or sexual enthusiasm quickly. But they can gradually help the person reconnect with deeper feelings of appreciation and sentiment, and find calmness, physical beauty, and better sleep. As we shall see, often the fast-working sexual remedies treat the mind and spirit.

WHAT CAN *YIN* DO?

Useful long-term remedies for sexual weakness caused by *internal heat* treat anxiety, irritability, and loss of moisture and body fluids. They ensure the health of organs and the smooth functioning of hormones. Primarily they build what Chinese doctors call *yin,* thus ensuring fewer inflammatory symptoms. The anti-inflammatory or moisture-building reactions depend upon the herbs chosen. For example, some *yin-*building herbs reduce thirst, while others treat insomnia or palpitations. The most important herbs affecting sexual capacity increase the *yin* (retention of blood) of the kidneys and liver. Thus they can also build bone marrow and blood. They ensure strong muscles, young skin, lustrous hair, and healthy fingernails because all of these require adequate blood. As you read this book, you will realize that the origins of physical and spiritual beauty lie very deep.

FOR SPEEDY "LIVE WIRES"

You may not have the usual signs of *internal heat* affecting the kidneys—sparse, dark-colored urine, thinning hair, or a ruddy and dry complexion—but inflammation may show up in other ways. I saw an example recently.

A young couple came to one of my classes on Chinese herbs. During our tour of a Chinese food market, the young husband pulled me aside to ask if I knew of any herbs that lengthened lovemaking. He said he "came too fast." He was perhaps a bit embarrassed to ask, but he was not depressed or overly anxious. Very likely it was simply a physical problem brought on by dehydration of body fluids. I asked if he needed more semen, thinking I could recommend he shou wu (polygonum multiflori), an herb known to increase sexual fluids. (See chapters 24 and 29.) That was not his problem. He said he just "came too fast."

Upon looking at his tongue, I saw that it was red over its entire surface, with small bumps. I didn't have time to do a full diagnosis with pulses or case history, so I just asked a few questions. I wondered if his *internal heat* was caused by illness, bad habits, or stress. He was not diabetic. If he used cocaine, he wouldn't tell me. I knew I had to recommend a safe effective *yin* (moisture-building) tonic that could relieve the *heat* condition that covered his entire red tongue.

Did he have *internal heat* symptoms that applied specifically to the kidneys? I wondered. He reported that his urine was not especially dark or odorous. His urination was not painful. That eased my concern about possible infection. The muscles at the kidneys, near the waist, and behind the knees felt tight. This indicated he needed a *cooling, yin*-building tonic that could relax tight muscles specifically in that area—for example, fructus lycii. The muscles there would become "softer" because of more retention of blood in the kidney-adrenal area. That would relieve inflammation or spasm in the lower back. It would also let him experience less hyper-adrenal nerve irritation. His problem was the opposite of Martha's (see page 409); she needed adrenal strength and stronger muscles.

Cooling, *moistening diet and herbs*

The first thing I advised him to do was give up oily, fried, and hot, spicy foods for a while to ensure smoother circulation. The foods and herbs most helpful are *cooling*, such as those found in section II of chapter 13. He looked to heaven as if to say, "God, what can I eat? Hot spices are my favorites!" I knew I was on the right track.

Then I added a *yin-* and blood-building tonic to address his overall moisture deficiency caused by inflammation: **Liu Wei Di Huang Wan** (see chapter 24). Its ingredients include rehmannia, cornus, dioscorea, moutan, poris (fu ling), and alisma. It is also called "Six Flavor Rehmannia Pill." According to Jake Fratkin's *Chinese Herbal Patent Formulas,* it is recommended for "nourishing kidney, liver and spleen *yin* and tonifying kidney and spleen *chi.* Accompanying symptoms include weakness or pain in lower back, restlessness, insomnia, burning soles or palms, mild night sweats, dizziness, tinnitus, sore throat, impotence and high blood pressure due to kidney *yin* deficiency."

The young man did not have diarrhea or any other sign of weakness, so I recommended he start with a higher dose, as they usually do in China. He would take 15 pills twice a day between meals, along with drinking extra American ginseng tea, and call in two weeks to let me know the results. He would also monitor his tongue changes. His dark red tongue should turn smoother and healthy pink. When he called to report the herbs' success, I could almost hear him grinning. "Everything is great," he said.

Moistening, blood-building tonics such as **Liu Wei Di Huang Wan** are not for men alone. There is an equivalent with women for "coming too soon." We may not show it as dramatically as men, but nervous tension or restlessness can harm sexual focus. Have you ever found it hard to remain interested or engaged during sex because of vague complaints, worries, or irritations? Have you felt cranky when you "came too fast"? You may need to build *yin.*

Yin is at the core of our deepest feelings. It nourishes our organs with blood, the essence of life. It helps maintain healthy hormone balance. It is the lubricating "glue" that holds us together. Without adequate moisture, we become dry, wrinkled, brittle, or "burned out." *Yin* is what makes a kiss wet. *Yang* is what makes it hot.

Here is another example of a person who needed *yin:*

Alvin came over to study herbs. He had been self-prescribing for some time and needed to clarify his herb choices. He did not know about Asian tongue diagnosis, so he chose herbs according to symptoms alone, and was getting confused. He was thirty and still living at home. His mother and he were at odds about several things, so he shut himself in his room all night to study. He was nervous, insomniac, and hot-tempered, so he took heart-calming pills, which made him sleepy. He felt they were not enough.

After observing his bright red, dry tongue, I could see the source of his irritation: inflammation. Something was far too hot. It affected the whole body. He didn't speak of any friends or family other than his mother. He seemed to obsess about her attachment to him. If he had a girlfriend, I imagine his nervousness would have been extreme. Was this more than anxiety? He reported no diabetes, ulcers, prostate problems, or painful urination. I needed to establish the source of his inflammation.

Did he take ginseng? That is always my first question to an herb enthusiast with *internal heat*. I found he not only took Chinese ginseng, a *warming* stimulant, every day, but also cayenne pepper and miso soup, a salty stimulant. His body fluids and nerves were worn thin. He seemed ready to leap like a tiger. His hands shook and perspired. His eyes and face were red. He was driving himself full speed ahead in the wrong direction.

It is in extreme cases such as this that we can see the mind-body connection in action. Alvin's misuse of stimulants and hot foods sent his body into high gear and his mind into a state of imbalance. The more stimulants he took in an attempt to ease his nervous depression, the more unbalanced he became. *Warming* is not always strengthening. Too hot can become too fast, too destructive.

We gradually reversed his symptoms by eliminating the ginseng, pepper, and miso. We added many healthy green vegetables in the cabbage family, as well as alfalfa, aloe, and dandelion. They improved his acid-alkaline balance, which had nearly evaporated. We added an herbal combination for grounding and centering: **Xiao Yao Wan** with meals, because his imbalance came from being unhappy in his center, unhappy at home. He took this along with **Lung Tan Xie Gan Wan** to cleanse his liver, quiet his nerves, and resolve his anger. The liver-cleansing remedy helped resolve the emotional aspects of Alvin's *internal heat.* Then we worked to rebuild his body fluids with diet and herbs.

COOKING TO BUILD *YIN*

What do you cook for the nervous loved one with a red tongue? *Cooling,* moistening green vegetables build *yin.* They balance excess acid conditions. Serve salad and cooked dark, leafy greens. These *cooling* foods are cleansing, so they help irritable persons who have reddish tongues with a yellow or dark coating. Other *cooling* foods are moisturizing, and indirectly increase sexual fluids—for example, oysters and asparagus. Moistening grains such as white basmati rice and oatmeal help retain moisture throughout the body, as do almonds. You can add peeled almonds that have been parboiled or soaked overnight to many dishes. This supplies several minerals and protein in an easy-to-digest form.

MOISTENING HERBS TO INCREASE SEXUAL FLUIDS AND COUNTER DRYNESS

One of the best herbs to replace body fluids lost from fever, chronic illness, or smoking is American ginseng. Boil a piece of it in soup or drink the instant tea. It adds moisture to the skin, as well as preventing dry cough. This anti-inflammatory form of ginseng helps replenish all other body fluids (see chapter 32). There are other herbs that have even more specific action in replenishing needed fluids and hormones.

The long-term remedy of choice for persons who require more sexual fluids is called *he shou wu* in Chinese (in Latin, *radix polygonum multiflori*). It "nourishes the blood and benefits *jing,*" according to Chinese medicine. What does this mean in English? It means he shou wu gives men more semen and women more vaginal lubrication. But the herb doesn't stop there: It also helps reduce other signs of blood deficiency and dehydration. These can include dizziness, blurred vision, prematurely gray hair, weak lower back and knees, or insomnia. It comes as a loose herb that is boiled as a decoction, or in pill form. The herb is also very often an ingredient in patent formulas used to prevent signs of aging such as **Wan Nian Chun Zi Pu Ziang,** which is translated as "Thousand Year Spring Nourishing Syrup."

Another tonic, **Ren Shen Shou Wu Jing** ("Ginseng Polygona Root Extract") contains 60 percent polygonum (shou wu) and 40 percent ginseng. It is recommended for dizziness, poor memory, poor appetite, fatigue, aching joints and tendons, and diminished sex drive. It clearly works as a nutritive tonic, not as an irritant aphrodisiac, since its ingredients are a blood tonic and another herb to help its absorption.

INTERNAL HEAT AND EMOTIONS

So far the herbs I've discussed for *internal heat* conditions in this chapter have been used to treat *dryness* or inflammation. Certainly, having enough sexual fluids is very important, but there is another aspect of *heat* symptoms that affects sexuality. Irritability, anger, fear, and anxiety are considered "hot" emotions by Asian doctors. In other

words, they tend to occur more frequently in cases of *internal heat.* In the Indian medical tradition they are called signs of excess *pitta,* the *humor* used to describe inflammatory conditions, among other things.

Although these problems can be longstanding, there are many useful remedies that Chinese herbalists use to "calm the *shen.*" The *shen,* literally "spirit," helps maintain mental balance. It is observed as our degree of alertness, mental clarity, courage, and appropriateness of actions. If our *shen* is not healthy, we may lose our mental and emotional balance. Often, herbs used to calm the *shen* work by stabilizing the heartbeat. The results are reduced anger, irritability, palpitations, anxiety, and fear.

Here is a special recipe for rice pudding using herbs that can calm troubled *shen.* The recipe serves two persons.

WHITE RICE AND RED DATES

1½ cup white basmati rice

8 red jujube dates

*1 dose (one tube or tiny spoonful)
    powdered pearl*

a few drops culinary rose oil

1 package **Essence of Tienchi Flowers**
    sweetener

Cook the rice as you normally would. White basmati rice is recommended for *heat* conditions because it is more moistening and *cooling* than brown rice. Add a handful of red Chinese dates, semen ziziphi spinosae. They "nourish the heart and liver, calm the spirit" to treat irritability, insom-

422 ASIAN HEALTH SECRETS

nia, palpitations, and anxiety. For extra calming, add a dose of powdered pearl to the cooked rice. This often comes packaged in small tubes available at Chinese herb shops. For sweetening, add culinary rose oil. You can also use **Essence of Tienchi Flowers Instant Beverage** as a sweetener. (See the section of chapter 5 on sweeteners for tea.)

A CALMING TEA

For a major case of jitters, use a teaspoon of **Wuchaseng,** Siberian ginseng liquid extract. **Wuchaseng** liquid is more calming than powdered Siberian ginseng capsules sold in health-food stores, which are used by bodybuilders to increase testosterone. The milder liquid **Wuchaseng** is recommended for restlessness and anxiety.

CHINESE PATENT REMEDIES TO COOL AND CALM

A Chinese patent remedy known for its soothing, tranquilizing effect is **An Sheng Pu Shin Wan** ("Peaceful *Shen* Tonify Heart Pills"). It contains mother-of-pearl, polygonum (shou wu), ligustrum, eclipta, salvia, albizia bark, cuscuta seed, schisandra fruit, and acorus rhizome. It treats "weakness in kidneys and heart causing dizziness, restlessness, excessive dreaming or heart palpitations." By helping to normalize heart action, it reduces atherosclerotic plaque, which causes hardening of the arteries. (It proves that love and healthy lovemaking

begin with the heart.) Sometimes one dose of such remedies used for "calming the spirit" can quell nervousness.

Other useful remedies are **Jian Nao Wan,** "Healthy Brain Pills," used for agitation, mental and physical exhaustion, and insomnia; also **Pai Tzu Yang Hsin Wan** ("Biota Seed Support Heart Pills"), for anxiety, palpitations, and restlessness with dry mouth or lips. When treating anxiety, we use less of these remedies than the normal dose used for insomnia.

THE OPTIMUM DOSAGE OF SEXUAL TONICS

The dosage used in Asian herbal medicine is always an individual matter. In the case of sexual tonics, I recommend the smallest effective dose. The usual dosage is the recommended number of pills, often stated in English, taken twice or three times daily. Try one dose of the recommended number of pills and watch the results. Add the other doses throughout the day as needed.

Asian sexual tonics will profoundly affect your energy and vitality. If you need more *yin* and take enough moisturizing, blood-building herbs, your health, mental stability, and calmness will improve, as will your sexual fluids. But if you have enough moisture and add too much more, your dinner party may turn into a slumber party.

If you need more *yang* and take enough *warming, drying* stimulant herbs, your sexual drive and strength will im-

Sex and Emotions: Helpful Hints

These hints come from ancient Chinese medical texts. I also include a few suggestions of my own.

According to one antique source, sexual problems can arise, along with eye and ear disorders, when a person is exhausted by intercourse, after long abstinence from sex, or from "mistaken sexual techniques."

These techniques refer to practices common among early philosopher/doctors as well as among current advocates of Tantric sexual practice, whereby sexual partners are advised to delay or eliminate sexual climax in order to enjoy sex longer and protect youth and beauty by protecting *jing*. The prohibition, therefore, includes hasty or harsh sexual behavior and loss of sperm.

Other ancient prohibitions included making love at the beginning and the very end of the moon, at full moon, or during an eclipse, also following eating, urinating, strenuous exertion, or a bath, because this might weaken the semen.

Here's my advice: Aside from avoiding sex after eating, bathing, etc., I would recommend it should be avoided after arguments. Meditate together first in order to create a common ground for love. Sandalwood incense will help clear the air; so will drinking a warm tea made from catnip herb, one pinch of saffron, dried rose petals, and mint leaves. If you still need to relax, soak your feet in hot water and fresh lemon juice, then massage your partner's feet.

Making love during the menstrual period causes *stagnant chi* circulation for women, resulting in weakness, menstrual pain, and irritability. If you indulge, take a capsule of myrrh afterward in order to reestablish smooth circulation.

If you feel very tired after sex, eat a few blanched almonds with warm soy milk, rub the bottoms of your feet with sesame oil, massage the lower back, and take sexual tonic herbs. Rest quietly for a while.

---

prove, but so will your energy and outlook. You will be able to take a deep breath and look on the bright side of things. But if you have enough *internal heat* and add too much more, the party might go on for days and you could end up with a headache, insomnia, irritability, or high blood pressure.

THE GREAT ADVANTAGE IN USING HERBS FOR BETTER SEX

When we balance *chi* and blood by taking herbs, we build health and well-being. Some so-called sex experts and doctors have perfected other methods: exercises using variations of thrusting or tensing muscles, or counting thrusts, or pinching one's penis to slow ejaculation. What a shame! With all that work going on, no one dares think of love. Lovemaking becomes like a football match. The emphasis is put on performance, not on the depth and beauty of union.

The remedies we have studied in this chapter help us regain sexual strength as well as mental calm. The *yang* tonics used to treat so-called impotence and frigidity actually strengthen the adrenal glands and thereby support vitality and immune defenses against disease and depression. The *yin*- and blood-building remedies that replenish moisture and circulation soothe agitation and weariness of the heart. They replenish the blood supply of the liver and kidneys, thus ensuring smooth circulation, healthy nerves, and emotional balance. Harmonizing these fundamental energies brings about happiness, compassion, and love.

FOR INFECTIONS AND PAIN

Although I have covered *yin*-building and moistening herbs for dry or parched sexual organs and deficient sexual fluids, there is another category of *cooling* herbs for sexual problems. They are the anti-inflammatory, antiseptic, or antibiotic herbs used in vaginal infections and prostatitis. I will discuss some of the most commonly used ones.

For leukorrhea and trichomonas

Leukorrhea is the term used to describe the sticky vaginal discharge women some-

times get from yeast infections, or when they are run-down or stressed, and have abused their diet. It can be thick, creamy, and yellow, and burn and have an odor, which indicates *internal heat;* or it can be thin and runny, indicating *internal cold* and weakness. Thick yellow or dark discharge and pain can also indicate infection or other problems that require testing.

Usually the discharge is not transmitted sexually unless it is caused by a yeast infection. Then you have to take special steps to kill the yeast and change your diet. If the discharge is frequent or if you have recently taken antibiotics, a major cause of yeast infections, it is best to take herbs for yeast infection (also popularly called *candida*).

Trichomonas is an infection that can affect men and women and is transmitted sexually, though I have heard of cases in which women have gotten it from unclean swimming pools when the women were weak or had their period. The symptoms can include a smelly discharge, pain, pus, and internal lesions for women and few, if any, symptoms for men until advanced stages. The disease can result in infertility if untreated.

Herbal treatment for infections and discharge

Chien Chin Chih Tai Wan is a Chinese patent remedy recommended for leukorrhea, trichomonas, and vaginal infections. It clears inflammation and stops infection, normalizes *chi* and blood circulation in the sexual area, and stops pain. It treats deficiency or *heat* symptoms, either *internal heat* or *internal cold* discharge, strengthens kidneys and adrenal glands, and reduces lower-back pain, fatigue, and abdominal bloating and pain.

The formula contains a major antibiotic herb, indigo (isatis), and other herbs to build strength such as codonopsis, tang kuei, atractylodes, oyster shell (a source of calcium, to help bloating), and corydalis, for treating pain. Fennel is added for digestion, and for improving circulation in the lower body. This vegetarian formula can be used by men or women. The recommended dose is 10 pills once a day. When taking this or any antibiotic formula, add daily capsules of acidophilus, or eat yogurt, to ensure proper digestion and prevent further yeast infections.

Prostate pain

Prostate pain feels like sitting on a bulge, or tightness under the scrotum, or painful, straining urination. In Asia it is often treated as an unresolved infection, with antibiotic herbs. But there are also energetic causes of the problem. Two patent remedies address those problems well.

Qian Lie Xian Wan ("Prostate Gland Pills") treats prostate pain caused by poor circulation, clears pus and inflammation, and can be used for chronic or acute infection or swelling. The usual symptoms are dribbling or painful urination, and painful testicles. The formula also works for urinary-tract infections with lower-back and abdominal pain.

The vegetarian formula contains vaccaria seed, moutan root, paeonia, astragalus, patrina, peucedanum root, saussaurea, akebia, and licorice. The recommended dosage is 6 pills three times daily, but it can be increased to 10 pills three times daily.

Kai Kit Pill, another Chinese patent formula, treats prostate swelling and pain due to weakness. (Look for a pale tongue and lethargy.) The formula builds *chi* and moisture, promotes urination, and dries excess discharge. It reduces painful urination, pain in the groin, and chronic or pronounced swelling.

The formula contains rehmannia, astragalus, codonopsis, ligustrum, plantago, achyranthes, salvia, alisma, cuscuta, and mantis egg case. Dosage is 3 to 6 pills three times daily.

Health-food store capsules for prostate pain

Two traditional Western herbal remedies recommended for prostate pain have anti-inflammatory, diuretic, and hormonal properties. They are sarsaparilla and saw palmetto. For painful or dribbling urination and prostate pain, you can take up to a dozen pills per day of either remedy. Avoid hot and spicy or excess cold, raw food.

SEXUAL PROBLEMS

What makes them worse?

Heavy, rich, or cold, raw diet; alcohol or drug addictions; sedatives; excessive stimulants, including caffeine and loud noise; medications for high blood pressure and diabetes; chemotherapy; chemical poisoning; infections and pain; stress, fatigue, including fatigue from excessive sex, hormone irregularities, menstruation, jet lag, anxiety, depression, fear, anger, grief, worry, indifference; cold weather, cold showers.

What makes them better?

Nourishing but light diet (fruits, vegetables, grains, fish, soy products, green tea); rest, adequate sleep, vacations in the tropics, massage; tonic and stimulant herbs; deep, slow breathing; soothing perfumes or incense; meditating together.

	INTERNAL HEAT	*INTERNAL COLD*	*PHLEGM*
TONGUE	red, dry, yellow-coated	pale, large, scalloped, excess saliva	gray-coated
SEXUAL ENERGY	urgent sex drive	tepid interest, fear	too busy digesting food or reading
SYMPTOMS	premature ejaculation or nervousness	"impotence" or "frigidity"	tired or overweight
	stiff, sore back	muscle weakness	sinus congestion
	hot temper	vulnerability	
	high blood pressure	low immune strength	
	diabetes	hypoglycemia	headaches
	inflammatory arthritis	rheumatism	dull aches
	rashes, allergies	colds and flu	stomachaches
BEHAVIOR	aggressive or nervous	timid, restrained	drowsy
REMEDIES			
TONICS	*cooling*, nourishing, moisturizing	*warming*, stimulant	digestive
	he shou wu	tang kuei	**Xiao Yao Wan**
	royal jelly	damiana	
GINSENGS	American (white) **Wuchaseng**	Chinese (red)	tienchi

	INTERNAL HEAT	*INTERNAL COLD*	*PHLEGM*
KITCHEN HERBS	cumin, coriander, fennel, parsley, mint, cilantro, sarsaparilla, red clover	clove, fenugreek, cinnamon	ginger, orange peel, cinnamon
CHINESE PATENT REMEDIES	**An Sheng Pu Shin Wan**	**Tzepao Sanpien Wan**	

Chinese nonpatent remedies by Seven Forests

    For anxiety: **Fu-Shen 16**

    For male or female weakness and "impotence": **Antler 8**

    For aching legs and back, poor circulation: **Millettia 9** with **Salvia Shou Wu**

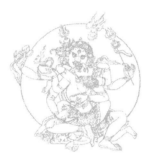

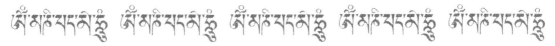

PART FIVE

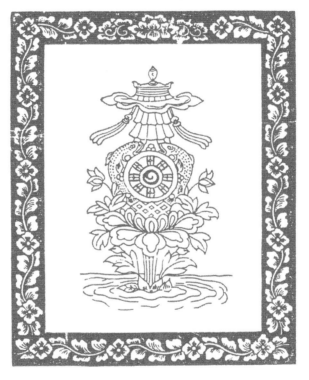

Herbs and the Mind

"The nature of Mind is a coalescence of Clarity and Emptiness." That is the essence of Tibetan Buddhist teaching. The mind is clear, empty, and calm. How can you achieve it? Think of a glass. A glass holds many liquids: sweet juices, bitter lemons, or water for flowers. It does not love or hate the liquid. It's only the container. Any liquid the glass contains, or any thought or feeling you have, can be emptied like water. Your mind is an empty glass. What do you most often put into it?

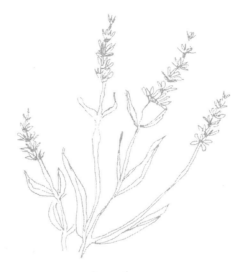

Lavender

Healing Body, Mind, and Spirit

Belinda sat before me, holding back tears and shredding a tissue as she spoke. She hoped to find a husband, but did not go to parties or out with friends because she was overweight. For one year she had taken Prozac, which caused her to gain eighty pounds. She wanted to stop taking the drug so that she could lose weight, but she'd lost the willpower and clarity of mind necessary to change her life. Now she felt addicted to antidepressant medicine. Sad, bewildered, lonely, she desperately needed help, but didn't know where to start.

The initial causes of her imbalance had not been addressed by the mind-altering drug: It affected her brain chemicals without improving her energy. Her slow metabolism and poor digestion gave her a tendency to put on weight. That condition, combined with the drug, curbed her vitality and oppressed her spirit. She felt trapped in a body that she did not want, in a life situation that she could not endure. Worse yet, Belinda did not claim any responsibility for creating or maintaining her health, so she felt victimized.

Belinda's situation is not isolated. Many people addicted to mind-altering drugs expect the medicine to do the work of their minds. Drugs cannot give you insight into the circumstances that created your problems. At best they can only temporarily dull the pain created by your situation. What is needed, instead, is a real look at the source of your inability to move forward, to pursue the life that you want in the most appropriate ways.

Herbs used to treat mental and emotional problems are nourishing and energizing tonics, and also purifying cleansers. They enhance peace of mind, productivity, and clarity of thought by promoting health and balance. Herbs help you take charge of your life because they improve your vitality.

The herbal route is a more experienced one than new drugs that control brain chemicals or up-to-the-minute theories about genes. Used correctly, herbs are body and brain foods that can bring your health into balance. Herbal medicines realign you with the healing powers of Nature, our fountain of life and positive change. Chemical control of your emotions and behavior may pacify your complaints temporarily, but do they enhance the quality of your life? Mind drugs are suited to maintaining society's delusions, enslavement, and social injustice. Who among the advocates of medical drugs would admit that mental and emotional problems stem from poverty, ignorance, and abuse? Merely changing our brain chemicals fails to address such issues.

癲狂 癲狂 癲狂 癲狂 癲狂　癲 癲 癲 癲 癲 癲 癲　狂 狂 狂 狂 狂 狂 狂

[diānkuáng] Depressive-maniac insanity　　[diān] Insanity with emotional depression　　[kuáng] Mania with emotional excitement

35
Blue Mondays: Depression

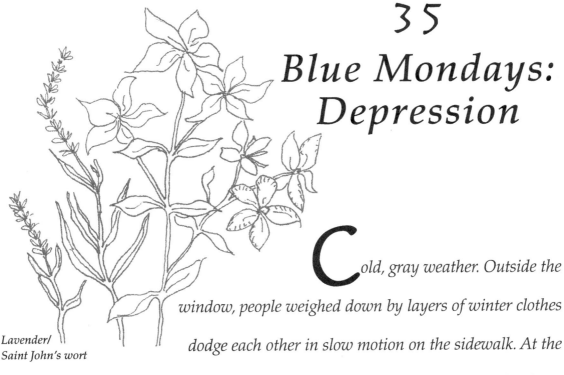

Lavender/
Saint John's wort

Cold, gray weather. Outside the window, people weighed down by layers of winter clothes dodge each other in slow motion on the sidewalk. At the corner, a young woman with a baby holds a sign no one reads. The homeless have moved somewhere indoors, except for a few men warming their hands over a fire they've made in a garbage can. Near the supermarket, young Canadian lumberjacks wearing red plaid shirts are selling Christmas trees for fifty dollars and up.

The air is sharp, as the smell of evergreen mixes with burning garbage and bus fumes. I've slept badly for weeks, awakened by numb fingers and *ringing ears. My tongue is pale, with deep scallops around the edges: deficient chi and chest pain. Time to take herbs from Chinatown to smooth my heart's rhythm and to prevent the winter blahs. I've shut myself in to write late into the night. My cat, Silky, lounges close by, her paw fondly stroking the computer.*

We fly off together. This time it's the Thai jungle. I remember a summer night under a starry canopy, the Milky Way spread out like a blanket high above my head. I'd decided to sleep on the porch to escape close quarters and fleas in the cot. My host's grass hut was about fourteen feet square with a dirt floor in the cooking area. A small fire lit the inside, and smoke escaped through a hole in the roof.

I jumped from a noise near the porch. Cows were mingling nearby. A woman strolled past, shooing them with a stick. She carried one baby on her back and another inside. I watched the outline of her body by fireglow, the cloth skirt and hat she'd woven, her thin bare breasts. White smoke from her pipe curled around her face. I tried to hear every sound like a pattern: crackle of fire; shuffle of cows; people far away, laughing. Late that night a mother pig moved under the porch with her piglets. Eden, squealing and swarming with life, lay all around me. Warm, dank air became my blanket as I watched the approach of dawn.

Silky is asleep. Back at my desk, I'm struck by the contrast of the city where I live and the jungle I visit. This summer's trip and others over the past dozen years have been rich reward for my interest in Asian herbs. How much better they are than any drug to lift my spirits!

When we use Asian medicine, we swallow more than plants grown on hillsides or in jungles. We partake of a living culture, a healing tradition that raises us out of the position of a patient who quietly waits to be sedated or punished for being sick. In this chapter we'll study a traditional Chinese view of depression, a health problem that has become part and parcel of a modern lifestyle. Many persons suffering from depression also experience weight gain or low sexual energy and vitality from addictive psychiatric drugs. They don't know whether to cry about their depression or about their drugs' side effects.

In this chapter we will examine several formulas used in Chinese hospitals today that address the mental and physical problems associated with depression. They are easily available in Chinese food and herb markets in the West, and by mail order from sources listed in the Herbal Access appendix. Herbal remedies for depression are of special value to us now, at a time when funds for patient care are threatened more every day, when drug therapy is too frequently applied, and when electroshock treatments have reemerged as "progressive medical care."

A Different Approach to Depression

Western medicine's answer to depression is drug therapy that affects certain brain chemicals—most often serotonin. That is a narrow and ultimately dangerous approach, because we are more than merely brain chemicals. Prozac, the current drug of choice, has been known to increase insomnia, anxiety, agitation, irritability, nausea, sexual dysfunction, and rates of suicide; and it is only one in a line of such medications that affect serotonin level.

However, there are other sources of serotonin—sunshine, for instance. Sunshine builds *chi*, but so do herbs. Certain digestive and energy tonic herbs are *warming* and *drying* like the sun.

HOW ANTIDEPRESSION HERBS WORK

Chinese remedies used to treat depression are not sedative drugs. Herbs for mental problems improve mental function by enhancing blood quality and blood circulation to the brain. Some also reduce cholesterol and treat indigestion. Mental problems, using a Chinese medical approach, are defined and treated as physical problems. Indirectly, hormones and brain chemicals may be affected, resulting in improved vitality, circulation, and so on. With Asian medicine we treat the whole person, not just brain chemicals. This approach is safe, effective, and nonaddictive. Because the herbs are nourishing and energizing, as your general health improves, so does your depression.

TREATMENT OF DEPRESSION IN CHINESE HOSPITALS

I spent the summer of 1993 studying acupuncture and herbal treatments for depression at Shanghai's College of Medicine, Research Institute of Acupuncture and Meridien (RIAM). Dr. Chao, my instructor and head of the Department of Traditional Medicine, had employed acupuncture and herbal treatments as standard hospital care for over forty years. A cheerful, rosy-faced man, he was typical of many Chinese doctors I've met. Dressed casually in shorts and sandals, he drank green tea all day, directly from a little teapot. His mentor, a lady doctor, had practiced acupuncture and prescribed herbs into her eighties. Supervised by Dr. Chao, I applied acupuncture weekly to several persons diagnosed as depressed and schizophrenic. Some had hallucinations and delusions and suffered from poor concentration and low energy, but all of them improved with herbs and regular treatments of acupuncture.

THE ENERGETIC BASIS OF DEPRESSION

Interestingly, both depression and schizophrenia are related to mental cloudiness, poor concentration, spacey feelings, and certain physical imbalances, including poor spleen/pancreas function, irregular heartbeat, and weak or stuck *chi.* This means that appropriate acupuncture and herbs would strengthen and regulate digestion; eliminate nervous tension and liver inflammation leading to anxiety and heart palpitations; and move stuck circulation to regulate hormones, life energy, and eliminate vague pains. This presents a two-sided approach: strengthening weakness and anemia while

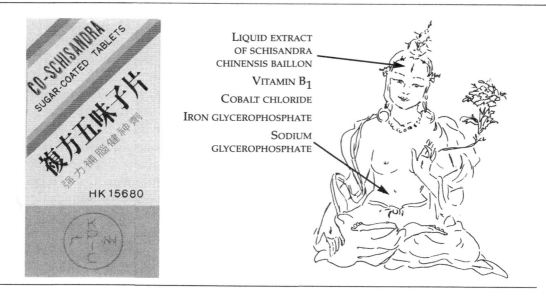

CO-SCHISANDRA SUGAR-COATED TABLETS

复方五味子片

强力补脑健神剂

HK 15680

LIQUID EXTRACT
OF SCHISANDRA
CHINENSIS BAILLON
VITAMIN B_1
COBALT CHLORIDE
IRON GLYCEROPHOSPHATE
SODIUM
GLYCEROPHOSPHATE

easing physical and emotional irritation and burnout. You can apply this general method to yourself after you've grasped the energetic origin of your depression.

BEGIN BY RECOGNIZING YOUR REAL PROBLEM

Are you in a depressing situation that you cannot change? At least you have the advantage of knowing you are depressed. Most people don't realize when they're depressed. They may admit that things could be better in their lives, but they don't consider indigestion, agitation, irritability, insomnia, or mood swings to be anything other than symptoms of temporary stress. Even if you are unable to resolve your negative situation entirely, with herbs you can enhance your energy and protect your health and vitality so that you can work toward positive change.

Are you depressed because you feel as though you absorb other people's problems or moods, that you no longer have the strength to distance yourself sufficiently from them? This may be related to exhaustion or poor digestion. You must strengthen your own *chi* before you can gain the mental clarity necessary to deal with your surroundings. The information in this and the following chapter, concerning herbs for mental clarity, will help you.

Do you fear the responsibility of preventing and treating your depression? It may seem easier to point at a doctor, parent, boss, or spouse and say, "It's your fault," or "I'm guilty. Drug me, shock me." But you will feel the pain of your depression more if you refuse to help yourself. Milder versions of this attitude include the sentiments expressed in such statements as "I don't have time to take care of myself"; "I don't know enough to treat myself"; "Nothing as imprecise as herbs is safe anyway." Those excuses won't work because you have already learned a great deal about how herbs affect your body, mind, and spirit. Your emotions are just another part of your energetic being.

To prevent depression, you need an approach that's more effective than verbalizing your emotions or swallowing a hundred pills. This chapter will help you to know when and how to use herbs, and also how to combine good nutrition with herbal treatment. You can begin to heal your depression by observing your *chi*.

OBSERVE YOURSELF

When preventing and treating depression, you need to reverse the underlying energetic factors. Please answer the following questions to observe them in yourself.

DIGESTIVE CAUSES OF DEPRESSION

Are you "fed up"? "Sick of it"? Have you "had it up to here"? We often use digestive terms to describe frustration or depression. There is a good reason for it. Deficient *chi* (weakness), indicated by a pale tongue,

DEPRESSION AND WEAK DIGESTION

WEAK KIDNEY AND SPLEEN CHI

- Is your tongue large, pale, coated, or spotted?
- Do you often sit in a chair obsessing about something or someone?
- Do you always have the same troubling thoughts or emotions?
- Do you lie around, sadly ruminating about past problems?
- Do you have chronic watery diarrhea?
- Do you feel weakened or injured by an emotional situation?
- Do you have chronic low energy with indigestion?
- Do you need to take an afternoon nap?
- Do sad movies or stories always make you cry?
- Are you lonely or worried most of the time?

- Do you procrastinate about your house chores, or avoid work?
- Have you neglected yourself, your beauty, your clothes?

EXCESS PHLEGM

- Is it hard to concentrate or think clearly?
- Do you have abdominal bloating and pain in the ribs?
- Do you have edema or feel puffy?
- Do you have irregular periods and mood swings?
- Do you have poor appetite or frequent nausea?
- Do you crave ice cream, pastry, candy, alcohol, or drugs?

hinders processing of food as well as ideas and emotions.

A coated tongue indicates troubled digestion and excess *phlegm*. *Phlegm* (the *humor*) "obstructs the senses." It clouds perception and thinking. This implies hormones, brain chemicals, and all subtle physical reactions that affect emotions. Excess *phlegm* makes thinking cloudy, concentration poor; it makes us moody and obsessive. With an excess *phlegm* condition, you may become too confused to move forward. You may also crave foods that aggravate the problem. Sweets, fried foods, fats, and oils increase *phlegm*. Alcohol and drugs, like sweets, can make everything cloudy.

INCREASE DIGESTIVE *CHI* FOR BETTER NUTRITION

By reversing *phlegm* with pungent, *drying* foods and herbs, we reverse one underlying cause of depression. Eating the right foods is important, but without enough digestive *chi*, all benefits are lost. Ensuring sufficient vitality from digestion, respiration, circulation, and immune strength is the basis of energetic medicine. What that means is that in treating depression (or any illness), there is no long list of supplements that will work for everyone. Capacity for absorption varies. We first must address our digestive weakness, then impediments to healthy body/mind/spirit will begin to dissolve.

ACTIVITIES AND DIET FOR WEAK DIGESTION AND *PHLEGM*

The following activities and recipes are designed to move stuck energy and build strength. They involve taking charge of your diet and participating in a compassionate way with those around you. It is this involvement that can ultimately save you from self-absorption, self-doubt, and low spirits. The cure comes from doing and giving, not from thinking, analyzing, or promising yourself that someday things will improve.

Cook the following easy-to-make soups and teas each day, infusing them with positive thoughts and good wishes for all those who are suffering. Daily put canned foods on the street, where they can be found by someone more hungry than yourself. Or put some money on the street each day. Soon you will feel the results. As your energy and activities become more expansive and generous, you will feel stronger and more confident and loving. Record your progress in a journal or with artwork, or write letters to people involved. Do not send any letters until they express positive aspirations.

A DIET FOR WEAKNESS, *INTERNAL COLD*, AND *PHLEGM*

If you feel sad, weak, and chilled, if you have a pale, coated tongue, reverse the production of *phlegm* by eating at least one bowl of barley soup per day. Boil raw barley until it is soft, and season it with fresh parsley, sliced ginger, orange peel, and salt and pepper to taste. Also eat radishes to spark appetite and digestion.

Drink a tea daily between meals made from ½ teaspoon each of powdered clove and basil leaves per cup of hot water. Clove raises your energy, and basil lifts low spirits away. These foods reduce congestion and improve breathing and energy. (*Caution:* Avoid all warming foods and spices if you have headache, fever, hot flashes, or hot temper. See the section below on stuck chi and internal heat.)

REMEDIES TO ENHANCE MENTAL CLARITY AND COMFORT

If weeping or sinus congestion obscures your senses so that you develop a headache or cloudy thinking, sniff an opened capsule of gotu kola like snuff. Your congestion will dissolve immediately so that you'll be able to breathe and think clearly.

If you can't sleep, try taking a warm bath, adding Epsom salts and essential oil of lavender to the water. After the bath, place some essential lavender oil on your chest and abdomen. (See remedies for mental clarity in the following chapter and in section I of chapter 13.)

Herbs for Depression Caused by Anemia

❧ Do you get depressed around your period time?

❧ Is your depression worse before the period (PMS)?

❧ Is it worse after your period (blood deficiency)?

Digestive weakness can result in poor blood production. Because of that, the following remedies are suited for depression related to menstrual irregularities as well as indigestion. Either men or women can take these herbal pills.

If you have a pale tongue or hypoglycemia, take **Xiao Yao Wan** in a dose large enough to reduce *phlegm* and improve appetite and energy—for example, 8 to 10 pills after meals. Start with a smaller dose and increase it as it feels comfortable. Avoid excessive cold, raw foods, white sugar, coffee, and alcohol.

Co-Schisandra Tablets, a potent tonic for the brain and a mental stimulant, are recommended for depression associated with weakness, fatigue and blood deficiency caused by illness, poor nutrition, or emotional problems such as anxiety, fear, and neurosis. If you feel depressed after your menstrual period or if your lips are pale, this remedy can help. Other symptoms may include headache, dizziness, blurred vision, and insomnia. The Chinese indications on the box require some clarification. In addition to the uses I've already mentioned, these pills are recommended for "brain-fag [fatigue and mental cloudiness] and alcoholism." The herbal combination contains Schisandra chinensis baillon, which improves respiration and circulation to enhance the functioning of the cerebral cortex. Also included in the pills are vitamin B$_1$, cobalt chloride, iron glycerophosphate, and sodium glycerophosphate.

FOR ANXIETY AND HORMONE IMBALANCES

Crystal Star Herbal Nutrition manufactures several Western herbal combinations that are helpful for depression because they address many related symptoms at once. They are available in health-food stores and by mail. Follow the company's directions for dosage.

Depress Ex liquid extract contains skullcap, ashwagandha, trifala, valerian, rosemary, hops, catnip, wood betony, peppermint, celery seed, cinnamon, and lime essential oil in a base that is 45 percent alcohol.

Depress Ex combines nervines such as valerian with digestive herbs, including catnip and celery seed, along with those that break apart stuck *chi*, such as cinnamon. Rosemary builds and balances *chi* of kidney and heart. The combination originally contained lady's slipper, but the company substituted the two Ayurvedic herbs ashwagandha and trifala when they heard lady's slipper was endangered. Good show! The combination is suited for men or women who are weak, tired, or overwrought, and who experience digestive problems. Add the drops to water and drink between meals.

Crystal Star also makes **Relax Caps** for exhaustion, anxiety, and insomnia from weakness and deficiency. They contain ashwagandha, black cohosh, skullcap, kava kava, black haw bark, hops, valerian, European mistletoe, wood betony, lobelia, and oatstraw. Ashwagandha is similar to pseudoginseng in that it normalizes energy. Although it's a neutral stimulant that rebuilds adrenal strength, it also treats exhaustion, insomnia, and blood deficiency. Black cohosh is added in this combination to ensure hormone balance. Mistletoe, valerian, hops, and skullcap are nervines to soothe anxiety and insomnia.

Depression from Stuck Chi, **Internal Heat,** *and* **Phlegm**

- Do you often feel angry, frustrated, or stuck?
- Do you experience chest or abdominal pain, burping or nausea?
- Do you have palpitations or anxiety?
- Do you become so agitated that you can't sleep?
- Do you crave hot spices or rich foods and drinks?
- Do you have nightmares?
- Are your sexual needs unsatisfied?
- Are you going nowhere in your job?
- Do you wish you could end a relationship?

DEPRESSION FROM BEING STUCK

Depression from stuck *chi* is often accompanied by indigestion, chest pain, and weary or fearful agitation. This is because emotions as well as blood and energy circulation are stuck. Uneasiness can simmer under the surface, leading to procrastination and avoidance, or erupt into major explosions when bottled up too long. Hiding or holding in rage is like lighting dynamite in a bottle. The vessel will break with the explosion. The charge must be adequately cooled and redirected in order to avoid damage.

ACTIVITIES AND DIET

To help smooth your digestion, do one half hour of gentle bend-in-the-middle exercise, or take a walk after dinner.

Persons with a reddish, coated tongue should eat a *cooling,* antiphlegm diet. You can accomplish this by alternating the recipes from section II of chapter 13, the anti-inflammatory diet, with those in section I, the antiphlegm diet. Barley soup is a fine dish for anyone with *internal heat* as long as you avoid hot spices such as garlic, pepper, ginger, and clove. Instead, try cumin, coriander, fennel, saffron, mint, and dill, which work better. Try to have at least one bowl of seasoned barley soup or white rice pudding per day. Add *cooling* vegetables such as broccoli, asparagus, and green beans, and enjoy a *cooling* tea.

A *COOLING,* HARMONIZING TEA

Drink mint, green, or chamomile tea daily, adding up to ¼ cup of aloe vera juice or gel to cool *internal heat.* If your circulation is poor, add one pinch of turmeric powder per cup of tea. If you have arthritic pain that feels better with heat and movement, take 1 capsule of myrrh with green tea between meals.

A SPECIAL SPLASH TO QUIET YOUR BRAIN

To cool off a hot head, soak your hair and scalp with olive oil for at least ten minutes before you wash. Then splash on essential rose oil afterward. Fragrances that cool and calm your nerves are pure essential oil of green apple, apple blossom, or sandalwood. Put a drop under your nose.

Does your brain chatter nonsense? Put pure essential sandalwood oil in a line in front of each ear, toward your jaw. It relaxes jaw tension and stuck circulation that provoke constant rumination.

HERBAL RECOMMENDATIONS FOR STUCK *CHI* DEPRESSION

If you are depressed, herbal combinations that treat *stagnant chi* will always help you. This is because depression is by nature an illness caused by being stuck in a bad situation. Stuck *chi* leads to anxiety, insomnia, and pains. *Stagnation* can result from being either too weak or too angry to move. Often they come together, along with unexpressed negative feelings. For that reason, Asian herbal combinations for depression are built with both *cooling* and grounding or tonifying herbs in order to break apart stagnant *chi* circulation. That helps the body and mind to heal themselves.

I'll explain several of the ingredients in the following depression remedies that treat stuck liver *chi*. Take those containing nervines (nerve sedatives) only when experiencing excess nervousness and insomnia.

DEPRESSION REMEDIES THAT CLEAR FRUSTRATION AND EMOTIONAL STUCKNESS

None of the formulas listed below are sedative or habit-forming. You may have to increase the recommended dose to suit your needs. Don't feel embarrassed to take a handful of herbal pills (for example, 8 to 10 pills) after meals or anytime you need them. Like healing foods, these herbs improve your digestion, circulation, and outlook very quickly. The following formulas free stagnant liver *chi.* You can choose any one and stay with it for as long as you need it.

Green Tiger—Liver Harmony, by Turtle Mountain products
Relaxed Wanderer—Stagnant Liver Qi, by Jade Pharmacy
Wood Constitution, by Nature's Sunshine
Jie Yu ("Bupleurum and Cyperus Eighteen Combination"), by Nature's Sunshine

This last combination is similar to a Chinese patent remedy: **Xiao Chia Hu Tang Wan.** Both treat depression, excess *phlegm,* and digestive complaints.

OTHER RELAXING HERBS FOR DAILY USE

- Do you think and talk so fast that you wear yourself out?
- Is it hard to slow down?
- Do you have stomach pain, bad breath, or blemishes from nerves?
- Is it hard for you to fall asleep or stay asleep?
- Are you taking final exams, or are you under lots of stress?

If you answered "yes" to those questions, you will need daily help to find your balance. The following herbs are easy to use and very safe for stress, anxiety, or excess acid conditions.

Aloe vera cools and cleanses excess acid from the liver, spleen/pancreas, stomach, and blood. It treats nervousness, anxiety, bad breath, and skin rashes. Persons with severe *internal heat* can use as much as ½ cup daily, in apple juice, tea, or water, adding lemon juice as needed for taste. If diarrhea or chill results, reduce the dose.

Siberian ginseng extract (**Wuchaseng**) nurtures nerves and brain to reduce agitation and insomnia. Take one teaspoon at a time during the day and before bed to reduce nervousness. The correct dosage is one that is comfortable for you. Do not take **Wuchaseng** indefinitely; it is a brain and nerve tonic. After it relaxes you, reduce and eliminate the herb because excess use can stimulate nervous agitation.

Cerebral Tonic Pills help reduce mania, poor concentration, and faulty memory. The remedy lowers unhealthy cholesterol and "phlegm that obscures the senses." It is not a sedative, but enhances circulation in the brain to reduce stress and mania. Follow the directions. If none are given (or if they are not in English), take 10 pills three times a day between meals. Certain ingredients, such as red dates and lycium fruit, tend to slow digestion. This herbal cure has worked well for persons I've known who were agitated from emotional upset and extreme fatigue, several of whom were unable to sleep for as many as ten days straight.

Depression and Rage

When stuck *chi* turns to rage, take the Chinese patent remedy **Lung Tan Xie Gan Wan,** a liver/gallbladder cleanser, in dosages large enough—for example, 10 pills three or more times a day—to eliminate headache, constipation, herpes, or vaginal discharge; enough to cool anger, agitation, and mania. This can be combined with half as much **Xiao Yao Wan** for pain in the chest or rib cage, or sinus congestion. Neither is a sedative, but both work to aid digestion and circulation. They are available in Chinese herb stores and by mail.

At the Shanghai teaching hospital where I studied acupuncture and herbal treatments for mental problems, Dr. Chao said large daily doses of **Lung Tan Xie Gan Wan** could be used to curb violent behavior. I've recommended it successfully for angry PMS. The correct dosage is one that works to relax you. Start with 10 pills three times daily for a day or two, then adjust the dosage. Reduce or stop the remedy when you feel relaxed and calm. The remedy itself will not weaken you. **Lung Tan Xie Gan Wan** has as a main ingredient 20 percent gentian, an herb recommended for shortness of breath, fatigue, depression, blood-sugar swings, and chronic diarrhea. It will not cause weakness, but improves mental clarity.

HOMEOPATHIC REMEDIES FOR DEPRESSION: A TEMPORARY "QUICK FIX"

Homeopathic and Bach Flower Remedies from the health-food store also treat emotional imbalances quickly and effectively. They can strongly reduce stress. The trouble is that sometimes a problem is so ingrained that such remedies are only a bandage. They should be used temporarily in conjunction with diet, herbs, and other therapies. Homeopathic remedies are used by the body at varying speeds; therefore the dosage varies. The usual dose is once every four hours, but acute problems require frequent doses, for example, once every fifteen minutes. When switching from one homeopathic remedy to another, wait a couple of hours until the first one wears off, or cancel the first with one cup of unsweetened decaffeinated or regular coffee. Then wait about fifteen minutes before taking the second remedy.

Homeopathic remedies are subtle

and powerful cleansers. They bring negative emotions to the surface. Be prepared to process what comes up. I recommend that you take them with the guidance of a healer or the sympathetic ear of a trusted friend. Be sure to give yourself time to deal with emotions that are freed.

Sadness

For excess *phlegm* and sadness, take homeopathic pulsatilla (30c potency). Add 10 or 12 pills to a pot of green tea. Sip a cup or more of hot tea during the day. Or add the same amount to one liter of springwater and sip as needed throughout the day. Each sip is considered one dose. Do not expect to finish the liter during one day, but keep it fresh in the refrigerator. Avoid coffee, or start the remedy one half hour after drinking coffee.

Panic

To reduce fear, anxiety, or panic, take homeopathic aconite (30c potency). Add 4 pills to one cup of water. Sip it every twenty minutes, and stop the remedy when it causes sweating. I recommend homeopathic aconite for persons with serious diseases, and for those who fear death or have hysterical trepidation of harming others. Using this remedy will temporarily cause anxiety to surface. This usually passes with the second or third dose.

Several case histories come to mind that illustrate how homeopathic aconite works. One woman was grieving over the death of her father. She said she disliked her father, but mourned the end of her family name. She feared she might get the same disease, and then no one would be left. Her depression was not from grief so much as from the fear of death. Homeopathic aconite eased her neurotic panic.

Another woman, a nurse, was given charge of her mother's health. The mother's condition was serious, and her daughter's feelings toward her were ambivalent. Fear and guilt approaching panic proportions kept the daughter from sleeping, but the nurse found relief with homeopathic aconite.

I gave another friend homeopathic aconite the day he learned that he'd tested positive for the HIV virus. He didn't speak or cry, but he looked gray, green, and yellowish all at once. He felt nauseated and horrified. After taking aconite 30c, he could breathe more deeply and seemed more present. He listened as I told him about the success that Chinese herbal remedies have had over the past sixteen years in treating AIDS; many people diagnosed with HIV have never developed symptoms of AIDS because they kept themselves strong with herbs.

Homesickness

For melancholy, homesickness, lovesickness, and loneliness, the Bach Flower Remedy honeysuckle is recommended. Perhaps the sweet, calming nature of that delicate flower soothes a spirit that yearns for love and peace. Add 6 drops to a glass of water and sip several times daily. Some people add Bach Flower Remedies to baths, but I prefer adding herbs or essential oils. Honeysuckle, worn as a fragrance, is sedating. I prefer lavender for aromatherapy to treat loneliness, because it stimulates stuck energy. But perhaps the best fragrance for one who longs for home is made from the flowers that grow there, the perfume that reminds us of home.

Hatred and revenge

For held-in feelings of hatred and revenge, try the Bach Flower Remedy holly. Hatred is sharp and prickly, like a holly leaf. The homeopathic dose of holly will remove the sting that wounds both giver and receiver. Add 6 drops to a glass of water, and sip it throughout the day.

Tibetan doctors believe a way to overcome hatred is by helping others. I once knew a selfish woman who was depressed most of the time. When she had her Tibetan astrology chart done, the monks advised her to overcome her negative karma by saving the lives of dying animals. But she had no pets of her own, and when given the chance to care for someone else's pets, she let them die and remain unburied. Her karma seemed irrevocable, but she finally started up an animal rights newsletter. I don't know if she took Dr. Bach's homeopathic holly regularly, but she used it as her logo.

Dread

A dear friend told me, "Money is energy. It can be used for good or bad, depending upon your intentions." He was blessed with talent and a fine artistic sensibility, but he always felt scared and nervous, pacing the floor miserably for days before performing a concert. He overpracticed to the point where, during a performance, he was unable to enjoy it or even hear it. This excessive worry is a form of depression.

I recommended that he take homeopathic gelsemium (30c potency), traditionally used for anxiety over an upcoming event, including stage fright. He told me that when he took the remedy three times daily during the week before the performance, it worked very well. He also sent a sum of money at that time to a music school for disadvantaged children, and imagined that he was performing the concert for them. He knew that a gift intended to help others opens a door of forgiveness in our psyche.

Herbal remedies for depression can help you either for long-term or quick-fix problems, because they regulate your vital energy, digestion, circulation, and all other factors that build health. They improve the quality of your life and give you the chance to take the bull by the horns.

DEPRESSION

What makes it worse?

Hunger, poverty; drug, alcohol, or smoking addictions; medications; cold, raw, and sour foods and congesting, phlegm-producing foods (fats, cheese, milk); mental, physical, and sexual exhaustion; worry, grief, stress; hormonal irregularity, PMS, menopause; stuck emotional situations; sexual dissatisfaction; feelings of failure and defeat; unacceptance of yourself.

What makes it better?

Herbs to build and move stuck *chi,* clear phlegm, and build energy; good nutrition, rest, exercise, massage; satisfying love, work, and family relationships; positive work to help others; funny movies.

	INTERNAL HEAT	*INTERNAL COLD*	*PHLEGM*
TONGUE	reddish, spotted	pale, spotted	coated
SYMPTOMS	anger, rage	sadness, obsession	cloudy thinking
	insomnia	insomnia	too much sleep
	palpitations	arrhythmia	stupor
	chest pain	joint aches	irregular menstrual period
	fever	chills	delirium
	mania	catatonia	
	hallucinations		

REMEDIES

Digestive disturbance, obsession, allergies, and anger: **Xiao Yao Wan** and **Lung Tan Xie Gan Wan**

Depression and blood deficiency (worse after your period): **Co-Schisandra Tablets**

After childbirth: **Shih Chuan Ta Bu Wan** (see page 344)

PMS: **Xiao Yao Wan, Relaxed Wanderer, Depress Ex**

Insomnia, anxiety: **Wuchaseng** (Siberian ginseng extract)

With excess *phlegm,* sinus congestion: homeopathic pulsatilla

Violent rage: **Lung Tan Xie Gan Wan**; holly (Bach Flower Remedy)

五志過極 五志過極 五志過極 喜 喜 喜 怒 怒 怒 憂 憂 憂 思 思 思 恐 恐 恐

(wǔzhì guòjí) Five emotions in excess: excessive joy,   anger,   melancholy,   anxiety,   and fear may influence the normal circulation of Qi (vital energy) and blood.

36

Herbs for Memory and Mental Clarity

A growing number of physicians recognize that a state of emotional balance and sense of well-being are necessary for easing stress and reducing illness. A few, like Dr. Andrew Weil, have noted how some of their patients, although suffering from cancer or other terrible illnesses, have spontaneously healed after accepting themselves and their lives completely, including their illnesses. Although it does not seem likely that this will become a trend in Western medical practice (rendering the physician essentially unnecessary), it certainly has great value. For one thing, it points out that the body/mind/spirit, viewed as an energetic totality, has great capacity to heal itself.

Many traditional Asian and Native American healers go even further and believe that healing the mind and spirit can actually prevent illness and misfortune. In this chapter we'll explore herbs used to facilitate memory and improve mental clarity. In the next chapter we'll cover useful herbs for high achievement and emotional growth. Such herbs, which enhance well-being, can be used in conjunction with Western drug therapies because they speed physical recovery and emotional rebalancing.

You might want to use the remedies covered in these chapters along with a personal cleansing routine or psychotherapy. You may take advantage of the calm and clarity gained from the herbs to focus your attention for work or to prepare yourself for a giant step forward in your career and personal life. This part of the book, Herbs and the Mind, will help you with important transitions such as birth, marriage, and death. In previous chapters we have considered remedies for clearing the ill effects of *phlegm,* inflammation, and nervous exhaustion; now we'll study herbs for corresponding mental and emotional states. Depression and mania are covered in more detail in the preceding chapter.

Although some of the remedies in this chapter and in chapter 37 have been

discussed previously because they are also used to treat physical ailments, they will be described here in terms of their ability to facilitate mental acuity and emotional balance.

A Multidimensional Approach

Asian-trained herbalists view the mind and emotions as changing *energetic* phenomena. What this means is that foods and herbs that affect *chi,* circulation, and blood also affect the mind. Emotions are a part of our energetic and physical make-up, and are described by such concepts as *shen* (in Chinese medicine) and *sattva* (in Ayurveda). First I'll describe a few formulas used to address various mental issues, including deficiencies in memory and concentration, then I'll discuss emotional problems by considering herbs that treat the *shen,* or spirit.

HOW HERBAL BRAIN TONICS WORK

Problems of poor concentration and memory are usually treated with nourishing, stimulant remedies that are combinations of blood-building herbs and energy tonics. These reverse weakness and anemia, build strength, and stimulate circulation. In addition, the herbs coordinate the functioning of the heart and adrenal glands.

Take, for example, **Cerebral Tonic Pills,** a Chinese patent remedy that is used for poor concentration and memory; it also reduces manic episodes by facilitating blood circulation and reducing cholesterol and hardened arteries. In other words, **Cerebral Tonic Pills** are not a brain sedative; instead they free stuck circulation, thus ensuring the brain's supply of oxygen and nourishment.

The formula contains schisandra, zizyphus, cistanche, and juglans, used to enhance energy; tang kuei and lycium, which nourish blood; acornus, to improve circulation; arisaema, to resolve *phlegm;* and gastrodia and succinum to calm anxiety, seizures, forgetfulness, and insomnia. In addition, the formula contains "dragon tooth," a calcium source, along with biota seed and polygala root acting as nourishing sedatives. It is interesting to note in this formula that both anxiety and forgetfulness are treated with blood- and energy-building herbs. This proves again that having adequate *yin* and *yang* normalizes physical and mental processes.

POOR MEMORY CAUSED BY WEAKNESS, FATIGUE, AND STRESS

The physical states most often associated with chronic poor memory are fatigue and weakness caused by a variety of factors, including those listed here. Accompanying such weakness will be signs of weak *chi,* including puffy face or body, poor appetite or nausea from excess *phlegm* conditions, and low energy and enthusiasm.

Internal cold symptoms are possible,

CAUSES OF POOR CONCENTRATION AND MEMORY

Low *chi*:

- 🌿 Do you feel tired, chilled? Are you over sixty, chronically ill?
- 🌿 Are you pale, listless, depressed?

Weak heart:

- 🌿 Do you have insomnia or palpitations from a weak heart?
- 🌿 Are you restless and nervous, with shortness of breath and low appetite?

Weak adrenal energy:

- 🌿 Do you have restless sleep, back pain, no sexual energy?
- 🌿 Are you often tired, with weak muscles?

Profound fatigue:

- 🌿 Have you recently been very sick, or given birth?
- 🌿 Do you have global edema, heart palpitations (congestive heart failure), insomnia, asthma with wheezing, or low immune strength?

Internal heat and nervous exhaustion:

- 🌿 Do you have nightmares, throbbing head, tinnitus, irritability?
- 🌿 Do you have skin rash, bloodshot eyes, or flushed appearance?
- 🌿 Do you have memory burnout?

including a pale tongue and low pulse, if you have been ill or exhausted, or have been chilled by cold diet or climate.

Internal heat poor memory is also possible, if you have been burning your brain at both ends with work, play, stimulants, hot spices, emotional upheaval, stress, fever, or drugs.

POOR MEMORY CAUSED BY *INTERNAL COLD*

When pale tongue and complexion accompany poor memory, it is best to take a *warming* energy and blood tonic such as those listed below. Since brain tonics are not meant to aid digestion, but are general nourishing restoratives, it is best to take them between meals for months at a time. You will know they have done their job when you look and feel better and you can remember their long list of ingredients in Latin. Here are a few examples of *warming* blood- and *chi*-builders. For a more complete list, see chapter 31.

POOR MEMORY CAUSED BY WEAK *CHI*

Ginseng Polygona Root Extract (Ren Shen Shou Wu Jing) contains he shou wu (fo ti) and ginseng. It treats weak-*chi* insomnia, poor appetite, fatigue, aching joints, and low sex drive. You can take 2 cc twice daily.

Ren Shen Yang Ying Wan contains a dozen plant-derived blood and energy tonics. It's recommended as a general tonic taken over long periods for weak heart of the elderly or others. It treats insomnia, palpitations, fatigue, and poor memory. You can take 10 pills three times daily, or one large herbal ball daily.

Angelicae Longana Pills (Gui Pi Wan) is recommended for poor memory caused by weak heart. It contains codonopsis, fu ling, zizyphus, atractylodes, longan, astragalus, polygala, tang kuei, and saussurea. The usual dosage is 8 pills three times daily.

For poor memory caused by weak kidney and adrenal energy, please refer to chapter 34. Also traditionally recommended are **Ching Chun Bao** ("Recovery of Youth Tablet"). The recommended dose is 2 to 5 capsules per day. It is a *heating* tonic, though not all the ingredients are listed.

Duzhong Bu Tian Su is recommended for weak heart and adrenal glands with edema, difficult breathing, and insomnia; for congestive heart problems, urinary incontinence, heart palpitations, poor memory, or dizziness following male sexual ejaculation; and also for fatigue after childbirth. It is brain food for exhausted, overweight, or elderly persons, and for those who have long-standing poor diet and exercise habits.

The formula contains eucommia, lycium, astragalus, codonopsis, tang kuei, rehmannia, morinda, cornus, cistanche, biota, and lotus seed. The recommended dosage is 2 to 4 tablets twice daily.

POOR MEMORY CAUSED BY *INTERNAL HEAT*

I have already recommended gotu kola several times, among other places, in chapters 31 and 33, on fatigue and insomnia respectively, also in the anti-inflammatory section of chapter 13, Achieving Balance. Gotu kola works by balancing the hemispheres of the brain and rebuilding the nerves. The herb is well suited for people who are chronically overheated to the point at which they are burning up their memory and concentration. It works well for menopausal women and for students who take too many *heating* stimulants. You can take 6 to 8 capsules or more daily, depending upon your energy and tongue observations. Remember, it is a *cooling* remedy; it is not meant for those with a pale, scalloped tongue.

Healthy Brain Pills (Jian Nao Wan) is another *cooling* formula recommended for severe insomnia with nightmares, palpitations, and restless, scattered energy. You can use it during stressful periods for mental exhaustion, dizziness, poor memory, and fatigue. It quiets inflamed liver and *wind* and is therefore useful for anger and muscle twitches. It improves memory and clarity of mind by calming inflammation (so you can remember who is giving you a headache).

Other anti-inflammatory herbs worth mentioning are ginkgo leaf, yellow dock, and evening primrose oil. These improve memory by increasing blood circulation and oxygen in the brain.

Yellow dock is a natural source of iron that increases blood circulation in the brain. Take 4 to 8 yellow dock capsules daily if you are anemic, weak, and have poor memory.

Evening primrose oil increases oxygen content in the body because it is detoxifying. In previous chapters I have recommended evening primrose oil for menstrual pain and PMS because it reduces inflammation and increases circulation. If your poor memory is accompanied by these problems, or by headache and acne, evening primrose oil will solve many problems at once. Its detoxifying action may also help prevent a serious, prevalent disease that is related to dehydration, poor circulation, and blood toxins: Alzheimer's disease.

ALZHEIMER'S DISEASE AND THE *HUMORS*

Autopsies done on Alzheimer's patients have revealed brain tissue that is withered, as well as a buildup of plaque. This corresponds to two *humors* described by Chinese medicine. The kidney essence, or *jing*, nourishes the brain; therefore, when the *jing* is deficient, brain tissue can deteriorate more rapidly. Excess plaque can result from obstruction of *phlegm* and from poor circulation.

Based upon this understanding of *humors*, the herbs most appropriate for prevention of Alzheimer's disease are nourishing *jing* tonics, formulas that resolve *phlegm* and those that enhance circulation—for example, **Eleuthero 10+,** **Cuscuta 15,** and **Acornus Tablets,** respectively. These are available for herbalists from Health Concerns.

Eleuthero 10+ is used to inhibit deterioration associated with aging. It enhances mental and sensory functions and treats general weakness. **Eleuthero 10+** contains eleuthero ginseng, polygonatum, lycium, crataegus, epimedium, rehmannia, astragalus, alpina, acornus, broussonetia, eclipta, cuscuta, cornus, and licorice as a tonic to build *jing*. This formula contains many moisturizing tonics, along with hawthorn (crataegus) and licorice as digestives.

Cuscuta 15 treats frequent urination, incontinence, premature ejaculation, amnesia, and dry skin. The formula contains cuscuta, dioscorea, cornus, fu ling, rehmannia, alisma, astragalus seed, plantago seed, cynamorium, rose fruit, lycium, lotus, schisandra, euryale, and rubus.

Acornus Tablets are recommended for hyperactivity and poor memory and concentration. The formula contains acornus, polygala, fu shen, alpinia, curcuma, rehmannia, dragon bone, dragon teeth, oyster shell, bamboo, tortoiseshell, and succinum.

Your herbalist will be able to differentiate which other remedies may be necessary to suit your current needs. There are a number of herbal tonics that enhance *jing*—for example, remedies that feature he shou wu, a moistening blood tonic (see chapter 25 for moisturizing and *cooling* herbal combinations).

A Chinese patent remedy that is especially good for improving memory and mental functions is called **Co-Schisandra Tablets.** It is a combination of blood-building herbs along with an astringent herb, schisandra. The astringent herb is added in order to prevent the kidney organ system from losing too much *jing*. In this combination, schisandra keeps the blood tonic herbs in the appropriate energy circuit to be able to affect the brain. You can find these pills in Chinese herbal stores and supermarkets. Take 6 three times daily between meals, if you are under stress and suffering from mental exhaustion, poor memory, and poor concentration.

A DAILY OUNCE OF PREVENTION

I recommend that, if you feel at risk of Alzheimer's or of age-related memory and concentration problems, or if your work or lifestyle "burns your brain at both ends," you can add some of the *jing* tonic and astringent herbs listed above to your daily diet. This is easy to do, either by taking a dose of *jing* tonic herb pills before bed or daily as a stock used for tea or soups. Here is a possible recipe:

Good Memory Soup (very moisturizing and nourishing)

I recommend a soup made of the following herbs simmered in two quarts of water for forty-five minutes: Two pieces of eleuthero ginseng and a handful each of polygonatum, lycium, cornus, dioscorea, schisandra, acornus, polygala, fu ling, hawthorn berries, and dried licorice root. You can drink 2 cups per day, preferably between meals, along with mixed trace minerals pills that include 1,000 mg of calcium with each cup of soup stock.

Individual variations

The great advantage of making your own "brain brew," such as the one above, is that you can vary the ingredients according to your needs. This soup stock is very moisturizing; therefore it slows digestion. If you don't need the extra moisture, it can give you nasal congestion and abdominal bloating. You know you need the soup if you have dehydration symptoms.

For example, if your tongue looks dry and reddish, indicating *internal heat* and dehydration, eventually that *yin* deficiency can affect your nervous system and brain. Because of that dehydration, you will be able to use the Good Memory Soup more often without feeling too sedated or moisturized.

But if your tongue shows pallor and a white or gray coating, you may have to add one tablespoon of chopped raw ginger and ½ teaspoon of powdered cardamom to the soup stock to ensure proper digestion.

The Mind and Emotions

Our memory and thought processes are greatly influenced by our emotions. They overlap in such a way that it is hard to distinguish exactly why we're confused or indecisive. This section deals with herbal remedies for troubled emotions because, once you have cleared the air of inner turmoil, all mental functions can improve. When you've realized which emotional issues are applicable, you will be able to add the appropriate herbs to the work you will do in the next chapter.

INTEGRATED BODY, MIND, AND SPIRIT

One primary distinction between the Eastern and Western views of mental health lies in the understandings of the innate relationship of body, mind, and spirit. In practice, the Asian-trained doctor does not view the body, mind, and spirit as discrete, separate entities.

Traditional Chinese doctors describe thoughts and emotions as being influenced by *chi* and spirit, which makes them an integral part of human anatomy and physiology found in acupuncture meridians and organ systems. Because of this, emotional states are represented in the Correspondences. Thus, we can view the emotions (the spirit, or *shen*) by observing the body. This is unlike Western medical practice, in which mind doctors treat the mind, a brigade of specialists tend to various parts of the body, and care of the spirit is relegated to the clergy.

This essential difference of approach in treating mental problems becomes more than philosophical speculation when you are choosing herbal remedies. In effect, herbs can treat physical, mental, and emotional problems all at the same time, although we often do not recognize it. Western medicine's high degree of specialization ultimately results in misperception. This is because the body, mind, and spirit work in an integrated manner to produce health. It is when we cut ourselves into parts that we get a false understanding.

WHERE DOES WESTERN MEDICAL WRONG THINKING LEAD?

Because Asian remedies regulate vital energy and balance the *humors,* many have broad-ranging effects. Much important information has remained "secret" because we've been unaware of the simultaneously physical and emotional effects of herbs. Our culture is not set up to handle this concept. For example, I might suggest capsules or tea made from the herb gotu kola as preparation for meditation, even though gotu kola is also recommended for nerve-related skin rashes such as eczema. The herb quiets and nurtures the nervous system. That would be unthinkable for the Western medical establishment because it steps on the turf of both psychiatrist and dermatologist at once.

When dealing with the mind/body question, where does the difference in Eastern and Western approaches ultimately lead? I've met persons diagnosed as schizophrenic who are addicted to psychiatric drugs. They cannot sit still while telling me they want to stop medication because they're also addicted to coffee and cigarettes. It's as if their doctors have told them, "Take this drug and you'll be okay.

There is no connection whatsoever between your illness and your diet or lifestyle."

Our Emotions and Chi

I once had a big fight with a loved one after a nice day on a hot beach and a dinner of spicy ratatouille. Was the argument a result of our unresolved feelings, the hot weather, or the ratatouille? It was all of the above! We cannot separate our emotions from our bodies because we cannot separate our emotions from our energy. Ponder that . . .

Our *chi* varies with diet, the weather, and the seasons.

When are the times that you most often suffer severe conflicts with family or co-workers? Is it during spring's allergy season? Is your reaction to them and to stress as though you were allergic? Do you try to get them out of your life?

When do people tire you, bore you? Are you already fatigued by autumn's faded bloom or winter's cold? This section will help you make sense of the parts of the Correspondences that apply to your emotions. Throughout this book you have been getting to know your *chi* better. You have observed your tongue many times, and have applied that information to chapters dealing with illness. You have answered questionnaires, tried special diets, and in many ways, come to recognize which of the Five Elements speak to you.

Now you can begin to understand how your weak or stuck *chi*—your internal imbalances—also pertain to your emotions. Your emotions are an energetic phenomenon. They are strongly influenced by *chi*, blood, and circulation. When *chi* is stuck, we feel stuck. When it is weak, we lack acuity, clarity, and good memory. When we lack adequate healthy blood, we lack oxygen, which gives us calm and insight.

WHAT IS MENTAL CLARITY?

When I studied psychology in France, I met students who had worked at a revolutionary hospital called La Borde. There the doctors and nurses dressed as patients and ate and worked alongside patients, so that no one stood out as an expert. One of them said that sanity was knowing how to act in a given situation, without always being stuck in the same patterns or kinds of thoughts or reactions. In other words, to be sane is to be flexible, to be able to judge a situation on its merits alone and react in an appropriate manner. I take that now as a definition of mental clarity.

Freedom from mental hang-ups—your usual way of reacting to a given situa-

THE FIVE ELEMENTS AND THEIR CORRESPONDING EMOTIONS

ELEMENT	EMOTION	REMEDY
Fire	Anxiety	**Fu Shen Tablets**
		Wuchaseng
		Ding Xin Wan
Earth	worry, obsession	
	depression	**Xiao Yao Wan**
	repressed feelings	**Shu Gan Wan**
Metal	grief	homeopathic pulsatilla 30 c
	depression and	**Albizzia 9** along with
	chronic fatigue	**Compound GL**
Water	fear	
	(dread, weakness)	**Ding Xin Wan**
	(panic, *internal heat*)	**Niu Huang Ching Hsin Wan**
	(manic behavior)	**Cerebral Tonic Pills**
	(drug withdrawal)	**Ardisia 16**
Wood	anger, irritability	**Lung Tan Xie Gan Wan**
	indecisiveness, low enthusiasm	**Bu Zhong Yi Qi Wan**

Note: **Fu Shen Tablets, Albizzia 9, Compound GL,** and **Ardisia 16** can be ordered by health practitioners and health-food stores from mail-order sources. (See Herbal Access appendix.) The others listed are Chinese patent or homeopathic remedies available in herb shops.

tion—requires self-knowledge. As a tool for self-knowledge, we can use the Correspondences. In a number of chapters, you have used the Correspondences to observe imbalances in your body. Now you can begin to see how those same imbalances can affect the mind and emotions.

EMOTIONS AS PART OF THE BODY: A CHINESE VIEW

In chapter 9 we learned that each of the Five Elements houses a corresponding spirit that guides its emotions. The spirits are located in and depend upon the health of the internal organs of each element. When the element is unbalanced, the corresponding negative emotion surfaces to announce illness. In the chart on page 455, the Five Elements are shown, indicating their associated negative emotions and a recommended remedy for each.

How to use the chart

If you often experience emotions related to imbalances in the Five Elements, either because of your constitutional type or temporary stress, you will benefit from using the listed remedies. If you feel that such emotions endanger your mental clarity or work performance, you may wish to spend a couple of weeks adding the appropriate remedies from this chart to those you'll study in the following chapter, which covers herbs for high achievement. They will help you cross your emotional barriers.

HERBS FOR EMOTIONS AND MENTAL CLARITY

Although the chart indicates emotions traditionally associated with the Five Elements, it is not written in stone. The emotions and herbal choices are relative, because I chose the herbs according to energetic principles, not simply based on emotions. That is because there is no one correct herb or combination for anxiety, fear, grief, or other emotions. When I thought of the emotions, I thought of how specific emotions might affect *chi* or blood in the body. I had to ask myself, "With this emotion, what is stuck, what is weak, *hot, cold,* and so on?" in order to imagine how that emotion might affect the circulation, quantity, and quality of *chi*. Here I'll explain each herbal choice in order to help you decide if it's best for you.

The Fire element is associated with anxiety because that is often what is experienced when the heart and pericardium are agitated. Other symptoms might include palpitations, nightmares, or insomnia. The remedies I chose address those issues. **Fu Shen Tablets,** available from Health Concerns, contain natural sources of calcium, blood-builders, and *warming* and *cooling* herbs. The remedy can be combined with **Ardisia 16** for severe anxiety caused by drug withdrawal. For anxiety, the usual dosage is 3 to 5 pills three times daily of **Fu Shen Tablets.** For drug withdrawal, add the same amount of **Ardisia 16** for at least two months or until anxiety is resolved.

The other recommendations are **Wu-**

chaseng, an extract of Siberian ginseng, and **Ding Xin Wan,** both useful for insomnia and anxiety. The dosage I recommend of **Wuchaseng** is 1 teaspoon before bed. The dosage of **Ding Xin Wan** is 5 pills three times daily, or as needed.

The Earth element, our emotional as well as digestive center, is prone to feelings associated with malnourishment. You may feel spacey, weak, ungrounded, or off balance because your food is not being well utilized. Depression results, with poor circulation and undernourishment, when your food does not calm and strengthen you. For that I have recommended a remedy used by traditional Chinese medicine that treats hypoglycemia and depression, **Xiao Yao Wan.** For depression and poor circulation, take at least 10 pills three times daily if you have a pale tongue. If you have a red tongue, take **Shu Gan Wan,** 8 to 10 pills, three times daily. Also for repressed feelings, I've recommended **Shu Gan Wan** because it moves stuck *chi* in the abdomen.

The Metal element, including the lungs and large intestine, is prone to weakness and its resulting emotion, grief. With excess mucus discharges, breath and energy suffer. For that I have recommended an antiphlegm, antidepression remedy, homeopathic pulsatilla 30c. For weeping, shortness of breath, and feelings of suffocation (along with a pale tongue), add 10 pills of pulsatilla 30c to one quart of springwater, and drink a few sips at least five times during the day. Wait twenty minutes after eating or drinking coffee.

For weakness and depression associated with chronic fatigue, I've recommended two modern Chinese herbal remedies, available through Health Concerns and other mail-order sources: **Albizzia 9,** along with **Compound GL.** You can take 5 pills of each between meals.

The Water element controls the interaction of energy and blood with the adrenal and pituitary glands and heart. When Water is unbalanced, the resulting emotions can be anxiety or fear. I've recommended calming sedatives that improve energy and circulation. **Ding Xin Wan,** 5 pills three times daily, is recommended for weakness, fatigue, and poor memory and concentration. It is suited for *internal cold* conditions, while **Niu Huang Ching Hsin Wan** is suited for *internal heat* with panic, palpitations, vertigo, convulsions, and constipation. It is recommended for children's fever. The usual dosage is 1 large gummy pill twice a day. See other details on the box. The formula has been changed to eliminate rhino horn, which may affect the dosage.

The Wood element affects decision making and carry-through of plans. Persons addicted to marijuana, alcohol, or other *heating* substances may eventually have problems with mental clarity or aggression. Also, many medications harm the smooth flow of *chi,* causing subtle physical and emotional problems. For that reason, remedies that heal the Wood element ensure smooth circulation of *chi.* **Lung Tan Xie Gan Wan** is recommended for anger and aggressive behavior because, as a liver cleanser, it reduces inflammation and toxins. The usual dosage of **Lung Tan Xie Gan Wan** is 6 pills twice daily, but that is for headache and simple constipation. For rage, or at least angry PMS, you may have to take 10 to 12 pills instead of 6, three times daily.

Bu Zhong Yi Qi Wan strengthens energy in the digestive organs and emotional center, and thus helps reverse chronic weakness, diarrhea, and feelings of low enthusiasm or indecision. The dosage depends upon the severity of the problem. The usual dosage of **Bu Zhong Yi Qi Wan** for weakness is 8 pills three times daily, but for severe emotional vulnerability with collapsed *chi,* you may need to take more, depending on how well you tolerate it. But use caution: It can be constipating or cause headache or irritability in higher doses.

The next chapter describes herbs useful for high achievement. Your goals and methods must be individualized. Once, at a graduation banquet given after I'd completed some studies in China, I asked the hospital administrator what he did to ensure the health of his body, mind, and spirit. He told me that each day he made a plan for his work that he could surely accomplish, and carried it out. Another doctor, a dedicated and amiable man, smiled brightly and bantered that he drank Chinese beer. He was the sort who'd never missed a day's work in the clinic for forty years, went home to the same wife for lunch every day, and loved his patients.

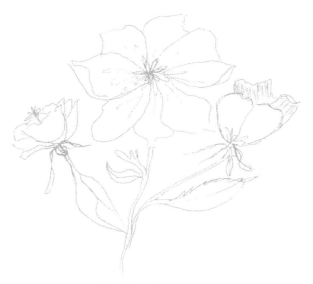

Evening primrose

MEMORY AND CONCENTRATION

What makes it worse?

Dehydration of *jing* from undernourishing diet, pollution, chemical toxins, drugs, alcohol, stimulants such as caffeine and cocaine; depressants such as marijuana; jet lag, sexual exhaustion; emotional upset.

What makes it better?

Blood-building *yin* tonics, along with astringent herbs that affect brain function, nourishing brain foods such as walnuts and sesame seeds; herbs that ensure healthy brain function (detoxifying, anti-inflammatory, nourishing, circulatory stimulants); rest and mental calm.

	INTERNAL HEAT	*INTERNAL COLD*	*PHLEGM*
TONGUE	dry, red, with dots	pale, scalloped, dots	large, coated
SYMPTOMS	dizziness	depression	cloudy thinking
	headache, insomnia	weakness	confusion
	anxiety	exhaustion	apathy
	irritability	shortness of breath	indigestion
	dry skin, thirst	backache	edema
	deficient short-term	poor long-term	confusion
	memory	memory	
	anemia, depression		
REMEDIES	**Co-Schisandra Tablets**	gotu kola capsules	**Xiao Yao Wan** homeopathic pulsatilla

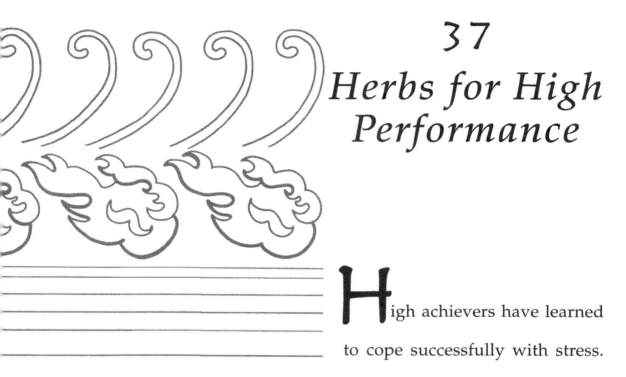

ཧང་རྒྱས་ ཧང་རྒྱས་ ཧང་རྒྱས་ ཧང་རྒྱས་ ཧང་རྒྱས་

Awakened, developed. The Enlightened One has awakened from the sleep of ignorance and has developed his/her mind with knowledge. (Tibetan)

37
Herbs for High Performance

High achievers have learned to cope successfully with stress. Beyond correcting illness, you can use herbs to improve the quality of your life by reducing tension and emotional blocks. This chapter offers new herbal resources and methods to add to your familiar stress reducers. You may find that massage, dance, or Tai Chi is a relaxing way to clear your mind. When the body is free from physical tension, thoughts flow more freely. You may also gain insight into emotional problems by doing artwork, keeping a diary, engaging in psychotherapy, or using visualizations or meditation.

The information in this chapter can help you to achieve the mental calm and clarity you require to do your work, as well as providing insights for emotional growth. You will find that taking the herbs covered in this chapter will help you to feel areas where your *chi* is blocked, and will bring up emotional issues that are stored there. No matter what anti-stress methods you choose, your efforts will be fruitful because the remedies described in this chapter will uncover the source of your emotional blockage in order to facilitate recovery and growth.

YOUR INNER DIALOGUE IS UNIQUE

Although herbs have biochemical components that react more or less the same way, the emotional reactions among people are extraordinarily variable because the content of our minds and the songs of our spirit are unique. Our energetic and *humor* imbalances are another important factor. The same food, herb, or activity may encourage one person to be loving, another to be calm, and a third to fall asleep. To overcome stress and accomplish your goals, you must be able to *predict* your energy. For that reason I have included information on the *humors*, especially how they apply to high achievement.

VISUALIZATION AND HERBS

Deep breathing and visualization techniques are often used these days in performance training. Actors, athletes, and business executives have learned to visualize themselves in successful situations, thus ensuring mastery of their skills.

You can apply those techniques to clarify personal growth issues, as a tool of personal divination. With the method I describe, as you look deeper within, you will find emotions and memories that prevent your complete fulfillment and good health. But first there are some inherent problems in visualization we must overcome. First, the exercise requires quiet surroundings and a quiet mind. Some people can only fidget, troubled by nervous energy or memories. Therefore, I will suggest a remedy to help make visualizations possible.

THE ADVANTAGE OF USING HERBS

Using natural remedies along with mind-centering practices is better than using chemicals, because the result is healthier for the brain. It also facilitates performance. For example, a lot of mind drugs (tranquilizers and antidepressants) attempt to sedate painful thoughts and nervous tics without helping us understand or integrate them. Whether we use street drugs or prescription sedatives, their aim is to control behavior, not to develop clarity and insight. You need to *understand* your troubling thoughts and transform them, in order to improve your performance.

OUR METHOD

Our method will give you a sensitive tool to bring forth and express your emotions in a positive way. You will use natural remedies during three different sorts of visualizations in order to overcome emotional and energetic barriers to your achievement, define and refine your goals, and mentally accomplish them. This method does not involve meditation or any religious practice. It helps you to achieve your own definition of success. In the process, you will answer the following questions:

1. What are my energetic and emotional blocks?
2. What are my goals?
3. How can I accomplish my goals?

You will use a special homeopathic remedy in the first visualization, then add herbs for mental clarity, based on your self-analysis, in the later ones. In that way, your visualization will reveal tendencies that need improvement. By transforming negative emotions into positive ones, you can eventually improve performance and, some say, refine character. This is because when you can change your emotions about a troubling situation, your actions can also change.

Section I. What Are My Negative Emotions?

The following method includes a visualization that can facilitate emotional clearing. It will bring out underlying negative emotions so that you can look at them clearly. It requires some preparation and time. You may need to arrange a time when you can be alone or with supportive friends.

THE FIRST VISUALIZATION: EMOTIONAL CLEARING

First, create your healing space. I recommend a private corner of your home that will be used only for this purpose. During the visualization you will face a blank wall, either white or light blue, and eliminate all noise and distractions.

At a time when you will not be disturbed for at least one hour, add five pills of homeopathic ignatia 30c to a cup of hot water. Sip the liquid while breathing peacefully for twenty minutes or more.

Imagine yourself alone in a quiet, beautiful place. Melt into your surroundings and stare at the wall until you imagine persons or places that bring up emotions for you. You may experience temporary pain or tensions where the emotions are trapped in your body. These will dissolve in this way: When you feel discomfort, give it a name and tell it to relax. As you relax, you may need to mentally clear negative memories, emotions, or people. Imagine them on the wall in front of you, and mentally dissolve them.

THE REMEDY

Homeopathic ignatia 30c, a highly dilute form of Saint Ignatius' bean, has been used traditionally to overcome physical and emotional effects of worry, grief, and emotional ambivalence. It has been recommended for stress accompanying separation from a loved one, or other important life changes. When none of that is an issue, the remedy can clear the field of agitation that impedes visualization. Ignatia 30c brings the hidden content of your worries into consciousness in order to process it. As you take the remedy, the emotion will lessen so that the physical and emotional stress leave you.

I remember once having had a particularly hard workday. After I took ignatia, nothing happened. I took another dose in a little while—still nothing. The next day I started crying for no apparent reason, and realized it was six months of worry over my clients that was finally coming to the surface. What a relief to have it come out! I usually recommend to health practitioners, counselors, lawyers, and other professionals who must deal with everyone else's troubles that they use ignatia 30c on a regular basis. Taken regularly, it can help you clear your workday.

When using ignatia, it is important to take adequate time to deal with feelings that arise. They may be little everyday aggravations or old memories. You may have to forgive people who have hurt you, or face something you haven't wanted to remember. After several uses, the traces of the memory will no longer keep you from sitting still. More important, you will have recognized your painful issues and worked to alleviate them. Ignatia initiates a deep cleansing process that builds clarity and calm.

USE OF THE CLEARING VISUALIZATION FOR HIGH ACHIEVEMENT

This visualization may make you feel calmer and clearer, but you still need to observe your physical and emotional tendencies in a new light, so that you can overcome their limits. Notice the kinds of issues that arose during the visualization process. They will be related to imbalances of your *humors.* By understanding which of your *humors* need help, you can begin the process of emotional balance. Please answer the following questions.

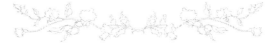

THE CLEARING VISUALIZATION REVEALS YOUR *HUMORS*

When you did the visualization:

WIND:

- ✺ Did your mind wander aimlessly?
- ✺ Did you become weak or depressed?
- ✺ Did you yawn a lot?
- ✺ Was it hard to sit still?
- ✺ Did you think of all the things you needed to do that day?
- ✺ Did you crave your addictions?
- ✺ Did your lower back and knees hurt?
- ✺ Did you become nervous or anxious?
- ✺ Did you remember fearful events?
- ✺ Did you feel your emotions in your shoulders, hips, or chest?
- ✺ Did you *hear* voices of people with whom you have problems?

BILE:

- ✺ Did you feel your emotions in your head, eyes, ribs, or back?
- ✺ Did you *see* the source of your unhappiness?
- ✺ Did you become flushed or hot?

- ✺ Did you feel angry or frustrated?
- ✺ Did you think of someone who makes you angry, jealous, envious?
- ✺ Did you burp or feel nauseated?
- ✺ Did you get a headache?
- ✺ Did your joints feel stiff?
- ✺ Did you crave rich food and drink?
- ✺ Did you think about trips or traveling?

PHLEGM:

- ✺ Did you fall asleep?
- ✺ Did you obsess about the past?
- ✺ Did you mentally count your money, friends, or clothes?
- ✺ Did you feel foggy and stuffed up?
- ✺ Did you ponder old grudges or worries?
- ✺ Did you blend into bliss?
- ✺ Did you *feel* pain or discomfort while remembering problems?
- ✺ Did you have indigestion?
- ✺ Did you become totally bored?
- ✺ Did you just not care?

THE *HUMORS* AND HIGH ACHIEVEMENT

Did you respond more often to one or more group? If so, that *humor* (*wind, bile,* or *phlegm*) needs help. Those *humors,* which we discussed in chapters 10 and 13, do more than determine your metabolism; they establish underlying physical and psychological tendencies we usually maintain during our entire lifetime. Without introspection, we will continue the same emotional bad habits we learned as children. Most people never realize what part of their experience and emotions they get secondhand from parents, schools, or friends.

In order to break old habits of failure or indifference, we can now look at the emotional aspects of the *humors.* This is valuable because imbalances of the *humors* can keep otherwise bright, ambitious, and talented persons from accomplishing their goals. Fortunately we can find valuable help from one of the world's oldest and most respected civilizations.

TIBETAN MENTAL GYMNASTICS

Among the Asian medical and philosophical traditions that have proven to be the most effective in changing attitudes is that of Tibet. I have met Tibetans who have accomplished miraculous feats of mental prowess under the worst conditions imaginable. For example, Tensen Choedok, a Tibetan doctor, survived seventeen years in a Chinese prison camp by literally eating scraps, his own wastes, and rodents in his cell. He managed to do this, using a form of Tibetan meditation called *tumo,* by imagining a fire and a deity within himself to purify his illness. (I adapted this meditation for our use in section I of chapter 13.)

During that time he also increased his efforts toward his enlightenment by urging his jailers to consider their actions carefully and treat others with kindness. He said that his daily meditation became breaking rocks. In other words, he turned his terrible imprisonment into positive mental work. In the end he not only survived his ordeal, but eventually went on to become the head of the School of Tibetan Medicine in Dharamsala, India, and the personal physician to His Holiness the Dalai Lama.

I chose this example not because I condone oppression, torture, or genocide, but because I see this man's behavior as a prime example of someone successfully overcoming stress.

Section II. Clear the Negative, Develop the Positive

What Tensen Choedok did was not essentially different from other Tibetan Buddhist practices designed to produce mental clarity. First, empty your mind of prejudices and negative emotions. Then focus on positive work to help others. Helping others is a key element because it opens all the "you are okay" doors within yourself that have been shut by old patterns of failure, self-doubt, hatred, and indifference inflicted on you by yourself or by other people. We shall expand upon this method by using herbal help at every step along the way.

YOUR EMOTIONS AND YOUR INNATE ENERGETIC AND EMOTIONAL PATTERNS

Your emotions do not fall out of the sky or happen completely by chance. They are, in fact, rather predictable. You can think of them as "How I usually feel about ———." High achievers know themselves. With that awareness comes the flexibility to be able to change your usual responses in order to improve your goals and actions.

First you have to recognize what your innate energetic and emotional patterns are. For that we have two resources, the *hu-*

mors and the Correspondences. Observing yourself in this way can help change your life, because knowing what your physical and emotional limits are, you can go beyond them.

EMOTIONS ARE RELATIVE AND CHANGEABLE

Though you may not realize it, the troubling emotions you most often express indicate an imbalance in the *humors.* Ancient theories concerning this notion formulated corresponding body types. For example, in the simplest terms, *wind* types tend to be anxious, *bile* types angry, and *phlegm* types indifferent. Those ancient theories were absolute: If you have a certain energy type, you must have a certain emotion.

But our understanding of this mind/body connection is relative, their expression being determined partly by the individual and partly by society. For example, "anxiety," in a *wind* person, may surface as heart palpitations, restlessness, or insomnia instead of as the emotion itself. Also, our notion of energetic types comes with the understanding that you can *change* your energy. It is not a body type you are born with and have forever.

To find your energetic weaknesses, notice the mental and emotional issues that surfaced for you during the Clearing Visualization. Did they apply more to imbalances in *wind, bile,* or *phlegm*? You might think of these as the emotions that come naturally to you because of your energy tendencies. The information on the *humors*

and mental clarity that follows will also help you make sense of your responses.

EMOTIONAL BLOCKS AND THE CORRESPONDENCES

To understand your emotional blocks, you can examine your prevalent negative emotions according to the Correspondences. Please refer to chapter 36. There I recommend a number of herbal remedies that traditionally treat such negative emotions as fear, anger, and anxiety. (See page 455.)

You probably noticed one or more of those emotions during the Clearing Visualization. The emotion that is blocking your progress will come up in various ways. For example, you may notice your troubling emotion associated with physical ailments that you have studied in previous chapters. That is because the emotion is related to physical energetic imbalances according to the Correspondences.

THE SECOND VISUALIZATION: BEGINNING THE HEALING PROCESS

This second visualization helps you directly process your troubling emotions, transforming a negative response to problem people or situations into a positive one. With this visualization you can transform illness into health, and anxiety, worry, grief, fear, or hatred into wisdom. It may take some time, but do not get stuck in this stage of development. You have another visualization after this one. Do not fall in love with processing your emotions or you will never reach your goals.

TAKE TWO REMEDIES: HOMEOPATHIC IGNATIA AND ONE FOR YOUR PROBLEM

When you finally decide what emotion or mind-set is currently blocking your way, then you can repeat the Clearing Visualization, taking homeopathic ignatia 30c along with the appropriate herbal remedy for emotional balance from chapter 36. For example, if you had angry thoughts during the Clearing Visualization, you should take 4 pills of ignatia 30c in a cup of hot water or under your tongue, along with 8 pills of **Lung Tan Xie Gan Wan,** a Chinese patent remedy that was recommended for anger. (See other emotions on page 455.) In that way you will evoke the negative emotional experience while taking the proper remedy. That gives you the opportunity to work on reducing the troubling emotional block in the following manner.

WATCH THE DRAMA OF YOUR EMOTIONS

During the visualization, imagine that the problem persons or events in your memory are on the blank wall in front of you. Watch them as though they were on television. Imagine that they need your help. You can think of ways to comfort them. You can watch yourself helping them on the screen.

If you are unable to help them because you are still too upset, then visualize them on the blank wall and mentally dissolve the memory, including the persons and events. You should repeat that process until the issue is resolved.

In that way, you can create a new mental reality. When I do this practice, I sometimes mentally eliminate everything in my healing space. I start from zero—with myself—empty of all experiences and associations with people. Then I am very selective about who and what I mentally invite into the visualization, so that the next time I have to deal with similar negative experiences, I can start fresh, from a different point of view. Eventually you will be able to do this sort of emotional clearing anywhere, in a matter of minutes.

HOW TO REFINE YOUR GOALS

Our final visualization involves your naming your goal and mentally acting it out with the help of your appropriate herbs. The individual herbs you need to use during the visualization will be determined by your emotions and your *humors*. The following information will help you make your herbal choices.

THE *HUMORS* AND YOUR ACHIEVEMENT GOALS

When you can determine which of your *humors* are out of balance, you can refine your achievement goals. You may be aiming too high, too low, or not at all, depending upon which of your *humors* needs help. I'll explain the *humors* according to Tibetan health practices.

Wind *and Nervous Exhaustion*

According to Tibetan medicine, the *wind humor* is light and dry in character. It encompasses movement and change. The several types of *winds* used in Tibetan medicine can be likened to a telecommunication system in the body. *Wind* is a metaphor used to explain circulation and nervous system functions. When we abuse this system, we might experience power failures or blowouts that correspond to nervous exhaustion, paralysis, depression, or hysteria. Also, our ideas and achievement goals may become muddled.

I defined *wind* in chapter 10, and referred to *wind humor* imbalances in chapters concerning pains such as neuralgia, arthritis, and nervous headaches; I've also discussed it in relation to insomnia and nervous exhaustion as they affect vitality and sexuality. An imbalance in the *wind humor* can scatter your energy and obscure your achievement goals.

IS THE *WIND* BLOWING ON YOUR GOAL?

🖎 Do you have too many projects to finish?

🖎 Is it difficult to know where to begin on your projects?

🖎 Do you get confused or depressed, unable to start?

🖎 Do you give up because of anxiety or fatigue?

🖎 Do you aim to "get it done," no matter what it takes?

🖎 Do you drive yourself beyond your energy capacity?

If your *wind humor* is out of balance, your goals may be many, imprecise, and impractical. That is because *wind* provides pure drive, not insight. Your *wind humor* needs to be grounded in common sense, experience, and benevolence. Otherwise your enthusiasm may carry you to extremes. This can take the form of what Tibetan doctor/philosophers call "delusion." Unfortunately, there is no herb to dispel delusion, but with certain grounding herbs, you can at least quiet your *wind* problem.

When Tibetan doctors speak of a patient's confusion or delusion, it refers to more than clarity of thought. More precisely, it is an inability to predict negative results from negative actions. An example is, "I can smoke or take drugs and still be perfectly well." Or "I can wreck the environment and remain unharmed." At the base of delusion is the misguided premise that we are completely alone, self-sufficient, and above natural laws.

People ruled by delusion may be depressed or spacey a good deal of the time. They may rush through life chasing entertainments, work projects, or lovers. If they guide their lives according to their unbridled desire for pleasure and experience, they may exhaust themselves without learning who they are. They may have high ideals but express them superficially, or they may base their lives solely on personal gain. If they do not learn to be wise with their energy and emotions, they may, according to Tibetan astrologers, choose their next lifetime to become a small flying creature. Wings are more economical than "frequent-flier miles," after all, and we need no more than a buzz to express simple thoughts.

EXCESS *WIND:* SIGNS AND SYMPTOMS

The person exhausted by work or pleasure may have a dry, reddish tongue with many dots around the edge, indicating toxins affecting the nerves. Urine will be clear light bluish, or like water with large bubbles. The radial pulse will be irregular and will disappear when the doctor applies pressure with the fingers.

The person may yawn and shiver excessively, or may feel cold chills, or pain around the waist or in the bones and joints and when hungry. Persons with excess *wind* energy cannot sit still long enough to meditate. Or if they manage to sit down, their minds jump from subject to subject like a grasshopper. This imbalance is aggravated by a light, cold diet—salads, black tea, orange juice, and white rice—and such stimulants as coffee and street drugs, including marijuana, as well as late-night work, sexual exhaustion, and jet lag. Have you ever felt you have turned into a bee after a long jet flight?

REMEDIES FOR *WIND* IMBALANCES

For depression and anxiety, put a drop of pure lavender oil at the heart. Its pungent, bitter fragrance both stimulates and quiets heart action at the same time, so the overall effect unblocks stuckness there. To quiet *wind* anxiety, put one drop of fresh raw sesame oil into each nostril with a dropper.

Rest and sleep will help clarify and focus your goals. If you cannot sleep, you very likely need one of the nourishing herbal formulas for insomnia covered in chapter 33, such as **Ding Xin Wan.** That combination will also help dissipate anxiety, fear, restlessness, and scattered thinking, each a nemesis for *wind*-type persons.

MENTALLY ACCOMPLISH YOUR GOAL, AND THEN WRITE IT

Then mentally act out your entire achievement plan step by step, correcting the details you have to improve. Take at least half an hour. Your *wind* tendency will make you race through your goals. After that visualization, slowly write down the steps necessary for your goal in as much detail as possible. Try to keep your goal simple and benevolent; that way it can become a high achievement.

Bile: *Anger and Frustration*

Bile is hot, oily, heavy, and sharp in character. It creates the heat of digestion and sparks our drives and ambition. When bile is adequate, we are hungry and digest well. Also our thoughts are clear and well organized. When bile is excessive or blocked, it stops normal digestion and circulation. We feel stuck and overheated from frustration or anger.

I defined *bile* in terms of Asian energetics in chapter 10, and referred to *bile* problems of *internal heat* and pain in chapters concerning inflammatory arthritis (19), headaches (20), insomnia (33), allergies (23), skin blemishes (25), inflammatory menstrual pain (26), PMS (27), menopause (29), blood-deficiency insomnia (33), and sexual problems such as premature ejaculation (34).

If you have *heat* symptoms from excess or stuck *bile*, your visualizations may be resentful or aggressive, and your goals may lack wisdom. You may be too nervous or angry to be able to make plans. You need to cool and refine your bilious emotions before you can move forward.

IS THERE A BITE AND SCRATCH IN YOUR GOALS?

𝒻𝔞 Do you procrastinate?

𝒻𝔞 Do you attempt only things you excel in?

𝒻𝔞 Do you become outraged at criticism?

𝒻𝔞 Do you become nervous when people watch you?

𝒻𝔞 Performing, do you become short of breath, or feel feverish?

𝒻𝔞 Do you lose sleep criticizing yourself?

𝒻𝔞 Do you always aim for control of a group or situation?

𝒻𝔞 Is it hard to work with other people?

𝒻𝔞 Performing, do you get hives, allergies, headaches, hiccups?

𝒻𝔞 What makes you angry, jealous, envious?

𝒻𝔞 Do you get angry at yourself if you fail at a task?

𝒻𝔞 Do you often get angry at people who make mistakes?

EXCESS AND STUCK *BILE*

If you experienced anger after taking homeopathic ignatia 30c, you may experience it often. Other bilious emotions are jealousy, envy, and arrogance. According to Tibetan doctors, bilious people have sharp tongues, quick minds, good memories, large appetites, and aggressive behavior. They may order the most expensive foods on the menu, wear rich clothes, and have sharp wits, but if they don't learn to be kind to others, Tibetan astrologers say, they may reappear in their next lifetime as furry animals with sharp teeth and claws. Presumably the claws could help them tear into their food and enemies.

EXCESS *BILE* SIGNS AND SYMPTOMS

Bilious persons often experience a bitter taste in the mouth; a yellow-coated tongue;

and malodorous, oily-looking urine that appears to steam if put into a clear glass. The radial pulse is thin and twisted from poor circulation. These people may angrily chew on their feelings, experiencing frequent headaches, pain in the upper body and neck, and high blood pressure; they may have thinning hair and a red complexion. Such *internal heat* tendencies are made worse by eating all the foods they love: oily foods, nuts, cheese, and tahini, hot foods such as garlic, onions, and meat, and alcohol; also by living in hot apartments and playing the stock market.

The clients I have described in this book with excess or stuck *bile* were those who suffered from broken capillaries, rashes, sciatica, and arthritis, as well as women with angry PMS, and people with ulcers and hypertension headaches. All of them need anti-inflammatory diets and herbs to free their stuck *bile* and improve their tempers. Bilious people cannot relax during a visualization because they chew on a grudge, plot a business deal, or organize their work when they need to put it aside.

HOW TO USE *COOLING* HERBS FOR THE VISUALIZATION

Put a drop of pure sandalwood oil at the third eye. It slows and cools body and mind. Put a drop of aloe vera gel into each nostril with a dropper. That cools all the nerves going from the sinus area to the brain. It takes the redness out of your eyes and cools your temper.

You may have to add another remedy for anger. In chapter 35 I suggested **Lung Tan Xie Gan Wan,** which also helps liverish headache. You can take 8 to 12 pills at a time, depending upon the level of your anger, frustration, jealousy, and other hot emotions.

In your visualization process, start with a personal goal that is fun, something that you know you can easily accomplish. Then you can add to this and refine your goal later. Mentally (and slowly) walk through your activity, while taking relaxing breaths or humming to yourself. When you have finished visualizing the pleasurable mental activity, imagine that you are doing the same thing with a problem person or in a problem situation until the whole process becomes smoother.

Phlegm, *Greed, and the Great Giant Sloth*

Phlegm is a by-product of digestion that is sticky and moistening. *Phlegm* as a *humor* helps hold us together. It is necessary to balance the lightness of *wind* and the heat of *bile.* But when the *humor phlegm* becomes excess or stuck, body and mind cannot effectively carry on the functions of *wind* and *bile. Wind* becomes heavy and clogged, so that thinking becomes cloudy and movements stiff. With excess *phlegm,* we cannot move forward in our thoughts. We become trapped in the past or in self-centered ruminations.

IS *PHLEGM* CLOUDING YOUR GOALS?

🦤 Do low energy and sleepiness slow your work?

🦤 Do poor digestion or overweight get in your way?

🦤 Do you suffer nausea often?

🦤 Is it hard to concentrate on your goal?

🦤 Is it hard to understand what is necessary for your goal?

🦤 Is it hard for you to get out of bed or up from the chair?

🦤 Have you given up caring about your achievements?

🦤 Do you blame others for the way things turn out?

🦤 Do you spend lots of time thinking or meditating on your goals?

🦤 Is your unhappiness your parents' or teachers' fault?

🦤 Do you think about the past a lot?

🦤 Do you hold grudges?

EXCESS *PHLEGM*

According to Tibetan doctors, people who experience attachment and greed will also have excess *phlegm*. This may translate into late-night rich meals that include cream, sweets, pasta, and gooey or oily foods and nuts, as well as blintzes, lobster, and chocolate mousse. Their habits are designed to slow them down. They love to collect things, read long novels, and watch TV. If they don't create good karma by helping others, Tibetan doctors suggest they might come back as the great giant sloth.

EXCESS *PHLEGM:* SIGNS AND SYMPTOMS

Hot, humid weather increases these *phlegm* symptoms: grayish, sticky coating on the tongue, cloudy urine, sunken and weak radial pulse. Food has no taste, and the stomach feels full even when empty. The person is frequently nauseated and can be overweight or thin with a large middle. Mind and body feel heavy, and thinking is confused. One feels cold internally and externally, and uncomfortable after eating. Pounding headaches with sinus congestion are another symptom. All this indicates what Tibetan doctors refer to as *phlegm*. It can result from poor food combining (meat with milk, fish with milk, or beer with creamy, rich food), causing mucus in the digestive tract and worms clogging the bile duct. Eating richly and then going to sleep increases *phlegm*. People with excess *phlegm* conditions need pungent wake-you-up remedies to warm their metabolism.

HOW TO USE PUNGENT HERBS FOR VISUALIZATIONS

Open one capsule of the herb gotu kola, and use it as snuff. It opens your sinuses, cures a sinus headache, and wakes you up with a bang. It will help clarify your thinking during your visualization. Then take a few deep breaths.

For your visualization, imagine what your goal is, and the actions you must take to accomplish it. Then act it out by moving or speaking your part just as though you were in the real situation. Working some-

A KEY: HERBS FOR HIGH ACHIEVEMENT

FIRST VISUALIZATION	Notice your emotions and memories
	Homeopathic ignatia 30c
SECOND VISUALIZATION	Process your emotions
	Homeopathic ignatia 30c
	One remedy for your emotional hang-up
Emotion	Remedy from page 455
Anxiety	**Fu Shen Tablets, Wuchaseng,** or **Ding Xin Wan**
worry, obsession	
depression	**Xiao Yao Wan**
repressed feelings	**Shu Gan Wan**
grief	Homeopathic pulsatilla 30c
fear	**Niu Huang Ching Hsin Wan**
mania	**Cerebral Tonic Pills**
drug withdrawal	**Ardisia 16**
anger, rage	**Lung Tan Xie Gan Wan**
indecisiveness, weakness	**Bu Zhong Yi Qi Wan**
THIRD VISUALIZATION	Refine and accomplish your goals
	One *humor* remedy, one for emotions
HUMOR	inhaler remedy:
Wind	sesame oil
Bile	aloe vera gel
Phlegm	gotu kola powder

how to end the suffering of others or to help protect nature is the most beneficial visualization and activity for you.

Balancing the Humors

The problems of nervous exhaustion, rage, and spiritual apathy are the emotional illnesses Tibetans describe as resulting from imbalances in *wind, bile,* and *phlegm.* We need the coordination of all these *humors.* Without the nervous drive of *wind* in our sails, we lack enthusiasm and new ideas.

Without *bile*—the heat of battle against our enemies or our imperfections and the drive to do our work—we lack vitality. Without the soothing effects of *phlegm,* we would incinerate. It is all a matter of balance.

THE THIRD VISUALIZATION: ACCOMPLISH YOUR GOAL

After you have determined your energetic and emotional hang-ups and worked to clear them, then refined your goals by considering your *humor* imbalances, you will be ready to begin with the final phase, which involves a visualization and activity.

This time you will take the proper inhaler remedy to heal your *humor* and, if needed, another herbal combination to heal your emotional hang-up, then visualize yourself successfully accomplishing your goal. Make sure to offer some benefit of your success to help others.

This book has helped you to understand your vitality. A *humor* is nothing more than how you would usually react in a stressful situation. But with insight and the help of herbs, you can change your energy so that you can adapt your responses. Here is an example: Observe your *humor(s)* by looking at your tongue.

Your tongue may be shaking (*wind*), your actions may be self-protecting or sporadic, so that your achievement (and good karma) are limited by nervousness and fear. But, even because of that *wind*, you can use your expansive, creative energy to start new directions and find new horizons. You already have the desire to change, which is the first step toward improvement.

Your tongue may be reddish-colored or yellow-coated (*internal heat* or *bile*), your actions may be forceful, dramatic, angry, or full of frustration. But your fire can also fuel your search for truth and enlightenment. You can find fulfillment by working for others. You already have the energy necessary to accomplish your goals. All you need is to clarify them.

Your tongue may be pale and wet (*internal cold* or *phlegm*), your methods may be indirect, or your projects may require time to ripen, but you can draw upon your sensitivity, insight, and capacity to love others to attain your wisdom. You already have the dedication that can help you achieve your ideals. All you need is to begin.

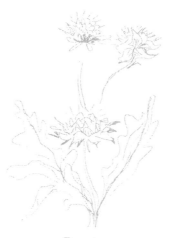

Desert sage

Epilogue

An Invitation to Thanksgiving

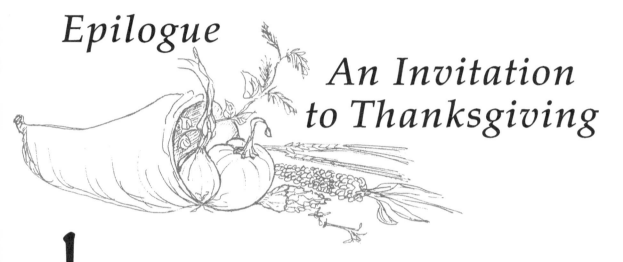

I awoke one morning to the smell of home-baked bread and roasting pumpkins in the oven. It was a dream of New England, of the old farmhouse on the pond with a hundred lazy acres of meadows and balsam, now covered with snow. I thought, "I'll give a New England winter's feast and invite friends from the city. You come too!"

We'll have fresh corn, squash, beans, grains, kale, cranberries, and a cornucopia of life-giving herbs that I've grown. Ginger, tarragon, and mint will ease digestion. Cinnamon that I'll add to punch will spark circulation. Astragalus and dang shen from Chinatown will build immune strength: I'll simmer a handful of each in a soup. Shiitake and reishi mushrooms will be magic because they help prevent cancer. I'll cook carrots with tang kuei and sweeten pies with lo han kuo. Who says herbs have to taste bad? We'll eat dinner by a roaring fire, then go out in the snow to feed the birds, our guests at a vegetarian feast.

Whose woods these are I think I know
Her apartment's in Chelsea, though
Take a train north, or a bus will go
To find the woods, now full of snow.
Here we are in New England,
Where Thanksgiving started long ago!

The afternoon I arrived, snow hung like a white sheet on a line, ready to fall from any loud noise. Escaped from the city's pressure cooker, I tore around town, buying squash jelly, extra-sharp cheddar, and tart apple cider, pausing only a moment to read a paper to see what I'd missed since summer—the annual Cow Appreciation Day with a milking contest, a guided tour of barns, and Fiddle Fern walks. Summers in the country have saved my life for years.

For Thanksgiving dinner we won't eat turkey. Native Americans named corn, beans, and squash "the trinity," a meal of complete proteins. These vegetables will star in a casserole brought to the feast by the Lafoes, Iroquois and Sioux friends from Brandon. Other friends have flocked from all parts at once.

Juan and Molly have finished a documentary in Peru; Jean-Claude's directing a play in Hawaii, but he'll be here soon. Fred has arrived from the Village. Luke and Don will fly in from Hollywood. Brian, Elma, and baby Juniper promise to sing! Our friends carry cameras, pens, and tunes instead of rifles. We'll send greetings to all those who can't come: Gad and François are tied up on a shoot for *Vogue,* and Scott is celebrating with friends in Rome.

My editor and I are discussing my next book, but we will soon put business aside. By late afternoon we are ready to start. A handful of sage fills the air with desert smoke as I light it with the kitchen hearth fire. Tenzin and Pema Lama, from Dharamsala, start to intone low-pitched Tibetan blessings, which bring us to the center of the room. We feel the pains of the year melt away as Ira sings "Amazing Grace" . . .

We had a "church suppa" Thanksgiving on a long wooden table decorated with evergreens. Off in a corner, Chinese and Iroquois guests were discussing ginseng and drinking green tea. My Darling and I gave thanks to each other with our eyes.

Those of us steeped in the Herbal Tradition practice a sort of religion. In times of worry, illness, or loss, we turn to Nature. We respect the power of plants. With sensitivity and insight, we find friends in our garden, kitchen, and in herb markets around the world. We turn to the children of the Earth, to our connection with all that lives, grows, and is capable of love. May you always find many such friends. The bounty of the Earth is the true cause for Thanksgiving.

CROSS-REFERENCE OF HERB NAMES

HERB NAME	PINYIN	DESCRIPTION (PART USED)	FUNCTION (USAGE)
Abutilon	dongguizi	seed	diuretic
Achyranthes	niuxi	root	circulation
Aconite	fuzi	root	*warming*
Acorus	chuanpu	rhizome	antiphlegm
Acronychia	jiangzhexiang	wood	regulate *chi*
Actinolite	yangqishi	mineral	*warming*
Adenophora	nanshashen	root	antiphlegm
Agkistrodon	baihuashe	snake	anti-numbness
Agrimonia	xianhecao	plant	anti-bleeding
Akebia	mutong	stem	diuretic
Albizzia	hehuanpi	bark	sedative
Alisma	zexie	rhizome	diuretic
Allium seed	jiuzi	leek seed	*warming*
Alpinia	yizhiren	fruit	*warming*
Andrographis	chuanxinlian	rhizome	antibiotic
Anemarrhena	zhi mu	rhizome	anti-fever
Angelica	baizhi	root	digestive
Apricot seed	kuxingren	kernel	moistening
Aquilaria	chenxiang	wood	regulate *chi*
Arca	walengzi	shell	dissolve mass
Arctium	niubangzi	seed	dissolve mass
Ardisia	jinniuca	plant	antitoxin
Areca seed	binglangzi	betel nut	removes worms
Arisaema	tiannanxing	rhizome	antiphlegm
Aristolachia	xungufeng	leaf	diuretic
Artemesia	aiye	leaf	stops bleeding
Artemesia apiacea	ching hao	plant	anti-parasite
Asarum	xixin	ginger	*warming*
Asparagus	tianmendong	root	moistens lungs
Astragalus	huang qi	root	tonify *chi*
Astragalus	shayuanzi	seed	tonify *yang*
Atractylodes	baizhu	rhizome	tonify *chi*
Atractylodes, red	cangzhu	rhizome	*drying,* digestive
Aurantium	zhupi	peel	regulate *chi*
Bamboo sap	tianzhuhuang	sap	*cooling,* antiphlegm
Belamcanda	shegan	rhizome	anti-viral
Benincasa	dongguaz	seed	antiphlegm
Biota	boziren	seed	sedative
Biota leaves	ceboye	leaf	anti-bleeding
Blue citrus	chenpi	fruit	circulation
Borneol	longnao	resin	opens orifices
Buddleia	mimenghua	bud	*cooling* (vision)
Bulrush	puhuang	pollen	circulation
Bupleurum	chaihu	root	digestive
Calamus gum	xuejie	resin	circulation
Capillaris	yinchenhao	leaf	*cooling* (jaundice)

HERB NAME	PINYIN	DESCRIPTION (PART USED)	FUNCTION (USAGE)
Carthamus	honghua	safflower	circulation
Cassia seed	juemingze	seed	*cooling*
Centipeda	wugong	whole	spasms, seizures
Cephalanopios	xiaoji	root	anti-bleeding
Changium	mingdangshen	root	cough
Chih-ko	zhiko	fruit	regulate *chi*
Chih-shih	zhishi	(unripe) fruit	regulate *chi*
Chrysanthemum	juhua	flower	anti-fever
Cibotium	gouji	rhizome	tonify *yang*
Cicada	chantui	slough	*cooling*, sedative
Cimicifuga	shengma	rhizome	*cooling*, diaphoretic
Cinnamon	guipi	bark	*warming*
Cistanche	roucongrong	top	tonify *yang* (kidney)
Clematis	weilingxian	root	clears *wind/damp*
Clerodendron	chouwutong	top	clears *wind/damp*
Cnidium	chuanxiong	rhizome	tonify blood
Codonopsis	dang shen	root	tonify *chi*
Coptis	huanglian	rhizome	*cooling, drying*
Cordyceps	chanhua	fungus	anti-*wind/heat*
Cornus	shanzhuyu	fruit	astringent
Crataegus	shanzha	hawthorn	digestive
Curculigo	xianmao	rhizome	tonify *yang*
Curcuma (turmeric)	yujin	tuber	circulation
Cuscuta	tusizi	seed	tonify *yang*
Cyperus	xiangfuzi	rhizome	circulation
Dandelion	pugongying	plant	clears toxins
Deer antler	lurong	antler	tonify *yang*
Dendrobium	shihu	stem	tonify *yin*
Dianthus	gumai	top	*drying*
Dictamnus	baixianpi	bark	clears toxins
Dioscorea	shanyao	rhizome	digestion
Dipsacus	xuduan	root	tonify *yang*
Dragon bone	longgu	whole	sedative
Drynaria	gusuibu	rhizome	tonify *yang*
Earthworm	dilong	whole	bronchodilator
Eclipta	hanliancao	top	tonify *yin* (liver)
Eleuthero ginseng	ciwujia	rhizome	tonify *chi*
Epimedium	yin yang huo	leaf	tonify *yang* (kidney)
Eucommia	duzhong	bark	tonify *yang*
Euryale	qianshi	seed	astringent
Evodia	wuzhuyu	fruit	*warming*
Fluorite	zishiying	mineral	sedative
Forsythia	lianqiao	fruit	clears toxins
Frankincense	ruxiang	gum	circulation
Fraxinus	qinpi	bark	*cooling, drying*
Fritillaria	zhebeimu	bulb	*cooling*, antiphlegm
Fu-shen	fushen	root	sedative
Galanga	liangjiang	rhizome	*warming*
Ganoderma	lingzhi	whole	nourishing, sedative

HERB NAME	PINYIN	DESCRIPTION (PART USED)	FUNCTION (USAGE)
Gardenia	zhizi	fruit	*cooling*, antiphlegm
Gastrodia	tianma	tuber	anti-spasm
Gecko lizard	gejie	whole	tonify *yang*
Gentiana	longdancao	root	*cooling*, (diarrhea)
Geranium	laohuancao	whole	anti-*wind/damp*
Ginger	ganjiang	rhizome	*warming*
Ginseng, Chinese	ren shen	root	tonify *chi*
Gypsum	shigao	mineral	anti-inflammatory
Haliotis	shijueming	shell	anti-*wind*
He shou wu	heshouwu	root	tonify blood
Hoelen (poria)	fuling	fungus	diuretic
Houttuynia	yuxingcao	plant	clears abscess
Hu-chang	huzhang	plant	clears toxins
Ilex (holly)	maodongqing	root	circulation (angina)
Isatis leaf	daqingye	leaf	anti-viral
Isatis root	banlangen	root	anti-viral
Kadsura bark	hongmuxiang	root	regulate *chi*
Kochia	difuzi	fruit	antiphlegm
Laminaria	kunbu	seaweed	antiphlegm
Lapis	mengshi	mineral	antiphlegm
Leech (dried)	shuizhi	whole	anticoagulant
Licorice	gancao	root	digestive, spasm
Ligustrum	niuzhenzi	fruit	tonify *yin*
Lily	baihe	bulb	tonify *yin*
Lindera	wuyao	root	circulation
Lithospermum	zicao	whole	*cooling*
Lonicera	jinyinhua	honeysuckle	antibiotic
Lotus node	oujie	node	regulate blood
Lotus seed	shilianzi	seed	astringent
Lotus stamen	lianxu	stamen	astringent
Lysimachia	jinqiancao	top	diuretic
Magnolia bark	houpu	bark	digestive
Ma-huang	mahuang	twig, node	diaphoretic
Malt	maiya	sprout	digestive
Melia	chuanlianzi	fruit	regulate *chi*
Millettia	jixueteng	stem	circulation
Morinda	bajitian	root	tonify *yang*
Morus (Mulberry)	sangbaipi	root bark	relieve cough
Morus fruit	sangshen	fruit	tonify blood
Mother-of-pearl	zhenzhumu	shell	sedative
Moutan	moudanpi	root bark	cools blood
Mume	wumei	fruit	astringent
Myrrh	moyao	resin	circulation
Nardostachys	gansongxiang	rhizome	antiphlegm
Nuphar	chuangu	rhizome	antiphlegm
Oldenlandia	baihuasheshecao	rhizome	clears toxins
Ophiopogonis	mai men dong	tuber	tonify *yin*
Oyster shell	muli	shell	sedative
Paris	zaoxiu	whole	clears toxins

HERB NAME	PINYIN	DESCRIPTION (PART USED)	FUNCTION (USAGE)
Patrina	beijiang	whole	clears toxins
Peony	baishao	root	tonify blood
Perilla leaf	zisuye	leaf	anti-*wind/chill*
Persica	taoren	kernel	circulation
Phellodendron	huangbo	bark	*cooling, drying*
Pinellia	banxia	tuber	antiphlegm
Piper	pibo	pepper	*warming*
Placenta	ziheche	human	tonify *yang*
Platycodon	jiegeng	root	antiphlegm
Polygala	yuanzhi	root	nourishing, sedative
Polygonatum	huangjing	rhizome	tonify *chi*
Pomegranate	shiliupi	rind	astringent
Prunella	xiakucao	top	*cooling* (thyroid)
Pteropus (squirrel)	wulingzhi	excretion	circulation
Pulsatilla	baitouweng	root, flower	clears toxins
Quisqualis	shijunzi	fruit	remove worms
Rehmannia	shoudihuang	root	tonify blood
Rehmannia, raw	shengdihuang	root	cools blood
Rhubarb	dahuang	rhizome	purgative
Rose fruit	jinyingzi	fruit	astringent
Salvia	danshen	root	circulation
San-she-dan	sanshedan	3 snake gallbladder	clears toxins, anti-numbness
Sargassum seaweed	haizao	whole	antiphlegm
Saussurea	muxiang	root	regulate *chi*
Schisandra	wuweizi	fruit	astringent
Scute	huangqin	root	*cooling, drying*
Scutellaria	banxhilian	whole	clears toxins
Seahorse	haima	whole	tonify *yang* (kidney)
Sesame seed	humaren	seed	moistening, laxative
Shen-chu	shenqu	whole	digestive
Silkworm	biajiangcan	whole	anti-*wind* (paralysis)
Smilax	tufuling	rhizome	cleansing, diuretic
Sparganium	sanleng	rhizome	circulation
Talc	huashi	whole	*drying*
Tang-kuei	danggui	root	tonify blood
Tienchi ginseng	sanchi	root	circulation
Tortoiseshell	guiban	shell	tonify *yin*
Tremella	yiner	fungus	tonify *yin, chi*
Trichosanthes	gualou	fruit	*cooling*, antiphlegm
Turmeric	jianghuang	rhizome	circulation
Uncaria	gouteng	stem	anti-*wind*
Vaccaria	wangbuliuxing	fruit	circulation
Viola	dihetao	flower	antibiotic
Vitex	manjingzi	fruit	*cooling*, anti-*wind*
Wasp nest	lufengfang	nest	clears toxins
Xanthium	cangerzi	fruit	anti-*wind/damp*
Zaocys	wushaoshe	snake	anti-numbness
Zizyphus	suanzaoren	seed	nourishing, sedative

HERBAL ACCESS

I am pleased to offer you resources for buying Asian herbs direct from Oriental food stores and herb retailers as well as from reliable mail-order sources. I have also listed referral services for qualified health practitioners who can assist you in ordering the herbal products that are available to professionals. Many of these people offer personal and phone consultations for a fee. Here are some general pointers that can guide your way.

What to Look For in Herbal Sources

If you decide to make one of my herbal recipes, buy a ready-made pill remedy, or replicate a Chinese patent remedy with raw herbs, here are what I consider to be important things to look for in an herbal source. Whether it is a supermarket or a specialized herb shop, the place should be clean and busy. Packaged herbs will move quickly off the shelves if the demand is high. Packaged or loose herbs should be kept away from heat and sunshine. The shelf life of most loose herbs is about three months, whereas pills and extracts can remain fresh for years.

The staff should be friendly, speak English, and offer help when necessary. You may need to consult them by phone for clarification after buying the herbs.

FOR INDIVIDUAL ATTENTION

Often, Asian herb shops have an herbal doctor on staff who can answer specific questions. For truly individualized care, it is best to make an appointment with the store's herbal doctor. Very often the consultation is free when you buy herbs in their shop. Ask for a copy of the herbal prescription, even if written in Chinese, so you can fill the prescription at any time, even elsewhere at a better price. You can always ask the store to substitute herbs in a given recipe—for example, less expensive or vegetarian ones instead of animal ingredients if you wish. Or you can insist on pills if you feel that cooking herbs is too much trouble.

If you have never bought Asian herbs before, it's a good idea to photocopy or fax the page from this book containing remedies for your problem. That way you don't have to worry about pronunciation and spelling. I have listed the ingredients of most herbal combinations so that if your herb shop or health practitioner does not have the herbal pills you need, they may be able to substitute others that are similar.

HOW TO SAVE MONEY

You will save quite a lot of money by choosing herbs instead of Western medicines. Unless you are buying the most expensive ginseng or rare herbs, the price should be no more than a few dollars per dose of raw herbs, even though a dose may contain a number of different herbs. Pills cost anywhere from two to twelve dollars or more per bottle. Chinese-made patent remedies are much less expensive than American-made herbal combinations. Many Ayurvedic herbs are sold at reasonable prices in East Indian groceries. There is usually little variation in price from one store to the next.

I am wary of herbalists who exclusively recommend their own high-priced formulas. The Asian herbal tradition is ancient and rich; no private formula can be completely new or unique. Although special processing or strongly concentrated herbal extracts may be more expensive than health-food store capsules and Chinese patent remedies, they should not cost a fortune.

COOK TWICE

As you know, herbal combinations can contain as many as ten to twenty or more ingredients per dose. When you use loose herbs, you can cook them twice, unless otherwise directed, to save money. Ask for specific cooking directions for your herbs. I always cook the herbs a longer time in less water at the second use. The softer, nice-tasting herbs can be eaten, except for woody ones like astragalus. In several chapters I have offered recipes for a few tasty, easy-to-make soup stocks. These can be reused, adding fresh herbs indefinitely.

If you can't stand their taste or smell, have the herb shop powder the herbs so you can fill empty capsules from a health-food store. For additional information on cooking and storing herbs, see chapters 3 and 4 of this book.

MAKE THE HERBAL REMEDY SPECIFIC

A traditionally trained herbal doctor in private practice, or in an herb shop, will perform the same kind of diagnostic inquiry you have studied in this book. It should include analysis of your radial pulses and tongue, along with questions related to your condition. You can expect to take the recommended herbs for some time if the problem is chronic, so it is best to consult periodically with the same herbal doctor who first gave you the recommendation. The herbs should change as your condition changes, accounting for variations of the seasons and other factors.

If you have a phone consultation with an herbalist, try to relate as much pertinent information about your condition as you can. This will include when you first got the condition and its particular circumstances, how long it has lasted, your symptoms, and your tongue observations and discomforts.

Keep in mind that some problems are constitutional and tend to recur, so it will be helpful to notice how and when your problem develops. Give the herbalist a brief physical description of yourself and your current lifestyle, or any other factors that you feel are important. Let the herbalist know what remedies you have used for the condition, and how they worked. Don't rush through this personal information. Anything you can say about your condition will help the doctor decide how to begin with herbal treatments.

KEEP IN TOUCH

Herbs need time to work. They might reveal underlying conditions you were not aware of. Let your herbalist know if you develop such odd symptoms as rashes, fever, nausea, or other discomforts from the herbs. It's very likely that the herbs are doing their job to free stuck *chi*, but a change of dosage or ingredients will help

things move along more smoothly. If you fall in love with the taste and effects of your herbs, remember that they must be changed if they are no longer needed. The following information will help you purchase herbal remedies and stay in touch with qualified practitioners in your area. Herbal sources listed here include the following:

- Selected food markets and herb shops in local areas
- Herb shops for mail-order loose herbs and pills
- Mail-order sources for professional herbalists
- Herbal practitioner referral services
- Herbal book distributors and correspondence courses

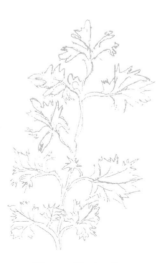

Cilantro/Coriander

Oriental Food and Herb Shops

These are stores or chains that feature Oriental foods including herbs. They are useful for local walk-in business, and offer a friendly atmosphere where you can get acquainted with Asian remedies. I've included the name of a contact person if necessary, and other helpful information on specialty stores. I have not listed anywhere near all the possible sources. For example, the Wild Oats chain has some twenty American locations and offers a help line (800-494-WILD), and Twin Labs, one of the largest manufacturers of vitamin and mineral supplements, also makes several lines of herbal products (Power Herbs, Nature's Herbs, etc.) available in local pharmacies. More new brands are appearing every day.

CALIFORNIA

Acacia Pharmacy
818 North Pacific Avenue
Glendale 91203
(818) 548-5157

All Ginseng Center
835 Washington Street
San Francisco 94108
(415) 982-8723
Fax: (415) 982-7786

Dynasty Herbs
250 26th Street
Santa Monica
(310) 917-1996

Great China Herb Company
857 Washington Street
San Francisco 94108
(415) 982-2195
Fax: (415) 982-5138

Hong Ning Company, Inc.
827 North Broadway
Los Angeles 90012
(213) 622-9542
(specializing in shark's fin and bone)

Javin Market, Inc.
1050 Grant Avenue
San Francisco 944133
Phone and fax: (415) 421-5257
Contact: Jack Wong

Rosemary's Garden
132 North Main Street
Sebastopol 95472
(707) 829-2539

Superior Trading Company
837 Washington Street
San Francisco 94108
(415) 982-8722
Fax: (415) 982-7786

Yao Hing Company
831 Grant Avenue
San Francisco 94108
(415) 989-0620
Fax: (415) 362-8877

COLORADO

Wild Oats
seven locations, including:
1668 Vultec Lane
Boulder 80301
(303) 499-7636

Also:
2260 East Colfax Avenue
Denver
(303) 320-1664
Fax: (303) 320-6489

GEORGIA

APP American Preferred Plan
710 Peachtree Street N.E.
Atlanta 30308
(404) 881-0838
Contact: Amanda Bell

KANSAS

Wild Oats
three locations, including:
5101 Johnson Drive
Mission 66205
(913) 722-4069

Also:
1040 Vermont
Lawrence 66044
(913) 865-3737
Fax: (913) 865-2940

MISSOURI

House of Hezekiah
4305 Main Street
Kansas City 64111
(816) 753-3312

NEVADA

Wild Oats
6720 West Sahara
Las Vegas 89102
(702) 253-7050

NEW MEXICO

Herbs Etc.
323 Aztec
Santa Fe 87501
(505) 982-1265

The Herb Store
107 Carlisle S.E.
Albuquerque 87106
(505) 255-8878
Fax: (505) 255-7901

Wild Oats
6300 San Mateo N.E.
Albuquerque 87111
(505) 823-1933
Fax: (505) 857-9221

Also:
1010 St. Francis Drive
Santa Fe 87501
(505) 983-5333
Fax: (505) 986-6087

NEW YORK

American Preferred Plan, Inc.
197 Eighth Avenue
New York 10011
(212) 691-9050
(Resist, Restore, herbs for
    AIDS, and Chinese patent
    remedies)

C. A. Trading Company
91 Mulberry Street
New York 10013
(212) 267-5224

Foods of India
121 Lexington Avenue
New York 10016
(212) 683-4419
(Indian herbs and foods)

K&F Trading Company
44 Bowery
New York 10013
(212) 619-3298

Lin Sisters
4 Bowery
New York 10013
(212) 962-8083
Fax: (212) 406-9211
Contact: Frank or Susan Lin

PENNSYLVANIA

Chung May Food Market
1017–1021 Race Street
Philadelphia 19107
Phone and fax: (215) 625-8883
Contact: Mrs. Mark

Fung Yuan Gifts
143 North 10th Street
Philadelphia 19107
(215) 592-4191
Contact: Tally

VERMONT

18 Carrots Natural Foods
47 Pleasant Street
Woodstock 05091
(802) 457-2050

Osaanyin Herb Cooperative
104 Main Street
Montpelier 05602
(802) 223-0888

The Herbal Alternative
24 Wales Street
Rutland 05701
(802) 747-0705

Meadowsweet Herb Farm
729 Mount Holly Road
Shrewsbury 05738
(802) 942-3565

WEST VIRGINIA

Open Hearth Herbs and Gifts
124 West German Street
Shepherdstown 25443
(304) 876-2569
Contact: Pearl Rohrer

Mail-Order Sources

HERB SHOPS

Lin Sisters Herb Shop
New York, NY
(888) LIN SIST
Fax: (212) 406-9211

MANUFACTURERS/ DISTRIBUTORS

American Preferred Plan
New York, NY
(800) 227-1195

Crystal Star
Sonora, CA
(800) 736-6015

East Earth Herbs, Inc.
Eugene, OR
(800) 827-HERB
(Jade Pharmacy, Jade Chinese
    Herbals, Jade Herbal, Jade
    Tonic, and Turtle Moun-
    tain)

Ganges Herbs
Chicago, IL
(800) AYU-VEDA
(Ayurvedic medicines)

Health Concerns
Oakland, CA
(800) 233-9355
Fax: (510) 639-9140
(Health Concerns, Seven
Forests, Turtle Mountain,
K'an Herbals, and Zand)

McZand Herbal, Inc.
Santa Monica, CA
(800) 800-0405
(Zand)

Nature's Herbs and Power
Herbs (Twin Labs)
American Fork, UT
(800) 437-2257

Nutritional Life Support
Systems
San Diego, CA
(800) 669-3954

Yogi Tea Company
Los Angeles, CA
(800) 964-4832

*FOR HEALTH
PROFESSIONALS*

Crane Enterprises, Inc.
Mashpee, MA
(800) 227-4118
Fax: (508) 539-2369
(Three Treasures, Health
Concerns, Heaven's
Essence, Lanchow Works,
MycoHerb Mushroom
Extracts, Phytotherapy
products)

Health Concerns
Oakland, CA
(800) 233-9355
Fax: (510) 639-9140
(Health Concerns, Seven
Forests, Turtle Mountain,
K'an Herbals, Zand
products and books)

Institute for Traditional
Medicine
Portland, OR
(800) 544-7504
(Seven Forests, Chinese
patent remedies, research
data on Chinese herbal
treatments)

Jiang Jing Herbs
Hebron, IN
(800) 404-JING
Fax: (219) 345-JING

Min Tong Herbs
Richmond, CA
(800) 538-1333
(concentrated Chinese herbal
formulas)

Pro Botanixx
Irvine, CA
(800) 909-HERB

Spanda Company
Belmont, MA
(800) 772-6320
(Heron Herbals, Golden
Flower, Chinese Modular
Solutions)

*HOMEOPATHIC
REMEDIES*

Boericke & Tafel, Inc.
Santa Rosa, CA
(800) 876-9505
Fax: (707) 571-8237

SunSource Health Products
Maui, HI
(800) 666-6505

Washington Homeopathic
Products
Bethesda, MD
(800) 336-1695
(homeopathic remedies for
humans and animals)

Homeopathy Works
Berkeley Springs, WV
(304) 258-2541
(homeopathic remedies for
humans and animals)

Asian Medicine and Acupuncture

The following organiza-
tions offer lists of compe-
tent professionals in Asian
herbal medicine. You can
call them for referrals in
your area. I have also included the names of sev-
eral individual herbalists
in various locations.

American Association of
Acupuncture and Oriental
Medicine
433 Front Street
Catasauqua, PA 18032
(610) 433-2448

Bastyr University Clinic
1307 North 45th
Seattle, WA 98103
(206) 632-0354

Institute for Traditional
Medicine (ITM)
2017 S.E. Hawthorne
Boulevard
Portland, OR 97214
(write for referrals of Chinese
herbalists in the U.S.)

Quan Yin Center for Chinese
Medicine
1748 Market Street
San Francisco, CA 94102
(415) 861-4964
(clinic for AIDS and referrals)

The Acupuncture Association
of New York
(800) 257-6876
(referrals to acupuncturists,
professional associations,
and schools)

The National Commission for
the Certification of
Acupuncturists
1424 16th Street, N.W.
Suite 501
Washington, DC 20036
(202) 232-1404

Individual Herbal Practitioners

Many excellent Asian herbal practitioners may not be on referral lists such as those above, because they are not affiliated with herb distributors or American health associations. You may have to consult the Yellow Pages in your area to find them. I have also listed a few individuals and clinics.

CALIFORNIA

Misha Cohen
30 Albion Street
San Francisco 94103
(415) 861-1101
(phone consultations for
AIDS and other health
problems)

COLORADO

Jake Fratkin, O.M.D.
3065 Center Green Drive
Boulder 80301
(303) 541-9055
(private practice and phone
consultations)

MASSACHUSETTS

Lonny Jarrett
Stockbridge Health Center
Main Street
Stockbridge 01262
(413) 298-4221
(acupuncture and herbs for
spiritual and emotional
balancing)

NEW JERSEY

Dr. Oreste Pelechoty
Aloha, Shorthills Plaza, 2J
636 Morris Turnpike
Shorthills 07078
(201) 376-4669

NEW YORK

Susan Lin
4 Bowery
New York 10013
(212) 962-5417, 962-8083
Fax: (212) 406-9211
(women's and children's
health)

Dr. Lili Wu
New York and Brooklyn
(718) 439-8805

Phyllis Bloom, D.Ac.
New York
(212) 675-1164
(phone consultations)

OREGON

An Hao Clinic
2348 N.W. Lovejoy
Portland 97210
(503) 224-7224
(office and phone
consultations)

PENNSYLVANIA

Yong H. Xu, O.M.D.
931 Arch Street
Philadelphia 19106
(215) 627-8209

FLORIDA

Dr. George Love
S.H.I.E.L.D. Wellness Center
450 N.E. 20th Street, #108
Boca Raton 33431
(407) 394-4660

Ayurvedic Herbalists (Indian herbs)

Ganges Herbs
Professional referral service
(800) AYU-VEDA

CALIFORNIA

Dr. Mary Jo Cravatta
Marin and Palo Alto
(415) 323-3241

Ayurveda Health and
Education Resources of
San Francisco
(415) 255-1928

NEW MEXICO

Dr. Vasant Lad
P.O. Box 23445
Albuquerque 87112
(505) 291-9698
(correspondence courses)

NEW YORK

Ayurveda Center
265 West 23rd Street
New York 10011
(800) 353-2772

Dr. Rudolph Ballentine
Center for Holistic Medicine
19 Dash Place
Riverdale 10463
(212) 243-6057
Fax: (718) 549-0975
(herbs and homeopathy)

Tibetan Physicians and Herbs

Most Tibetan physicians bring herbal pills with them when visiting from India. They can be reached through the Office of Tibet in your area. Here is the one in New York:

The Office of Tibet
241 East 32nd Street
New York, NY 10016
(212) 213-5010

Referrals to Homeopathic Health Professionals

International Foundation for Homeopathy
2366 Eastlake Avenue East, #301
Seattle, WA 98102
(206) 324-8230

National Center for Homeopathy
801 North Fairfax, #306
Alexandria, VA 22314
(703) 548-7790

Newsletters

The American Botanical Council
P.O. Box 201660
Austin, TX 78720-1660
(*HerbalGram*)

Gary Null's Natural Living Journal
P.O. Box 495
Huntington, NY 11743-0495

Publishers and Distributors

TRADITIONAL CHINESE MEDICINE

Blue Poppy Press
1775 Linden Avenue
Boulder, CO 80304
(303) 447-8372

China Books & Periodicals
2929 24th Street
San Francisco, CA 94110
(415) 282-2994
Fax: (415) 282-0994

Eastland Press
1260 Activity Drive, Suite A
Vista, CA 92083
Fax: (800) 241-3329

Mayfair Medical Supplies
204–206 Nathan Road, #501
Far East Consortium Building
Kowloon, Hong Kong
Fax: (852) 721-2851

Redwing Book Company
44 Linden Street
Brookline, MA 02146
(617) 738-4664

Spanda Company
8 Depot Street
Dalton, MA 01226
(800) 772-6320

AYURVEDIC STUDIES

Ayurvedic Institute
P.O. Box 23445
Albuquerque, NM 87112
(505) 291-9698

TIBETAN MEDICAL BOOKS IN TRANSLATION

The Office of Tibet
241 East 32nd Street
New York, NY 10016
(212) 213-5010

TIBETAN MEDICAL INSTITUTE

Khara Danda Road
Dharamsala, Dist. Kangra,
H.P. India

SELECTED BIBLIOGRAPHY

Anon. *A Barefoot Doctor's Manual*. Philadelphia: Running Press, 1977.

Beinfield, Harriet, and Efrem Korngold. *Between Heaven and Earth*. New York: Ballantine, 1991.

Bensky, Dan, and Andrew Gamble. *Chinese Herbal Medicine Materia Medica*. Revised edition. Seattle: Eastland Press, 1986.

Bin, Song Tian. *Atlas of Tongues and Lingual Coating in Chinese Medicine*. Strasbourg: Editions Sinomedic, 1986.

Chen, Ze-lin, and Mei-fang Chen. *A Comprehensive Guide to Chinese Herbal Medicine*. Long Beach, Calif.: Oriental Healing Arts Institute, 1992.

Connelly, Dianne. *Traditional Acupuncture: The Law of the Five Elements*. Columbia, Md.: The Centre for Traditional Acupuncture, Inc., 1979.

Dharmananda, Subhuti. *Chinese Herbal Therapies for Immune Disorders*. Portland, Ore.: Institute for Traditional Medicine, 1988.

———. *A Bag of Pearls*. Portland, Ore.: Institute for Traditional Medicine, revised 1993.

Donden, Yeshi. *Health Through Balance*. Ithaca, N.Y.: Snow Lion Publications, 1986.

Enqin, Zhang, ed. *Clinic of Traditional Chinese Medicine*. Ten volumes. China: Shanghai College of Traditional Chinese Medicine, 1990.

———. *Chinese Medicated Diet*. China: Shanghai College of Traditional Chinese Medicine, 1988.

———. *English-Chinese Highly Efficacious Chinese Patent Medicines*. China: Shanghai College of Traditional Chinese Medicine, 1988.

Flaws, Bob. *Arisol of the Clear*. Boulder, Colo.: Blue Poppy Press, 1991.

Fratkin, Jake. *Chinese Herbal Patent Formulas*. Portland, Ore.: Institute for Traditional Medicine, 1986.

Gaeddert, Andrew. *Chinese Herbs in the Western Clinic*. Dublin, Calif.: Get Well Foundation, 1994.

Gyatso, Tenzin, H.H. the 14th Dalai Lama. *The Union of Bliss and Emptiness*. Ithaca, N.Y.: Snow Lion Publications, 1988.

Hsu, Hong-yen. *How to Treat Yourself with Chinese Herbs*. Los Angeles, Calif.: Oriental Healing Arts Institute, 1980.

Hsu, Hong-yen, and Chau-shi Hsu. *Commonly Used Chinese Herb Formulas with Illustrations*. Long Beach, Calif.: Oriental Healing Arts Institute, 1980.

Hsu, Hong-yen, and William Preacher. *Chinese Herb Medicine and Therapy*. Long Beach, Calif.: Oriental Healing Arts Institute, 1976.

Jarrett, Lonny. "Myth and Meaning in Chinese Medicine." *Traditional Acupuncture Society Journal* 11:45–48, 1992.

———. "The Returned Spirit (Gui Ling) of Traditional Chinese Medicine," *Traditional Acupuncture Society Journal* 12:19–31, 1992.

Kaptchuk, Ted. *The Web That Has No Weaver*. Chicago: Congdon & Weed, 1983.

Keys, John. *Chinese Herbs: Their Botany, Chemistry and Pharmacodynamics*. Rutland, Vt.: Tuttle Co., 1976.

Lad, Vasant. *Ayurveda, The Science of Self-Healing*. Santa Fe: Lotus Press, 1984.

Lad, Vasant, and David Frawley. *The Yoga of Herbs*. Santa Fe: Lotus Press, 1986.

Lau, D. C. *Lao Tzu Tao Te Ching*. Middlesex, England: Penguin Books, Ltd., 1963.

Mills, Simon. *Out of the Earth*. London: Viking Arkana, 1991.

Requena, Yves. *Acupuncture et Phytothérapie*. Vols. I and II. Paris: Malonie S.A. Editeur, 1983.

Tsarong, T. J. *Fundamentals of Tibetan Medicine*. Dharamsala, India: Tibetan Medical Centre, 1981.

Veith, Ilza. *The Yellow Emperor's Classic of Internal Medicine*. Berkeley, Calif.: University of California Press, 1972.

Waley, Arthur. *The Analects of Confucius.* New York: Vintage Books, 1938.

Weed, Susan. *Wise Woman Herbal Childbearing Year.* Woodstock, N.Y.: Ash Tree Publishing, 1986.

Weil, Andrew. *Spontaneous Healing.* New York: Knopf, 1995.

Recommended Popular Reading

Articles or other information on herbs regularly appear in the following.

PERIODICALS

Gary Null's Natural Living Journal, P.O. Box 495, Huntington, NY 11743-0495.

MAGAZINES

Allure; East-West Journal; Family Circle; Fitness; Health; Health Care (London); *Healthy Living; Let's Live; Longevity; Muscle and Fitness; Natural Health; Natural Living; New Age Journal; Self; Shape; Vegetarian Times; The Yoga Journal*

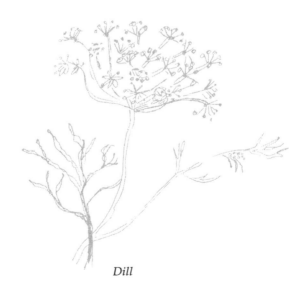

Dill

INDEX

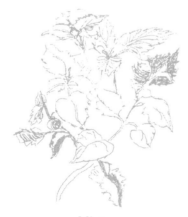

Mint